RESPIRATORY DISEASE AND INFECTION - A NEW INSIGHT

Edited by **Bassam H. Mahboub** and **Mayank Vats**

Respiratory Disease and Infection - A New Insight
http://dx.doi.org/10.5772/46040
Edited by Bassam H. Mahboub and Mayank Vats

Contributors

Fernando Saldias, Orlando Díaz, Pablo Aguilera, Anna Breborowicz, Irena Wojsyk - Banaszak, Carlos Cabello Gutiérrez, Maria Eugenia Manjarrez, Dora Patricia Rosete, Luis Horacio Gutiérrez-González, Isabel Hagel, Maira Cabrera, Maria Cristina Di Prisco, Jaume Torres, Wahyu Surya, Al-Jumaily, Iara Maria Sequeiros, Nabil Jarad, Sameera M. Al Johani, Javed Akhter, Sara E. Cruz-Morales, Jennifer Lira-Mandujano, M. Carmen Míguez-Varela

Published by InTech
Janeza Trdine 9, 51000 Rijeka, Croatia

Publishing Process Manager Iva Simcic
Technical Editor InTech DTP team
Cover InTech Design team

Additional hard copies can be obtained from orders@intechopen.com

Respiratory Disease and Infection - A New Insight, Edited by Bassam H. Mahboub and Mayank Vats
p. cm.
ISBN 978-953-51-0968-6

For EU product safety concerns:
IN TECH d.o.o., Prolaz Marije Krucifikse Kozulić 3, 51000 Rijeka, Croatia,
info@intechopen.com or visit our website at intechopen.com.

Meet the editors

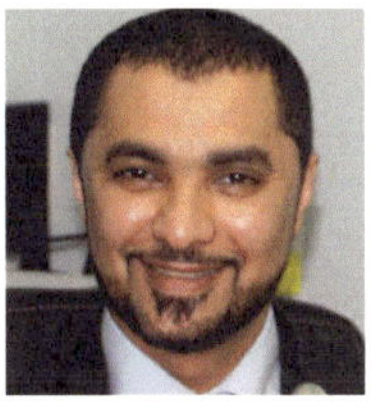

Dr. Bassam H. Mahboub is currently heading the department of Pulmonary Medicine and Allergy and Sleep Medicine, Rashid Hospital, Dubai & Assistant professor of Medicine and Chest disease, University of Sharjah, UAE. His main area of research and clinical interest includes asthma, respiratory allergy and COPD. Dr Bassam Completed his American Board of Internal Medicine, Pulmonology, American Board Allergy Clinical Immunology. Dr bassam got the fellowship of Royal college of physicians and Royal college Allergy & Clinical Immunology, Canada. Before that He was assistant medical director and Consultant and Head of division of Allergy/Immunology and Respiratory Medicine, Al Baraha Hospital, Ministry of Health, Dubai. Dr Bassam, is holding the position of Head and vice chairman of various medical professional societies in UAE & GCC countries. Dr Bassam has the credit of supervising graduates, postgraduates and doctoral students focusing on research in the field of respiratory medicine and allergy and immunolongy. He has authored many peer reviewed articles including original research, chapters published in international books and journals. He is presently also involved in numerous research projects undergoing in Gulf countries and the academic activities for the specialist doctors in UAE.

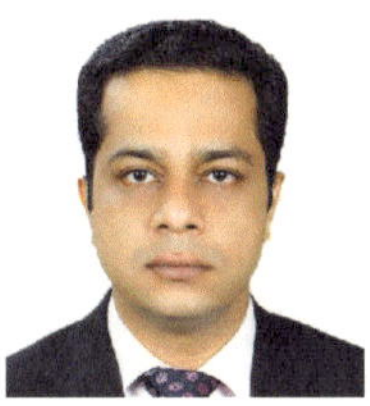

Dr. Mayank G. Vats is Senior Specialist in the department of Pulmonary Medicine and Allergy and Sleep Medicine, Rashid Hospital, Dubai. His main area of research and clinical interest includes asthma, respiratory allergy and COPD & Sleep Medicine. Dr Vats Completed his postgraduation (MD) in Pulmonary Medicine, then he did DNB in Respiratory Medicine & DNB in Critical Care medicine from the prestigious Escorts Heart Institute in new delhi, India and then served as Consultant Pulmonologist, Intensivist & Sleep Physician at Escorts Heart Institute & Apollo Hospital, New Delhi , India for More than 3 years. Dr Vats also got extensive Training in Sleep Medicine by American Academy of Sleep Medicine at LDS Hospital, Salt Lake City, UTAH, USA. Dr Vats got the Membership of Royal college of physicians and Surgeons of Glasgow, UK & was elected as fellow of American College of Physicians (FACP) & Fellow of American College of Chest Physicians (FCCP) & Holds the European Diplomat in Respiratory Medicine. Before that he provided his services as Specialist (A) in the department of Medicine and Chest disease, Al Qassimi Hspital, Sharjah, UAE. Dr Vats is the member in good standing of various medical professional societies viz. ERS, ACCP, AASM, APSR, ISCCM to name a few. He has authored many peer reviewed articles including original research, Case reports, Review articles & chapters published in international books and journals. He is presently also involved in many research projects in Gulf countries and the academic activities for the specialist doctors in UAE.

Contents

Preface

Medicine is an ever-changing science. Every day we are encountered with the new developments and knowledge in the pathogenesis, mechanism of disease, newer diagnostic modalities, treatment options and new challenges in the management of the various diseases. The same holds true for respiratory diseases with the emergence of new respiratory pathogens having significant impact on the respiratory system.

Respiratory Diseases are an important contributor to the morbidity and mortality of mankind since antiquity and its prevalence is on rise in with new disease are being recognized, however little importance has been given to the respiratory disease due to low level of awareness in physicians and general public.

This book has been designed to deliver the detailed knowledge about the various respiratory infections including viral, bacterial, and helminthic infections.

The first section covers the updated pathogenesis of the respiratory viral infections. The chapters covers the comprehensive view of the virology and molecular epidemiology of RSV, the commonest respiratory pathogen in children and in adults as well. In the same section detailed discussion has been done about the structural and functional aspects of viroporins.

The section on bacteriology primarily emphasize upon the very important but often overlooked cause of bacterial infection of the lung, the biofilm which acts as a persistent reservoir for the bacterial load and gives rise to frequent exacerbation in all population. Appropriate weightage has been given to the Clinical diagnosis and severity assessment of community acquired pneumonia which is a very common cause of morbidity and mortality in all age groups especially at extremes of age including the latest guidelines and recommendation from various professional societies.

Various challenges associated with the diagnosis and management of Helminthic infections and lung especially patients with asthma has been dealt in a very concise way.

As the prevalence of smoking has increased remarkably worldwide hence a dedicated chapter has been included on Smoking Cessation focusing on the Psychological approach to increase Smoking abstinence, which is very important component in any smoking cessation programme.

The authors and the publishers of this book have made sure that the contents and the knowledge delivered by the book is evidence based, updated and comprehensive and taken from the reliable sources.

The experience and knowledge of each of the editors have been directed to ensure that all specialized aspects of respiratory diseases and infection have been expertly covered and well presented in view of scientific content. After undergoing peer review, the book aspires to provide a readable and updated coverage of all the latest updates in respiratory diseases and infection.

The book Respiratory Disease and Infections- A New Insight has been intended for the internists, general practitioners and the respiratory physicians in order to broaden the horizon of knowledge about the respiratory diseases and infection.

We owe a great deal to all authors who worked hard to contribute the chapters in the book. We are greatly indebted to all and especially InTech publisher for their dedicated efforts and close collaboration with all the authors to publish the book for the advancement of knowledge and new insight in the field of Respiratory Disease and Infections.

Lastly, we owe a great deal to our family, who provided constant aspiration, encouragement, peace of mind and unwavering support to us to complete the editorial work of this book.

Editor:
Dr Bassam H. Mahboub
Director,
Department of Pulmonary Medicine and Allergy,
Rashid Hospital & Dubai Hospital,

Assistant Professor,
Dept of Medicine & Respiratory Disease & Allergy,
University of Sharjah, UAE

Co-editor:
Dr Mayank Vats
Specialist - A,
Pulmonary Medicine, Intensive Care Medicine & sleep Medicine,
AL Qassimi Hospital,
Sharjah, UAE

Section 1

Viral Infections

Chapter 1

Pathogenesis of Viral Respiratory Infection

Ma. Eugenia Manjarrez-Zavala, Dora Patricia Rosete-Olvera,
Luis Horacio Gutiérrez-González, Rodolfo Ocadiz-Delgado and
Carlos Cabello-Gutiérrez

Additional information is available at the end of the chapter

http://dx.doi.org/10.5772/54287

1. Introduction

Speaking of viral pathogenesis, it must describe the features and factors of viral pathogen, hosts and environment. Over its lifetime, an individual is exposed to many infectious agents, however, in most situations does not develop a disease thanks to factors such as physical and chemical host barriers. In other cases, pathogens circumvent these barriers and cause infection; however, a "biological war" will start between the determinants of pathogenicity and early host defenses. If the virus is able to overcome these first lines of defense, a type of highly specialized and specific protection will be activated. This defense will achieve, in most situations, the infection control and subsequent eradication of the disease. Furthermore, this process will initiate the generation of the immunological memory, enabling the individual with a more quickly and effectively response at the next contact with the same agent. On the contrary, if the foreign agent can overcome both defenses, the result is disease. In certain cases, the line of defense, when triggered, can also cooperate with the damage instead of healing, making the disease more severe. Thus, the immunopathology viral respiratory infection is a frequent consequence of the immune response against many of respiratory pathogens. Furthermore, if the infection is established, the factors or viral virulence determinants and physiological conditions of the host cell will determine which direction the infection will take. A virus is pathogenic when it is able to infect and cause disease in a host, while it is virulent when it causes more severe disease than another virus of a different strain, although both remain pathogens. Each virus can cause different cytopathic effects in the host cell, which may lead to several symptoms and disease. In addition, developing a disease reflects the existence of an abnormality of the host, either structural or functional, induced by the invading virus.

2. Viral pathogenesis

The term "pathogenesis" refers to the processes or mechanisms to generate an injury or illness, in this case induced by a viral infection. The results of a viral infection depend on factors related to the nature of the virus, the host and the environment. They include: number of infectious particles, the way to reach the target tissue, the rate of multiplication, the effect of virus on cell functions and the host's immune response. Three requirements must be satisfied to ensure the infection of an individual host [1]:

- Sufficient virus must be available to initiate infection,
- Cells at the site of infection must be accessible, susceptible, and permissive for the virus
- Local host anti-viral defense systems must be absent or initially ineffective.

To infect its host, a virus must first enter cells at a body surface. Common sites of entry include the mucosal linings of the respiratory, alimentary and urogenital tracts, the outer surface of the eye (conjunctival membranes or cornea), and the skin.

Among the factors that affect the infection process are:

1. **Virus-dependent factors.** They usually are dependent on the virus structure.

a. **Virulence.** Virulence is under polygenic control and is not assignable to any isolated property of the virus, but is often associated to characteristics that favor viral replication and cellular injury. For example, virulent viruses multiply themselves readily at high temperatures prevailing during the disease, block the synthesis of interferon and macromolecules related to immune system. Viral virulence is a quantitative statement of the degree or extent of pathogenesis. In general, a virulent virus causes significant disease, whereas an avirulent or attenuated virus causes no or reduced disease, respectively.

b. **Measuring Viral Virulence.** Virulence can be quantified in a number of different ways. One approach is to determine the concentration of virus that causes death or disease in 50% of the infected organisms. This parameter is called the 50% lethal dose (LD50), the 50% paralytic dose (PD50), or the 50% infectious dose (ID50), depending on the parameter that is measured. Other measurements of virulence include mean time to death or appearance of symptoms, as well as the measurement of fever or weight loss. Virus-induced tissue damage can be measured directly by examining histological sections or blood samples. For example, safety of live attenuated poliovirus vaccine is determined by assessing the extent of pathological lesions in the central nervous system in experimentally inoculated monkeys. Indirect measures of virulence include assays for liver enzymes (alanine or aspartate amino-transferases) that are released into the blood as a result of virus-induced liver damage [1].

c. **The amount of inoculum.** The impact of virus dose on the outcome of infection is poorly understood. It has been shown that, for rhinovirus, the size of the inoculum contributes to the kinetics of viral spread [2]. The amount of virus inoculated may influence or determine if it causes a mild or severe infection.

d. **Speed of replication.** Some viruses replicate so rapidly that they often cause acute infections, others are slow virus replication, or some have to travel greater distances, which slows replication.

e. **Viral Spread.** Following replication at the site of entry, virus particles can remain localized, or can spread to other tissues. Local spread of the infection in the epithelium occurs when newly released virus infects adjacent cells. These infections are usually contained by the physical constraints of the tissue and brought under control by the intrinsic and immune defenses. Respiratory infections are the typical example of local spread. An infection that spreads beyond the primary site of infection is called disseminated (for example: measles virus). If many organs become infected, the infection is described as systemic. For an infection to spread beyond the primary site, physical and immune barriers must be breached. After crossing the epithelium, virus particles reach the basement membrane. The integrity of that structure may be compromised by epithelial cell destruction and inflammation. Below the basement membrane are sub-epithelial tissues, where the virus encounters tissue fluids, the lymphatic system and phagocytes. All three biological environments play significant roles in clearing viruses, but also may disseminate infectious virus from the primary site of infection. One important mechanism for avoiding local host defenses and facilitating spread within the body is the directional release of virus particles from polarized cells at the mucosal surface. Virions can be released from the apical surface, from the basolateral surface, or from both. After replication, virus released from the apical surface is outside the host. Such directional release facilitates the dispersal of many newly replicated enteric viruses in the feces (e.g., poliovirus). In contrast, virus particles released from the basolateral surfaces of polarized epithelial cells have been moved away from the defenses of the lumenal surface. Directional release is therefore a major determinant of the infection pattern. In general, viruses released at apical membranes establish a localized or limited infection. Release of viruses at the basal membrane provides access to the underlying tissues and may facilitate systemic spread [1].

f. **Virulence genes.** Despite modern technology, identification and analysis of virulence genes is not easy. Part of the problem is that many of the effects of viral pathogenesis are the result of the action of the immune response mechanisms, including both innate and adaptive, and can not reproduce these effects in tissue culture assays. Another problem limiting the studies is that no one knows precisely what is being observed and what for. So, to address this field, most studies begin with the premise that if a virus has a defective virulence gene, it may not cause disease or, if at all, can only cause a weak disease, such that this reasoning can cause confusion. Molecular directed mutations has been a tool that, although difficult to control, has greatly contributed to the characterization of virulence genes. Thus, the reversion of mutations (mutations repair), the mixture of mutant and wild viruses, among others, have identified genetic defects in virulence. Some mutations lead to eliminated, reduced or increased protein function, whereas other proteins affect the level of transcription, translation or replication of the genetic information [1]. The viral genes that affect virulence status can be classified into four groups or classes: 1. those affecting the ability of the virus to replicate; 2. genes that modify the host's defense mechanisms; 3. genes that allow the virus to spread in the host, and 4. genes that codify proteins having toxic effects [1].

2. **Host-dependent factors.** There are factors that are innate to host such as: race and genetic load, sex, age, immunological and nutritional status, weight, etc.. These factors and the presence of specific cellular receptors for a given virus can determine resistance or susceptibility to viral infection. Subsequently, adaptive immune defense will enter into action and influence the success or the elimination of the infection.

Cellular virulence genes. Numerous studies have shown that certain cellular genes can be considered as virulence determinants [1]. Among the candidate genes are genes encoding components of the host immune response such as proteins required for T- and B-cell function, as well as cytokines. When these genes are altered, proteins do not perform correctly their function, which can have adverse effects during viral infection; thus, the disease may be more or less severe. Other candidate genes are cellular genes that encode proteins required for replication, translation, transcription and mRNA synthesis and are considered cellular virulence determinants; however, there are few studies that demonstrate this condition [1]. This field is still poor studied, but with the current tools and knowledge on the pathogenesis mechanisms, results are being achieved that in a near future will help us to learn more about the subject.

3. **Enviromental factors.** Environmental conditions such as temperature, moisture, pH, aeration, etc., can influence the viability of the virus before reaching their target organ and affect or facilitate its infectivity. A well-known example is the winter predominance of respiratory viral viruses and the summer propagation of enteric viruses.

3. Cellular level pathogenesis

Molecular interactions between the virus and the cell result in a phenomenon called pathogenesis. It can be analyzed at different levels ranging from the early interactions (cellular receptors) to the expression and suppression of cellular and viral genes, resulting in the production of inflammatory, pro-apoptotic or anti-apoptotic proteins, whose presence or absence induce the activation of complex networks of proteins that interact in cellular signaling pathways [3]. The sensitivity or resistance of a cell to viral infection is determined by early interactions with the virus, such as the adhesion and release of nucleic acids in the cell, and is strongly related to the characteristics of the cell, such as physiological maturation, genetic characteristics and specific receptors for a given virus [4].

Molecular gateway and viral spread. The site of entry of a virus is defined by the presence of specific receptors for a virus. Also, the gateway sets the path of its spread and consequently the disease process, which in some viral infections are not always predictable.

http://dx.doi.org/10.5772/54287

Usually, viruses that cause respiratory infections penetrate through the epithelium replicating at the site and causing localized infections. Sometimes, as in the case of herpes infection, virions bind to nerve endings in the nasopharyngeal cavity until they find the trigeminal ganglion and even spread to the brain, causing encephalitis; other viruses, such as measles, rubella, mumps etc., may enter through airways not being this site its target organ, so viral particles will be spread through various mechanisms.

Tropism. It is the ability of a virus to infect or damage specific cells, tissues, organs or specific cells. In some virus is strictly limited, other are pantropic and are able to infect and replicate in different types of cells and tissues. The tropism contributes significantly to the virulence and pathogenesis of viral infections, and is determined by several factors that intervere in the virus-host relationship such as the gateway and route of viral spread, the permissibility of the cell (receptors, cell differentiation), the nature of the innate and adaptive immune response of the host and specific tisular features.

Cell membrane receptors. A cell may be susceptible to viral infection if viral receptors are present and functional. In other words, if the viral receptor is not expressed, the tissue can not be infected. In epithelial cells from human respiratory tract, some receptors habe been identified such as N-acetyl neuraminic acid, glycosaminoglycans and glycolipids, ICAM integrin and molecules of the Major Histocompatibility Complex. In airways the sialic acid receptor that binds to the influenza virus has been identified. This receptor is found in several tissues of the body, although the infection in humans is restricted to the respiratory tract. Influenza A viruses infect a variety of animals. While viruses that infect humans bind to sialic acid type α-2,6, in birds they bind to α-2,3 type that is localized in the gastrointestinal epithelium where the virus replicates. In pigs, the virus can recognize both types, which facilitates the generation of gene arrangements between strains of different origin [1, 5, 6].

Virus-cell interaction. The interaction of a virus with its cellular receptor is mediated by one or more surface proteins. In enveloped viruses, the envelope glycoproteins (e.g. the influenza virus hemagglutinin); in naked viruses, the capsid proteins (e.g. exon protein of the adenovirus). Enveloped viruses have the ability to fuse directly to the cell membrane allowing the entry of the nucleocapside into the cytoplasm. Naked viruses and some enveloped viruses have the capacity to fuse to che cell membrane by means of endocytosis. Some viruses require co-receptor molecules to penetrate the cell as happens with Adenovirus [7].

Some viruses require cellular proteases that cut viral proteins to form an infectious viral particle. During an influenza virus infection, a cellular protease cuts an HA precursor generating two subunits in order to activate and allow the fusion between the viral envelope and the cell membrane. It has been described that alterations in the cleavage site of the HA of influenza virus causes changes in the pathogenicity of the virus, in fact, highly pathogenic strains of birds contain multiple basic amino acids at the cleavage site of the HA that is recognized by different proteases. As a result these strains are capable of infecting various organs such as spleen, liver, lung, kidney and brain. This same cutting activation procedure is performed with the F protein of the virus of the *Paramyxoviridae* family.

Sensitive cells. These cells have specific receptors on the cell membrane, capable of interacting with the virus antigenic proteins and to allow the infectious process. According to whether the cell allows or not the virus replication, it can differentiate them into permissive and non-permissive [8].

Permissive cells. Are those that allow the virus enter and allowing the complete viral life cycle, dividing, and producing offspring. So, the virus enters to the cell cytoplasm or nucleus, depending on the type of virus. In what is called early phase, several viral components are synthesized such as viral proteins. In the subsequent phase, these components are assembled and, in the final or lytic phase, cell death occurs, then freeing new generation virus. The infection becomes productive.

No permissive cells. These cells have viral receptors, but not allow productive infection. The infection is aborted at any step of the viral replication cycle. Upon access of the virus to these cells there is no synthesis of viral components. In some cases, if the virus is lysogenic, or it is an oncogenic virus, it can be observed the phenomenon of integration of the viral genome into the host ´genome.

Resistant cells. In all types of infection, the initial event is the interaction between the virus and the corresponding receptor present on the cell surface. If a cell lacks the appropriate receptor for a particular virus, is then automatically resistant to infection by that virus [8].

4. Cell damage caused by virus and cytopathic effect

Virus-induced cell damage. This damage may be a direct result of viral replication as well as the innate or adaptive immune response of the host; here we mention only those caused by viruses.

Direct effects on cells mediated by cytopathic viruses. Viruses cause morphological alterations known as cytopathic effect (CPE) and occur in both the cells of living organisms and *in vitro* culture cells. The alterations produced in virus infected cells ranging from those that do not immediately lead to cell death and those that destroy rapidly and kill the infected cell.

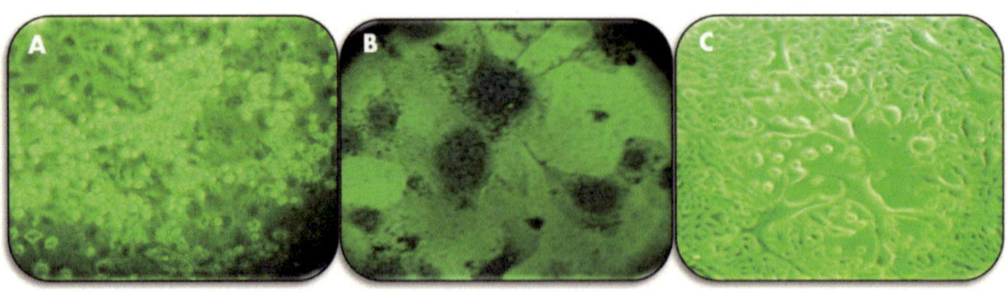

Figure 1. Diferent cytopathic effects in cell cultures. A) MDCK cells infected with influenza A H1N1 virus; B) A549 cells infected with respiratory syncytial virus, the virus includes syncytia formation; C) Vero cells infected with herpes simplex virus 1, the cytopathic effect of the virus is also the syncytia formation.

During the viral infection, cells may respond in different way, such that the ECP is different for each type of virus which might allow us to identify the virus. However, there are cases in which the cells show no apparent change. The ECP is a manifestation of the infectious process, and is defined as "morphological and functional changes of cells caused by a virus and is visible under the microscope, resulting in cell death". In cultures infected with influenza virus, cells were rounded and clustered like a bunch of grapes (Figure 1a) Adenovirus also rounded the cells but retract into a sphere. Respiratory syncytial virus (Figure 1b) and herpes simplex type I and II induce fusion of cell membranes forming syncytia or multinucleated giant cells (figure 1c).

Alteration of membranes. The plasmatic membrane is the first part of the cell with a virus contacts, this interaction occurs at the junction between the individual components of the cell surface proteins and the virus surface. After entry of the intact viral particle, and if penetration was by endocytosis, the genome is released into the cytoplasm after disruption of the membrane endocytic. In the case of paramyxovirus, a family of enveloped viruses and RNA genome, viruses contain two glycoproteins on its surface, one is the F protein that is able to initiate membrane fusion at acidic pH, the viral genome is introduced directly into the cell as a result of the fusion between the viral envelope and the cell plasma membrane. During the acute infection by cytolytic virus, especially the non-enveloped in the infected cell which finally releases large amounts of virus, the plasma membrane is damaged until to rupture. At this time, cytoplasmic proteins that are filtered, and ions such as Na + and K+ allow the entry of water and the development of cellular inflammation (cell swelling), which leads to cell lysis.

Cell lysis. Besides membrane damage by the entry of viral particles there are differene cell membrane alterations, including the nucleous and organelles that lead to cell lysis. Cell lysis is mainly due to the inhibition of cellular macromolecular synthesis by some viral proteins. DNA viruses inhibit early the cellular DNA synthesis and during late periods cellular RNA and proteins (e.g. adenovirus). RNA viruses inhibit the synthesis of RNA and proteins from earlier periods. The accumulation of viral products causes cell lysis and release of virions.

Effect on the cytoskeleton. Some viral and cellular proteins synthesized during infection act on the cell cytoskeleton. This alteration induces that cell is made round; this occurs mainly in cells infected with adenovirus. Other changes in the cytoskeleton are caused by oncogenic viruses that cause a cell morphology change (e.g. human papilloma virus in laryngeal papillomatosis). Cells that possess cilia, such as respiratory tract, lack their ciliary functionality during influenza virus infection [9].

Cellular fusion. Some viruses have structural proteins (e.g. F protein) which have the property of fusing cell membranes. In infected cells, same viral protein allows the fusion between neighboring cells, giving rise to multinucleated cells that are called polykaryocytes or syncytia. Among the viruses that show syncytia formation are RSV, measles, parainfluenza, herpes simplex, as they have fusion proteins and are able to move from one cell to another without having to leave cell.

Inclusion bodies. The inclusion bodies are intracellular granules consisting by virions or viral subunits. Its location is variable, can be intracytoplasmic as those induced by rabies virus, nuclear such as adenovirus or those caused by the virus of measles which are both nuclear and intracytoplasmic. Another example is the eosinophil corpuscles observed in cells infected by herpes simplex. Inclusion bodies break or change the cellular structure and function inducting cell death [1].

Induction of chromosomal aberrations. Viruses can cause changes at nuclear level that lead to the disintegration of the chromatin of infected cells as occurs in the herpes simplex virus infections. However, nuclear or chromosomal abnormalities can be as subtle to be detected by molecular methodologies, as example, as in the integration of viral genomes into the cellular genome during transformation mediated by certain viruses, in which the cell is alive, but altered in its properties. Other viruses that cause aberrations are mumps virus, measles, rubella, parainfluenza and adenovirus [10].

Cellular Transformation and cell proliferation. DNA and RNA viruses may integrate its genome into the cell, generating transformed cells that behave similarly *in vitro* to cancer cells. Cellular transformation corresponds to a phenomenon that occurs both *in vivo* and *in vitro* and has yielded valuable information regarding the etiology of certain cancers. Some viral proteins inactivate cell proteins which control the cell cycle and hyperplastic processes occur, inducing proliferation or cell growth, for instance, papilloma virus causing laryngeal papillomatosis that can lead to cancer [11]

5. Description and characteristics of virus

Viruses are microscopic infectious agents that are composed of genetic material (DNA or RNA), surrounded by a protein coat called capsid (naked virus), other viruses have a lipid membrane (enveloped viruses) showing glycoprotein spikes. The entire infectious unit is called virion. The proteins of the capsid of both, naked and enveloped viruses and the glycoproteins of enveloped viruses are the major antigens for inducing immune response of the host. The viruses replicate only in living cells, its genome contains the information needed to program the host cell to synthesize the virus specific molecules required for production of viral progeny [11, 12].

The pathogenicity of a virus is the ability to cause disease and is measured by the degree of virulence which in turn provides for determinants such as: ability to infect, replicate, invade cells, evasion of the host immune system and cause cellular damage. These virulence determinants are encoded by viral genes.

During the pathogenesis of an acute respiratory infection (ARI) are aspects that are shared by all the viruses that cause them:

Adherence capacity. Viruses must evade host innate immunity and defense mechanisms, such as mucociliary barriers, phagocytic cells and NK cells, and to adhere to achieve target.

Incubation period. Most ARI causing virus, have short incubation periods.

Viremia. Generally viruses causing the ARI do not cause viremia.

Immunity of short duration. As a result of the alteration of immunity mentioned above, usually the immune response shows short duration or it is incomplete.

Evasion of the immune response. The strategies used by viruses to evade the immune response are varied, from antigenic variation to the blocking of on inflammation process, and decrease of apoptosis levels [10-12].

Association with other microorganisms. Not much is known about this, but there have been some events that suggest it, for example, the bacterium *Staphylococcus aureus* produces a protease that can activate the influenza virus hemagglutinin, thus increasing the virulence level of the virus.

6. Types of infection

The interactions that occur between the virus and the host can take many forms, there are four basic patterns of infection:

1. **Subclinical infections.** Refers to infections that do not show clnical simptoms of disease in a host. They are very common in airways and are epidemiologically important because they represent an important source of transmission.

2. **Clinical infections.** These infections show symptoms and signs, the most common are acute respiratory infections which are characterized by quickly presentation with short incubation period as well as the duration of the disease. Usually, the virus is eliminated by the immune system and the physiological condition of the organism. Sometimes the disease becomes severe.

3. **Abortive infections.** Infection is interrupted in any step of the virus replication cycle. A clear example is the infection with poliomyelitis virus, which causes frequent abortive infections in early stages.

4. **Persistent infections.** After an acute infection, the virus is not eliminated and it can still replicate for long periods. The course of the infection can take one of three ways:

a. **Latent infections.** The virus remains most of the time hidden without replication, however, it can reactivate resulting in clinical manifestations. The organs or tissues where the virus remains dormant during respiratory tract infections are: The Herpes simplex virus in the trigeminal ganglion; varicella in sensory ganglia; Epstein Barr virus in B lymphocytes; Cytomegalovirus in renal and salivary cells; adenovirus in adenoids.

b. **Chronic infections.** After clinical or subclinical infection, the virus continues to multiply very slowly but continuously. Some viruses can integrate their genome into the cell, some not. Clinical manifestations may take years to develop but once manifest progress very fast. A typical example, although not a respiratory infection, is the Hepatitis B virus.

c. **Slow Infections.** This kind of infections have a long incubation period that lasts for months or years, symptoms usually do not occur during the incubation period. A well known example is the persistent infection showed by measles in the nervous system causing SSPE, usually conducting to death.

5. **Transforming infections.** Few respiratory viruses induce transforming infections, usually, the viral genome integrates into cellular DNA or remain as an episome. Some of the expressed proteins interact with genes and other cellular proteins, causing changes in cell growth rates. One example is found in laryngeal papillomatosis [10, 11].

7. Respiratory system

a. **Description of the respiratory system and functions.** The respiratory system consists of a set of organs that are grouped into upper respiratory tract (nasal cavity, pharynx, larynx, trachea) and lower airways (bronchi, bronchioles and lungs). The inner part of these organs is covered by epithelial cells which constitute an active physical barrier against pathogens being an important part of the innate immunity. Another structure of the respiratory amembrane is a mucociliary structure found from the nasal cavity to the distal areas of the lungs, consisting of a layer of mucus produced by goblet cells that maintain a continuous flow through the ciliary movement in the luminal surface respiratory epithelium. The lungs have not these structures, alveolar macrophages are the cells that are responsible for eliminating pathogens. These structures providing protection against respiratory viral infections. However, despite these protection mechanisms, respiratory system of a host may be infected by a virus by binding to specific receptors present in epithelial cells of the mucosa, thereby avoiding its removal by the mucociliary system or by phagocytic cells. Most viruses that infect humans enter into the body through the respiratory tract as in aerosols produced by coughing or sneezing of other infected hosts. Large particles are usually trapped in the turbinates and sinuses and could cause upper respiratory infections. Smaller particles can reach the alveolar spaces and cause infections in the lower respiratory tract [1, 13]. The viruses that cause respiratory infections in both upper and lower airways are distributed in different families: *Orthomyxoviridae, Paramyxoviridae, Picornaviridae, Reoviridae, Adenoviridae, Herpeviridae* and *Coronaviridae*. After penetration of the virus, they can cause local respiratory infections as with most respiratory viruses such as influenza, rhinovirus, respiratory syncytial virus, parainfluenza virus, coronavirus, bocavirus and metapneumovirus occasionally causing lower respiratory infections. Other viruses such as herpes, measles, rubella, mumps and varicella among others enter through airways but move to other organs.

b. **Viral infection in upper respiratory tract.** Infections of the upper respiratory tract usually present acutely and are the most common infections in humans, arise throughout the year but the incidence is higher in winter, are generally of low severity, however, are the main cause of medical consultation and, in consequence, school and work absenteeism is frequent. The virus originated 70-90% of these episodes and viruses that are associated with infections of the upper respiratory tract are: respiratory syncytial virus (RSV), rhinovirus (RV), parainfluenza (PIV), influenza A (IA), adenovirus (AD), human metapneumovirus (hMPV), human bocavirus (HBoV) and coronavirus (CoV). A virus can cause several syndromes, also too a syndrome may be caused by different viruses such that the clinical manifestations are variable. All individuals can be infected by these viruses, however, it has been observed that children are the most affected. The most common syndromes in upper airway are: nasopharyngitis, adenoiditis, pharyngitis, sinusitis, laryngitis and croup [14].

c. **Viral infection in lower airways.** Viral infections in lower respiratory airways occupy a smaller percentage, but with high mortality rates. The groups most at risk are young children and older adults. The disease is increased by several factors including anatomical disorders, immunological, metabolic or other diseases such as AIDS, asthma or chronic obstructive pulmonary disease (COPD).

In the next series of X-ray images are examples of lung damage caused by viral infections, upper and lower respiratory tract.

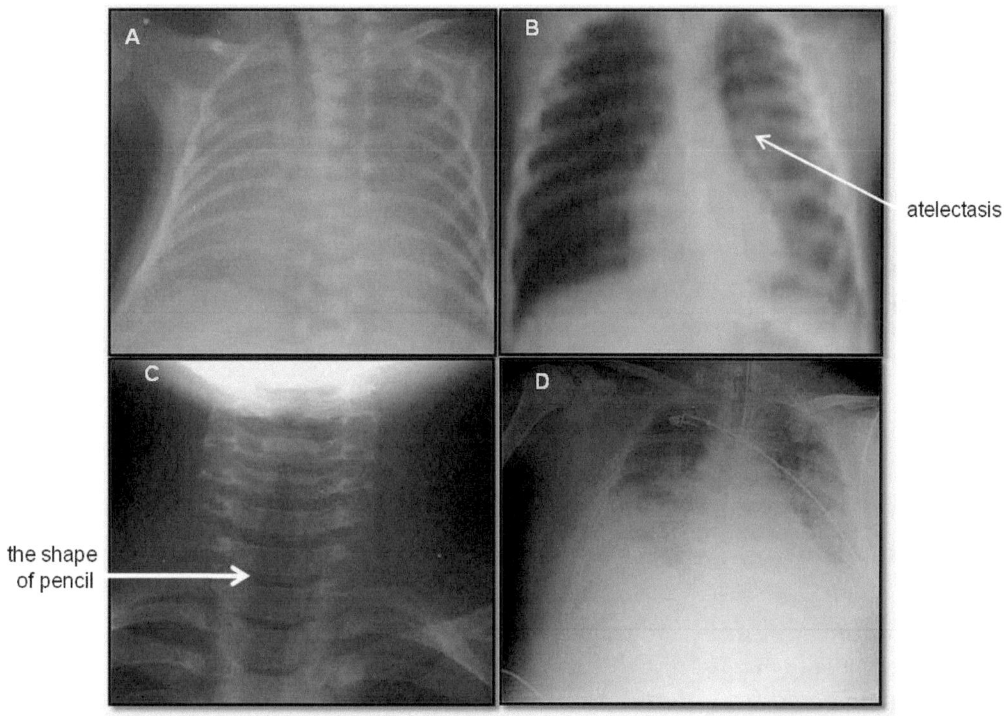

Figure 2. Radiographic images of airways infection by viruses A) pneumonia caused by respiratory syncytial virus; B) bronchiolitis in children caused by respiratory syncytial virus; Croup parainfluenza virus; pneumonia caused by influenza virus A (H1N1).

The main syndromes caused by viral infections at the lower respiratory tract are bronchiolitis and pneumonia. Bronchiolitis occurs primarily in young infants and preschool children, the most related virus to this syndrome is the RSV (50-75% of the cases). Pneumonia occurs most often in children younger than 3 years of age, as in bronchiolitis, the RSV virus are involved (50%), as well as the parainfluenza 1 and 3 virus (25%), other viruses participate with lower percentages. In elderly influenza A virus is the most important agent in causing severe pneumonia with high mortality rates [14], Figure 3.

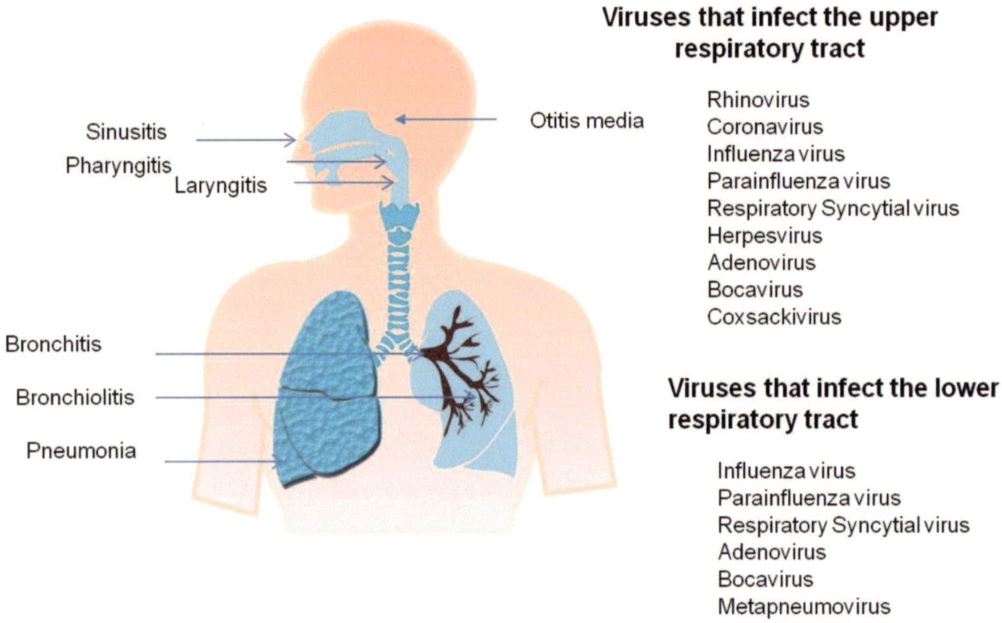

Figure 3. The Respiratory tract and the main syndromes caused by viral infections. The viruses can infect the respiratory tract upper and occasionally, some of them can cause infections in the lower respiratory tracts. Others enter trought the respiratory tracts but they move to other organs.

8. Immune response in the respiratory system (innate and adaptive), cells and mechanisms

The human immune system is divided in two defense mechanisms or responses: a) Innate or nonspecific response that lacks specificity and memory, is the first line of defense of the organism, its components are always present to act immediately and b) Specific or adaptive response. This response is more complex, has a memory and identifies the viral specific peptides processed by antigen presenting cells, which activate the humoral immune response mediated by B cells or a T cell mediated cellular response. An efficient immune response depends on a correct interaction between the innate and adaptive immune system.

Nonspecific or innate response. Airway use several mechanisms to recognize a virus and to mount a protective response. Cells of the innate immune system use a pattern recognition receptors (PRR) that are expressed on their surface and bind to pathogen-associated molecular patterns (PAMs), which are present in microorganisms. Viral PAMs can be: double stranded RNA or RNA produced during replication, surface proteins or glycoproteins. Toll-like receptors (TLR) represent a PRR family expressed in most cells of the organism, it have been identified 10 human types. The TLRs are formed by a binding domain ligand consisting of leucine repeats that interacts directly with viral antigens; a transmembrane domain and a cytoplasmatic domain responsible for initiating the extracellular signaling. Viral infections activate different TLR receptors (TLRs 3, 7, 8 and 9) that generally induce a protective immune response, however, also can be a part of pathogenic mechanisms. Recently, it has been shown that activation of TLRs in epithelial cells by viral infections participate in the regulation of expression of several genes encoding for cytokines, such as: tumor necrosis factor-alpha (TNF-α), Interleukin-1 (IL-1), IL-6, IL-8, IL-18, interferon alpha and beta (IFN-α and -β), chemokines (leukotrienes, prostaglandins) and antimicrobial peptides (α and β defensins), which are of great importance in the organization of the innate and adaptive immune response.

The components of the innate immunity are the physical and chemical barriers (epithelia and mucosae), the phagocytic process includes the participation of phagocytic cells (monocytes, macrophages and neutrophils), dendritic cells (DC) and natural killer cells (NK), also includes the production of soluble molecules (interferons, complement, acute phase proteins and antimicrobial peptides) [15- 19].

Epithelial cells. These cells are actively involved in the production of proteins (lactoferrin), enzymes (lysozyme) and antimicrobial peptides (defensins) which together eliminate or neutralize the virus. When the epithelium loses its integrity by the effect of viral infection, it can be observed the following consequences: exposure of sensory nerve endings, receptors found in the basal membrane is increased, the substances that modulate muscle tone and sensitivity are not working properly, finally, the active inflammatory response results in the alteration of inflammatory mediators.

Natural killer cells (NK). They are large lymphocytes with intracellular granules. An antibody binds to the surface of a cell infected by a virus, interacts with the Fc receptors and NK cells release proteins (perforins and granzymes) causing cell death. NK cells can be activated by the stimulation of IFN-β and α and other cytokines such as IL-12, IL15 and IL18 produced by infected cells, dendritic cells (DC) or macrophage (fig.3), [16, 17, 18, 19].

Dendritic cells (DC). DC are present in various tissues as skin, epithelium and mucosal. DC express MHC molecules on their surface localize the virus and migrate to the closest lymph node traveling through the lymphatic vessels eliminating the microorganism [17, 18].

Soluble molecules. Among the soluble molecules involved in innate immunity are: complement, interferons, antimicrobial peptides and acute phase proteins.

Complement. Complement is a system consisting of over 30 proteins that are activated by proteolysis in sequence. The complement is found in the human plasma as an inactive form and can be activated by three different pathways: the classical pathway, the alternative pathway and the lectin pathway; viral infections can trigger the three pathways. Complement is more efficient during the attack to enveloped viruses, because complement activation finished with the formation of a attack complex which is inserted in to viral membrane, causing the lysis of the virus [16, 19]. Complement anaphylatoxins (C3a and C5a) induce histamine, prostaglandins and leukotrienes release, promoting bronchoconstriction. C5a is a chemotactic factor for a variety of inflammatory cells. C3a and C5a have been found in high concentrations in the upper airways during infection by influenza virus. It has also been shown that RSV-infected cells activate complement [13, 15].

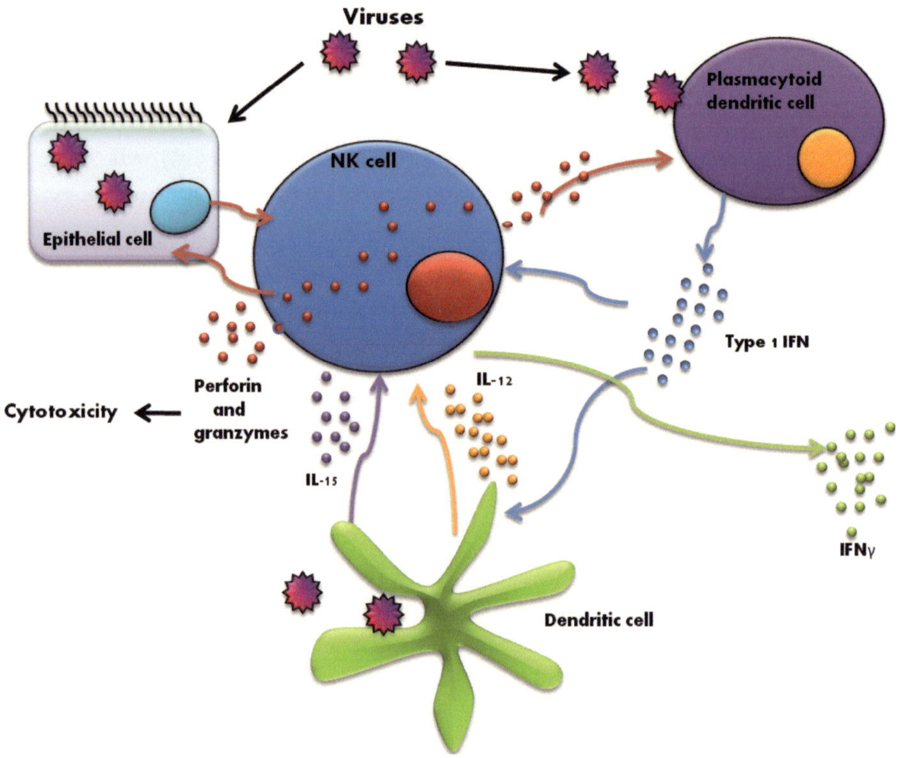

Figure 4. Activation of NK, dendritic cells and soluble molecules during virus infection. The viruses trigger the production of type – 1 interferons (IFNs) by plasmacytoid dendritic cells and other cytokines as interleukin – 12 (IL – 12). IL – 12 and IFN induce the production of IL – 15 by dendritic cells DC). IL – 15 is presented to NK cells, so that NK cells are activated. IL – 15 trigger other pro – inflammatory cytokines, including either the secretion of IFN – γ by NK cells or the release of perforin and grazymes, which leads to citotoxicity. Modified from: Lanier 2008.

Interferons (α and β). Interferons are cytokines that are produced in small amounts by cells infected with virus. Are efficiently induced by the presence of double-stranded viral RNA (viral replication intermediary), the process involves three antiviral proteins: protein kinase (PKR), Oas1 and RnasaL, which block the translation and degradation of viral and cellular RNAs. Interesntingly, influenza virus induces high levels of interferon with protective properties [20, 21, 22, 23] figure 5.

http://dx.doi.org/10.5772/54287

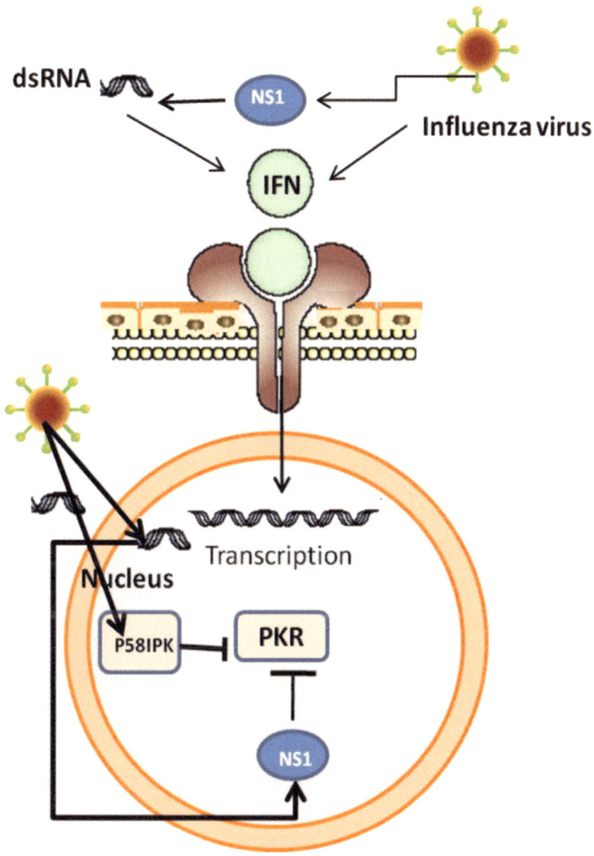

Figure 5. Influenza virus mechanisms to evade interferon action. The, NS1 protein encoded by the virus genome suppresses induction of IFNs-α/β. P58IPK is a cellular inhibitor of PKR that is activated by influenza – virus infection. Modified from: Katze 2002.

Defensins. They are cationic small peptides rich in arginine. They are syntethized in leukocytes, macrophages and epithelial cells constitutively, in response to infection or during inflammation. In humans, there are two types: α and β-defensins. Viral infections induce the production of defensins, which regulate the innate and adaptive immune response (positive and negative). The mechanisms of action and induction of defensins are multiple, generally depend on the type of infecting virus (enveloped and non-enveloped), defensin type and the target cell infected [18, 24].

The respiratory epithelium induces production of β-defensins, mainly of β-defensin-2. The mechanisms of action include: a) direct, when the peptide binds to the viral membrane by electrostatic attraction, form pores and cause lysis of the viral membrane. This mechanism occurs in the majority of enveloped viruses (influenzavirus, herpes, HIV); and b) indirect, when the defensin inactivate any signaling pathway in any step of the virus replication cycle (herpes, adenovirus). There are few studies on the mechanisms of induction of β-defensins in the respiratory epithelium. When rhinovirus infects the respiratory epithelium, the β-defensin-2 is induced by virus replication, mRNA activates the transcription factor NF-kB, and therefore, the gene that codifies for defensins; however, defensin has no direct effect on the virus. Influenza virus induces the expression of β-defensin-3, which inhibits the binding of the viral hemagglutinin with epithelium membrane. This same defensin inhibits viral fusion with the cell membrane during a RSV infection [25, 26].

Acute phase proteins (APP). APP are serum proteins whose its concentration increases or decreases when there is an infection. APP are induced by pro-inflammatory cytokines like TNF-α, IL-6 and IL-1 that are synthesized in the liver. Examples of APP are the lectin that binds to mannose, C reactive protein and surfactant proteins A and D. Acute phase proteins recognize PAMs viruses, activate complement and enhance the phagocytic capacity of immune cells [24].

8.1. Specific or acquired immunity

When the adaptive immune system contacts with a antigen it is developed a primary response that generates immunological memory, which at a second contact (secondary response) the response is more rapid and intense. There are two specific types of responses: humoral and cellular.

Humoral response. The humoral response has as a major component the B lymphocytes that differentiate into antibody-producing plasmatic cells. The antibodies are displaced by the body fluid to bind to antigens. When antibodies interact with phagocytic cells and complement, the viruses are neutralized. In humans, there are five classes of immunoglobulins (IgA, IgM, IgG, IgE and IgD). In viral respiratory infections, IgA is of great importance as it is secreted by mucous epithelia, preventing the establishment of virus. IgM is the first antibody that is synthesized and prevailing in a primary response, also fix complement. The IgG is found in greater concentration in serum and is the only one that can cross the placenta in humans. Presents an Fc fragment that binds to complement receptors on phagocytic cells. Most respiratory viruses induce such antibodies that persist, and when a second exposure to the same antigen, the disease is less severe; unfortunately, virus may have mutations that are not recognized by the antibodies, therfore, reinfections are common. IgE is the antibody with the lowest concentration in the serum, but is the most important in allergic disorders. It has been reported that some viruses such as RSV, influenza, bocavirus, parainfluenza and metapneumovirus produce bronchial hyperreactivity or asthma increasing concentrations of this immunoglobulin in blood and secretions. Basophils and mast cells have receptors for these antibodies, when the antigen-antibody binding occurs and consequently activate, these cells release inflammatory mediators that cause many manifestations of these respiratory diseases [27].

Cellular response. The cellular response has as its principal components the T lymphocytes, which are divided into two populations according to their surface markers and the pattern of cytokines produced: CD4+, also called helper T cells (Th) and CD8 +, the cytotoxic lymphocytes (CTL). These specialized cells can proliferate and differentiate into effector and memory cells.

In viral infections, CD8+ T cell response is essential for viral clearance. Lymphocytes are able to recognize through its receptor (TCR) by antigen processing performed by antigen presenting cells (dendritic cells or macrophages) associated with MHC molecules. For the differentiation and activation of T lymphocyte are required two signals are requare: the first is the specific recognition of the antigen on the target MHC class I-associated cel, and the second produced the cytokines produced by CD4+ T cells which recognize MHC-associated viral antigens class II. Cytotoxic T lymphocytes exert their antiviral effects by three mechanisms: producing lysis of infected cells, stimulate the production of enzymes that degrade viral genomes, and secrete cytokines. In severe viral infections including pneumonia caused by RSV, influenza and metapneumovirus, this type of response is important for the resolution of the disease; however, it has been observed that in severe cases this response has no effect and the pattern that develops is through cytokines produced by CD4 Th2 specialized cells that induce an inflammatory response increasing damage and thereby aggravating the condition.

9. Evasion of the immune response

Despite effective defenses, some virus can to evade it by using different mechanisms, for example, in respiratory tract infections influenza virus inhibits the production of interferon by the protein NS1, a non-structural protein that is abundantly expressed in the nucleus of infected cells. NS1 binds to double-stranded RNA by preventing activation of the dsRNA-dependent protein kinase (PKR) [28], commonly synthesized during induction of interferon (Figure 5). Another mechanism is the antigenic variation that occur mainly in the HA and NA proteins. PI and RSV respiratory viruses have a surface protein (F), which mediates the fusion of the viral membrane with the cell membrane. This mechanism enables the virus to spread from one cell to another without exposure and avoiding the effect of circulating antibodies. Another strategy is to make a latent infection. Viruses such as adenovirus and herpes employ transcription and replication strategies to maintain the viral genome in any cell type where the immune response is not efficient and viral particles are not produced for long periods. Other viruses interfere with antigen processing or complement. In summary, viruses use several strategies to evade the immune response [11].

10. Other mechanisms used by respiratory viruses in the pathogenesis

In most infections, the viruses cause upper respiratory infections, while others reach the lower airways, may even cause necrosis and cell death, also induce inflammatory processes such as wheezing and hyperreactivity, both important in the development of chronic diseases such as asthma and chronic bronchitis for which some mechanisms have been proposed. In summary, the strategies used by viruses that cause respiratory infections can be very varied; however, there are always some strategies are shared between different types of viruses.

Inflammatory cells. In viral respiratory infections has been observed recruitment of inflammatory cells such as eosinophils, neutrophils, basophils, monocytes, macrophages, mast cells and T lymphocytes. Thus, when activated, these cells release mediators, cytokines or other compounds that increase inflammatory response [29, 30]. **Macrophages.** Alveolar macrophages are one of the first lines of cellular defense against virus infections. During viral replication in macrophages antiviral mechanisms are activated by stimulating, by stimulating the release of interferons or other cytokines, for example, studies have shown that alveolar macrophage infection by RSV, causes increased secretion of tumor necrosis factor alpha (TNF-α), as well as interleukins IL-8 and IL-6. It has also been observed that the macrophages express high levels of intercellular adhesion molecule-1 (ICAM-1), receptor molecule specific for some virus [17, 31, 32].

Monocytes. Also express high levels of ICAM-1. When human monocytes are infected by viruses, monocytes are activated, producing and releasing IFN-α, IFN-β, IL-1β, IL-6 and TNF-α. The production of these cytokines (with the exception of IFN-β) potentiates the production of granulocyte macrophage-colony stimulating factor (GM-CSF) [33].

T Lymphocytes. T lymphocytes act as immunomodulators and as producers of cytokines. According to the pattern synthesis of cytokines, helper T cells (Th) are classified into two types: Th1 cells secreting IL-2, IF-γ and lymphotoxin, while Th2 cells secrete IL-4, IL-5, IL -6 and IL-10. The Th1 response is associated with the antiviral immunity. The RSV G protein stimulates Th2 type response and this would explain the symptoms of lower respiratory tract caused by this virus [34].

Neutrophils. In viral respiratory infections, neutrophils are activated and recruited into the airways and probably generate oxygen metabolites or other metabolites or inflammatory cytokines that cause damage and late hyperreactivity 36. They are found in high concentrations in bronchial secretions of children infected with RSV, with parainfluenza virus and in nasal biopsies of subjects with rhinovirus infection [34].

Eosinophils. Eosinophils release mediators such as leukotrienes (LTC4), platelet activating factor (PAF), major basic protein and cationic eosinophilic protein. When eosinophils are activated by virus are recruited into the airways causing damage and causing a late hyperreactivity reaction [35]. *In vitro* studies have shown that RSV in humans activates eosinophils [36].

Basophils.*In vitro* assays using basophils obtained from patients infected with RSV, adenovirus, influenza A, parainfluenza and rhinoviruses have observed an increase in the release of histamine [37, 38, 39].

Mast cells. These cells have a high affinity receptor for IgE and participate in hypersensitivity reactions, the release of histamine and leukotrienes, molecules that are increased in infants with respiratory wheezing [38, 39].

Stimulation of chemical mediators. It has been proposed that in the respiratory infections, viruses are able to originate the relase of inflammatory mediators, either directly or through viruses-activated cells. Whatever leads to a vigorous inflammatory response, airway obstruction induces exacerbation of asthma. Several mediators have been reported, which suggests that during infection can exist the interaction of more than one. Among the most mentioned are:

Histamine. Histamine is released from various cells as basophils, leukocytes, mast cells, among others. The secretion of this mediator is inflammation and airway is inflammation and airway obstruction. *In vitro* and *in vivo* studies with respiratory virus have demonstrated high concentrations of histamine in nasopharyngeal secretions and in the plasma of infected individuals. However, therapeutic success with antihistamines in asthma has not been confirmed so several authors have questioned the effect of histamine [36, 38].

Leukotrienes. Leukotrienes are inflammatory lipid mediators derived from arachidonic acid. Leukotrienes are released by primary inflammatory cells involved in inflammation, as well as endothelial and epithelial cells of the airways. They are very potent bronchoconstrictors that affect both the upper and lower airways. It has also been shown to increase vascular permeability and production of mucus, in addition, some evidence suggests that leukotrienes play an important role in the origin of wheezings. Respiratory viruses such as RSV, parainfluenza 3 and influenza A, induce the release of leukotrienes which are detectable in nasopharyngeal secretions. High concentrations of Leulotrienes have been found in infants with RSV infection [40-44].

Products of cyclooxygenase, arachidonic acid, prostaglandins and thromboxane. They are potent bronchoconstrictors and have shown an increase in the concentrations of the primary metabolite of prostaglandin type 2a in plasmatic cells from infants with RSV bronchiolitis and especially in those with recurrent wheezing. It is also reported that the prostaglandin E2 type has an inhibitory effect which may protect the airways of a bronchoconstrictor effect. It is suggested that viral epithelial damage may result in the loss of these protective prostaglandins. It was also found that complexes of RSV-antibody cause an increase in the release of thromboxane by neutrophils [36].

Platelet activating factor (PAF). Induces an inflammatory response and stimulates the production of mucus in the airways, alters mucociliary clearance and enhances pulmonary microvascular permeability. PAF is released by macrophages, eosinophils and neutrophils. *In vitro* studies have shown that mononuclear phagocytes upon RSV replication, stimulates the synthesis of platelet activating factor. From these results it has been suggested that this factor may play an important role in the inflammatory response caused by RSV [45, 46].

Kinins. These molecules are potent vasoactive peptides that are produced in tissues or fluids. Kinins may be involved in the pathogenesis of diseases such as asthma by its inflammatory and bronchoconstrictor action. Kinins are potent stimulus for C fibers, and therefore, improves axon reflex [34, 36]. In unmyelinated sensory nerves in the airways is found the P substance, potent neuropeptide belonging to tachykinin group which when released by local axon reflex, potentiate the cholinergic neurotransmission [47].

Nitric Oxide (NO). Nitric oxide has a mediator function with different effects such as: antiviral agent, increase bronchial blood flow, eosinophilic infiltration, epithelial damage, potent vasodilator, inhibit the proliferation of Th1 cells due to a Th2 phenotype change, and, in asthma patients, it has been observed that after a experimental rhinovirus infection, no increase in exhaled NO levels [48].

Cytokines. They are small proteins that act generally in cellular processes such as differentiation, activation and immune defense. All cytokines are secreted by cells due to the interaction with infectious agents and mechanical actions (e.g. cell stress). They interact through a complex network during the immune and inflammatory responses. There are a variety of cytokines and others are continually identified. There are cytokines showing chemotactic properties, therefore, these cytokines are called chemokines. In viral infectious processes it has been described the participation of various chemokines as a pathological characteristic of the infection process, so that it has been established that chemokines are directly responsible for the inflammatory processes that occur in respiratory viral infections [49]. Among the viruses that induce the release of chemokines may be mentioned: RSV, rhinovirus, influenza and parainfluenza viruses 3 [50]. It has been observed that, in cell lines, RSV increases the production of IL-6, IL-8, RANTES, macrophage inflammatory protein (MIP-1a), GM-CSF and IL-11.

Interleukin 8 (IL-8). IL-8 is a chemokine which promotes the recruitment of neutrophils and eosinophils that are responsible in part for the inflammatory process [49, 50].

RANTES. This eosinophil chemokine that induces exocytosis of the eosinophil cationic protein. It is also chemotactic for basophils and CD44 T cells [51, 52].

MIP-1α. Less potent than RANTES as eosinophil chemotactic, but it is important mediator in the inflammatory response during virus infection because it stimulates the release of histamine by basophils and mast cells. Its properties suggest that may be important mediators of asthma exacerbations induced by viral infections. In children, have been found in high concentrations in nasal secretions during asthma exacerbations associated with infection caused by RSV and rhinovirus [50,51].

Eotaxin. It is another chemokine with chemotactic activity for eosinophils. Eotaxin has additional functions such as endothelial migration, release of reactive oxygen, Ca+ ions mobilization, actin polymerization and is also chemotactic for basophils and Th2 lymphocytes. It is soluble in serum and has been found in high concentrations in patients with asthma and is associated with the severity of the disease [52, 53].

Intercellular adhesion molecule 1 (ICAM-1). This a receptor is located in the vascular endothelium, epithelium of the airways and in antigen presenting cells. Its ligands are found in circulating leukocytes [54, 55]. Several studies have shown that, *in vitro*, epithelial cells of human airways produce increased levels of ICAM-1. This ICAM-1 expression is observed also during the adhesion of eosinophils and neutrophils in response to inflammatory cytokines and in infection processes of various respiratory viruses such as RSV, rhinovirus and parainfluenza [53, 56, 57]. Rhinoviruses attach to the surface of cells via ICAM-1 receptor, suggesting that infection with rhinovirus leads to an increase in the expression of ICAM-1 in the upper airways. In this way, ICAM-I and induces the recruitment of eosinophils and neutrophils, thereby increasing and causing inflammatory activity and wheezing [58, 59, 60].

11. Pathogenicity and description of some viral respiratory infections

11.1. Infection with influenza virus A

The influenza A virus belongs to the *Orthomixoviridae* family, causes high morbidity and mortality. One feature of the virus is the frequent occurrence of new antigenic variants generated by both genetic mutations and recombination leading to epidemics and pandemics. Influenza viruses have a fragmented RNA genome (8 fragments). Among others, influenza virus has two glycoproteins, hemagglutinin (HA) and neuraminidase (NA), that are important in their biological activity and pathogenesis. The cellular receptor for this virus is sialic acid, which forms part of mucopolysaccharides found in glycoproteins and cell membranes. HA viral protein binds to the cellular receptor by endocytosis to enter the cell, allowing the virus to remain as an endosome, and is required to be activated so that the fusion peptide is exposed. This step is critical for virus infectivity and depends on both the virus and the cell. Once given membrane fusion, RNA migrates to the nucleus for replication, which is required for the cellular RNA polymerase II, as its polymerase is inefficient to generate mRNA, so viral replication depends on the help of the cell. Neuraminidase (NA) is the second virus glycoprotein. Its function is enzymatic and is important because once the new virions are synthesized, the glycoprotein is responsible for removing sialic acid residues from the infected cell membrane, which allows the newly synthesized virions can be released without auto aggregation. The viral M2 protein functions as an ion channel that allows the passage of protons into the virion and is the target for the action of the amantadine, its mutation or changes can lead to viral resistance to this compound.

The virus enters through the nasopharyngeal region, the target cells are mucus-secreting epithelial cells and ciliated cells, can be transmitted by droplets expelled by speaking, sneezing or coughing, by contact with contaminated material or hands. The cell binding is via the HA that binds to sialic acid receptor. The incubation time is 1 to 3 days. The virus multiplies rapidly and spreads to neighboring cells. It causes cellular necrosis and apoptosis, altering the ciliar activity and increasing mucus secretion. To exit and infect other cells, NA reduces the viscosity of mucus film breaking sialic acid residues. The damage to the epithelium causes respiratory symptoms and signs, stimulates the natural response of the tract and promotes bacterial incorporation. The inflammation process can damage bronchi, bronchioles and alveolar regions. All these events cause initial symptoms of infection like fever, chills, muscle aches, headache, anorexia and prostration. Local monocytes, lymphocytes and interferon are the main response to the virus. The virus induces an effective humoral response which is important in recovery, but it must be considered that the antibody response is specific for each variant of the virus, whereas the T lymphocytes and macrophage response is general and depends on the injury and the condition of the host to perform efficiently the epithelial repair (that can take up to one month).

In pandemics and severe cases, it has been observed that the immune response is exacerbated and may cause a greater damage [61].

The virus can evade the immune response in different ways. One is the constant genetic variation of HA and NA glycoproteins, which are the first that are recognized by antibodies. Another mechanism involves the NS1 Protein, which can block the role of interferon [15].

Until 2009, the origin of influenza pandemics was mainly due to the transmission of virus from birds to humans, by the transfer of genes from avian virus to the seasonal influenza virus that is recognized as human. When a new virus emerges, the body does not recognize it, which can lead to a pandemic. In April 2009, an epidemic arose from the emergence of a new influenza A virus. The first cases occurred in Mexico. Numerous patients with Influenza-like severe symptoms were attended at the Instituto Nacional de Enfermedades Respiratorias Ismael Cosio Villegas (INER), Mexico, and in many cases required hospitalization. Patients arrived in a serious, advanced conditions and, for this reason many of them died.

It has been observed that when an epidemic emerges and new viruses are detected, the human body quickly begins to produce the antibodies needed to contain the new disease. Some people develop these antibodies faster than others, so that the chance of infection in them is lower, because their immune system acts quickly creating antibodies, while those that fail to quickly develop antibodies start to develop the disease. Despite that, the viruses that cause ARI do not induce a good immune response. If after some time there is antibodies production, many patients will become before producing antibodies against the new virus. Other antibodies have neutralizing capacity.

We decided to carry out a study with the following objectives: To determine the titer of anti-influenza virus in serum samples from patients infected with influenza A (H1N1), as well as household contacts of patients infected with this virus by the method of inhibition of hemagglutination.

To determine the presence and titer of antibodies were used 196 samples of sera, of which 110 were in patients with influenza A H1N1 confirmed by RT-PCR assays and to household contacts 86 patients with influenza A H1N1. In this work, antibody titer of each sample was deyterming using the technique of hemagglutination inhibition.

The figure 6 shows the results of some sera, as can be seen, the positive titers appear as a red spot in the center of the well as a result of inhibition of hemagglutination while negatives occur in a uniform color of lower intensity.

90% of patients confirmed influenza A (H1N1) had antibodies, the highest title was 1:1024 and the lowest was 1:16. In the case of the sera of household contacts the highest antibody titer was 1:256 and the lowest was 1:4. In the case of the sera of healthy household contacts, antibodies are detected in only 84% of the sera.

In conclusion, the antibodies were detected during an acute late phase in the diseases acute phase but late in the disease, since patients usually arrived after two weeks of onset of the disease, and in serious condition. It is possible that after this stage titers have increased. Antibody synthesis is generally low at the beginning of the disease, and it is increased as the immune system responds to the infective agent, that is, after approximately two weeks. Up to that moment the antibodies could not stop the damage the virus had caused.

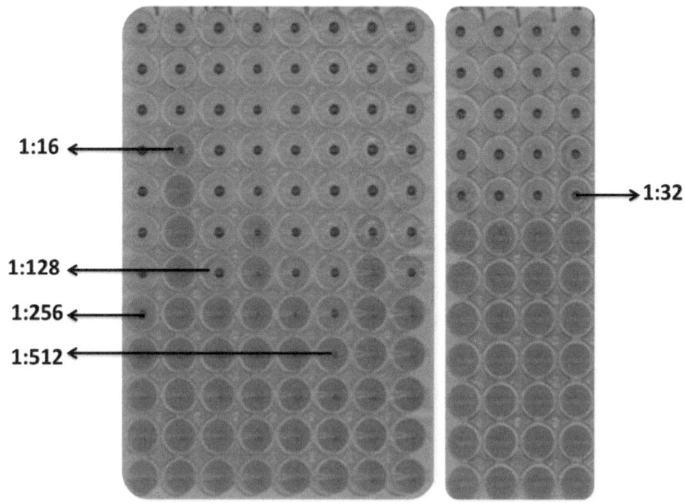

Figure 6. Hemagglutination inhibition test for the detection of antibodies against influenza A (H1N1) virus.

11.2. Respiratory syncytial virus (RSV)

RSV belongs to the *Paramyxoviridae* family is not segmented and is capable of performing polymerase mediated mRNA synthesis and is characterized by two glycoproteins, the F protein (which induces the formation of syncytia) and G protein.

In the case of RSV, this virus infects children under 2 years of age causing high rates of morbidity and mortality [61]. Usually, children between one and two years of age have had a virus infection [62]; however, reinfections are frequent, as the immune response is incomplete or immature. As all the respiratory viruses, RSV enters through respiratory airways, taking place the first replication in the nasopharyngeal region. For the ability to make syncytia, RSV virus can move from cell to cell without leaving, which prevents antibody attack. Thus, secretions or by dragging can reach lower airways, causing bronchiolitis and pneumonia with mucus production. As a child tracks are narrow, respiratory obstruction can be observed, which can be very serious. The most important mechanism of pathogenesis of the virus is its capacity to infect their terminal paths of the lung during childhood, when the diameter is quite small. The RSV virus has a propensity to infect the bronchiolar epithelium in comparison with the infection of the rest of the airways; even if the cause is unknown, pathological studies indicate that the inflammatory response is much greater in the area of the terminal airways that in the upper portions of the respiratory tract [63]. Besides, other factors are suspected important in the pathogenesis of the virus as immunological mechanisms, mainly by cytokines produced by Th2 lymphocytes. It has been suggested that the nature of the immune response to RSV, is determined by the pattern of cytokines produced sequentially by different cells [63]. There are high-risk groups such as immunocompromised children, premature infants, infants with heart, kidney and lung problems, where mortality is high.

11.3. Parainfluenza virus (PIV)

PIV is of the same family as the RSV, so that their characteristics are similar, except that one glycoprotein has the hemagglutinin and neuraminidase activities in a single structure. IN addition, PIV has an F fusion protein.

In the case of PI virus, and despite its freqeuncy, little is known regarding to their mechanism of pathogenesis. The PI virus also infects children causing the same syndromes. Small tracts of children, when ignited, conduce to the obstruction of the air flow allows the accumulation of secretions, so there are cases with severe obstruction [64, 65].

For either exist a vaccine, although in the case of RSV there is a monoclonal antibody which can be an important resource in the treatment of young children. However, but its cost, is only used in high-risk groups.

12. Conclusions

The viral pathogenesis represents a world of mysteries and extraordinary surprises, where apparently questions have not been able to answer. One of the main purposes of the pathogenesis study is to know and understand the molecular mechanisms by which viruses activate in the cells when generating a , and how they avoid the immune response; with that information, trying to eliminate or control the diseases that they provoke in humans.

Although there have been significant advances in different fields of medical virology, there are still many mysteries to solve, questions to answer and so many fields to explore in the pathogenesis of viral acute respiratory infections (ARI) and the viral pathogenesis in general. In spite of moving forward in the pathogenesis study, mainly in aspects such as: molecular interactions between viral factors and the host, and identification and comprehension of many of the biological, molecular, biochemical and even genetic mechanisms involved in the disease's development, many of these processes remain to be clearly understood. However, thanks to steady developments and improvements in many fields of biological sciences and technology, we hope to attain a deeper knowledge and comprehension of viral pathogenesis development.

Acknowledgements

The authors acknowledge the financial support from CONACYT (SALUD-2009-C02-126832).

Author details

Ma. Eugenia Manjarrez-Zavala[1], Dora Patricia Rosete-Olvera[1], Luis Horacio Gutiérrez-González[1], Rodolfo Ocadiz-Delgado[2] and Carlos Cabello-Gutiérrez[1]

1 Departamento de Investigación en Virología y Micología, Instituto Nacional de Enfermedades Respiratorias Ismael Cosio Villegas, D. F., México

2 Departamento de Biología Molecular y Genética. CINVESTAV, IPN, D.F., México

References

[1] Flint SJ, Enquist LW, KrugRM, Rocaniello VR, Skalka AM. Principles of Virology. Molecular Biology Pathogenesis and Control. ASM Press Washington D.C. 2000.

[2] Douglas RG Jr, Couch RB, Baxter BD, Gough M. Attenuation of rhinovirus type 15: relation of illness to plaque size. Infection and Immunity. 1974; 9(3) 519-523.

[3] Gottwein E and Cullen BR. Viral and cellular microRNAs as determinants of viral pathogenesis and immunity. Cell Host Microbe. 2008; 12; 3(6) 375–387.

[4] Ghosh Z, Mallick B and Chakrabarti J. Cellular versus viral microRNAs in host–virus Interaction. Nucleic Acids Research. 2009; 37(4): 1035–1048.

[5] Manjarrez ME, Rosete DP, Higuera A, Ocadiz-Delgado R, P{erez-Padilla JR, Cabello C. Start a Pandemic: Influenza A H1N1 Virus. In Respiratory Diseases. Mostafa Chanei, Intech Open Access Publisher, Rieja, Croatia 2012.215-242.

[6] Schneider-Schaulies J. Cellular receptors for viruses: links to tropism and pathogenesis J Gen Virol. 2000; (81):1413–1429.

[7] Corjon S., Gonzalez G, Henning P, Grichine A, Lindholm L, Boulanger P, Fender P and Hong S. Cell entry and trafficking of human adenovirus bound to blood factor X is determined by the fiber serotype and not hexon:heparan sulfate interaction. 2011; 6 (5): e18205.

[8] Landry ML , Mayo DR and Hsiung GD. Comparison of guinea pig embryo cells, rabbit kidney cells, and human embryonic lung fibroblast cell strains for isolation of herpes simplex virus.Journal Clinical Microbiology.1982; 15(5): 842-847.

[9] Albrecht T, Fons M, Boldogh I, et al. Effects on Cells. In: Baron S, editor. Medical Microbiology. 4th edition. Galveston (TX): University of Texas Medical Branch at Galveston; 1996. Chapter 44. Available from: http://www.ncbi.nlm.nih.gov/books/NBK7979/.

[10] Baron S, Fons M, Albrecht T. Viral Pathogenesis. In: Baron S, editor. Medical Microbiology. 4th edition. Galveston (TX): University of Texas Medical Branch at Galveston; 1996. Chapter 45. Available from: http://www.ncbi.nlm.nih.gov/books/NBK8149/.

[11] Knipe DM, Howley PM, Griffin DE, Martin MA, Lamb RA, Roizman B, Straus SE. Fields Virology. Lippincott Williams & Wilkins. Philadelphia, USA. 2007, pp 3091.

[12] López M J, Manjarrez ME and Zavala T J. Microbiología. Bacteriología y Virología. Méndez editores. México. 2010. 912.

[13] Shors T. Virus. Estudio molecular con orientación clínica. Editoria Mèdica Panamericana. Buenos Aires Argentina. 2009: 639.

[14] Dolin R and Wright PF. Viral infections of the respiratory tract. Marcel Dekker. New York, EU.1999, 432.

[15] Katze MG, He Y, Gale M. Viruses and interferon: a fight for supremacy. Nature Reviews Immunology. 2002; 2:675–687

[16] Pyzik M and Vidal SM. NK cells stroll down the memory lane. Immunology and Cell Biology. 2009; 87:261–263.

[17] Siamon Gordon and Philip R. Taylor. Monocyte and macrophage heterogeneity. Nature reviews immunology. 2005; 5: 953-64.

[18] Diamond G, Beckloff N, and Ryan LK. Host Defense Peptides in the Oral Cavity and the Lung: Similarities and Differences. Journal of Dental Research. 2008; 87:915-927.

[19] Lanier LL. Evolutionary struggles between NK cells and viruses. Nature Reviews Immunology 2008; 8: 259-268.

[20] Hasegawa K, Tamari M, Shao C, Shimizu M, Takahashi N, Mao XQ, Yamasaki A, Kamada F, Doi S, Fujiwara H, *et al.* Variations in the C3, C3a receptor, and C5 genes affect susceptibility to bronchial asthma. Human Genetics. 2004; 115:295–301.

[21] Barnes KC, GrantAV, Baltadzhieva D, Zhang S, Berg T, Shao L, Zambelli- Weiner A, Anderson W, Nelsen A, Pillai S, *et al.* Variants in the gene encoding C3 are associated with asthma and related phenotypes among African Caribbean families. Genes & Immunity. 2006; 7:27–35.

[22] Wills-Karp M. Complement Activation Pathways A Bridge between Innate and Adaptive Immune Responses in Asthma. Proccedings American Thoracic Society. 2007; 4.247–251.

[23] Silverman RH. Viral Encounters with 2,5 Oligoadenylate Synthetase and RNase L during the Interferon Antiviral Response, Journal of Virology; 2007; 81:12720–12729.

[24] Auvynet C and Rosenstein Y. Multifunctional host defense peptides: Antimicrobial peptides, the small yet big players in innate and adaptive immunity. FEBS Journal. 2009; 276:6497–6508.

[25] Ding J, ChouY Y, Chang TL. Defensins in Viral Infections. Journal of Innate Immunity. 2009;1:413–420.

[26] Kota S, Sabbah A, Chang TH, Harnack R, Xiang Y, Meng X, and Bose S. Role of Human β-Defensin-2 during Tumor Necrosis Factor α/NF-kB-mediated Innate Antiviral

Response against Human Respiratory Syncytial Virus. Journal of Biological Chemistry. 2008;283 22417-22429.

[27] Janeway CA, Travers P, Walport M, Capra JD. The immune system in health and disease. In Inmunobiolog. Mason, Barcelona España, 2000. 644.

[28] Hayman A, Comely S, Lackenby A, Hartgroves LCS,Goodbourn S, McCauley JW, and Barclay WS. NS1 Proteins of Avian Influenza A Viruses Can Act as Antagonists of the Human Alpha/Beta Interferon Response. Journal of Virology.2007; 81:2318-2327.

[29] Kobasa D, Jones SM, Shinya K, Kash JC, Copps J, Ebihara H, Hatta Y, Kim JH, Halfmann P, Hatta M, Feldmann F, Alimonti JB, Fernando L, Li Y, Katze MG, Feldmann H, Kawaoka Y. Aberrant innate immune response in lethal infection of macaques with the 1918 influenza virus. Nature. 2007; 445:267–268.

[30] Canoz M, Erdenen F, Uzun H, Mu°derrisoglu C, Aydin S. The relationship of inflammatory cytokines with asthma and obesity. Clinical Investigation of Medicine. 2008; 31:E373–E379.

[31] Peters-Golden, M .The alveolar macrophage: the forgotten cell in asthma. American Journal Respiratory Cellular Molecular Biology. 2004: 31, 3–7.

[32] Thepen, T., Van Rooijen, N., and Kraal, G. Alveolar macrophage elimination in vivo is associated with an increase in pulmonary immune response in mice. Journal Experimental Medicine. 1989. 170, 499–509.

[33] See H and Wark P. Innate immune response to viral infection of the lungs. Paediatric Respiratory Review. 2008; 9(4):243-250.

[34] Gotera J,Giuffrida M, Mavarez A,Pons H, Bermudez J, Maldonado M, Mosquera J and Valero N. Respiratory syncytial virus infection increases regulated on activation normal T cell expressed and secreted and monocyte chemotactic protein 1 levels in serum of patients with asthma and in human monocyte cultures.Annals of Allergy, Asthma & Immunology. 2012; 108(5): 316-320.

[35] Yoshizumi M, Kimura H, Okayama Y, Nishina A, Noda M, Tsukagoshi H, Kozawa K and Kurabayashi M. Relationships between cytokine profiles and signaling pathways (IkB kinase and p38 MAPK) in parainfluenza virus-infected lung fibroblasts.Frontiers in microbiology. 2010; 1 (124): 1-7.

[36] Lindemans CA, Kimpen JL, Luijk B, Heidema J, Kanters D, van der Ent CK and Koenderman L. Systemic eosinophil response induced by respiratory syncytial virus. 2006, 144: 409-417.

[37] Holt PG, Strickland DH and Sly PD. Virus infection and allergy in the development of asthma: what is the connection?. Current Opinion Allergy Clinical Immunology. 2012, 12(2):151-157.

[38] Kimpen JL, Simoes EAF. Respiratory syncytial virus and reactive airway disease. American Journal of Respiratory Critical Care Medicine. 2001;163:S1–S6.

[39] Ogra PL. Respiratory syncytial virus: The virus, the disease and the immune response. Paediatric Respiratoty Reviews. 2004; 5(1): S119-S126.

[40] Jose D R, Toro A, Baracat E. Antileukotrienes in the treatment of asthma and allergic rhinitis. Jornal de Pediatria. 2006; 82(5 Suppl):S213-21.

[41] Bisgaard H, Szefler S. Long-acting beta2 agonists and paediatric asthma. Lancet. 2006; 367: 286-288.

[42] McCarthy MK and Weinberg JB. "Eicosanoids and Respiratory Viral Infection: Coordinators of Inflammation and Potential Therapeutic Targets," Mediators of Inflammation, vol. 2012, Article ID 236345, 13 pages, 2012. doi:10.1155/2012/.

[43] Pavia AT. Viral infections of the lower respiratory tract: old viruses, new viruses, and the role of diagnosis. Clinical Infectious Diseases. 2011; 52(4): S284–S289.

[44] Greenberg SB. Viral respiratory infections in elderly patients and patients with chronic obstructive pulmonary disease. American Journal of Medicine. 2002. (112)6:28S–32S.

[45] Yokota S, Okabayashi T, Hirakawa S, Tsutsumi H, Himi T and Fujii N, Clarithromycin Suppresses Human Respiratory Syncytial Virus Infection-Induced *Streptococcus pneumoniae* Adhesion and Cytokine Production in a Pulmonary Epithelial Cell Line. *Mediators of Inflammation,* vol. 2012, Article ID 528568, 7 pages, 2012. doi: 10.1155/2012/528568.

[46] Carr MJ, Hunter DD, Jacoby DB, and Undem BJ. Expression of Tachykinins in Nonnociceptive Vagal Afferent Neurons during Respiratory Viral Infectionin Guinea Pigs.2002; 165(8): 1071-1075.

[47] Kenneth J. Broadley, Alan E. Blair, Emma J. Kidd, Joachim J. Bugert, and William R. Ford. Bradykinin-Induced Lung Inflammation and Bronchoconstriction: Role in Parainfluenze-3 Virus-Induced Inflammation and Airway Hyperreactivity. The Journal of Pharmacology and Experimental Therapeutics. 2010; 335(3):681-892.

[48] Reiss C and Komatsu T. Does Nitric Oxide Play a Critical Role in Viral Infections?. Journal of Virology. 1998; 72(6): 4547–455.

[49] Noah T and Becker S. Respiratory syncytial virus-induced cytokine production by a human bronchial epithelial cell line. Lancet.1993; 205 (5): L472-L478.

[50] Wan CT. Viruses in asthma exacerbations. Current Opinion in Pulmonary Medicine. 2005; 11(1): 21-26.

[51] Bonville C, Rosenberg H , Domachowske J. Macrophage inflammatory protein-1α and RANTES are present in nasal secretions during ongoing upper respiratory tract infection. Pediatric Allergy and Immunology. 2002; 10 (1): 39-44.

[52] Schaller M, Hogaboam C, Lukacs N, Kunkel S. Respiratory viral infections drive chemokine expression and exacerbate the asthamatic response. Journal of Allergy and Clinical Immunology 2006; 118(2):303-304.

[53] Kumar A and Grayson M. The role of viruses in the development and exacerbation of atopic disease. Annals of Allergy, Asthma & Immunology. 2006; 103 (3): 181-187.

[54] Boyd A, Wawryk S, Burnst G, and Fecondo J. Intercellular adhesion molecule 1 (ICAM-1) has a central role in cell-cell contact-mediated immune mechanisms. Proccedings of the National Academy of Sciences of the United States of America. 1988; 85(9): 3095-3099.

[55] Osborn L, Hession C, Tizard R, Vassallo C, Luhoswskyj, S Chi-Rosso G and Lobb R. Direct expression cloning of vascular adhesion molecule 1 a cytokine-induced endothelial protein that binds lymphocytes. Cell. 1989; 59 (6): 1203-1211.

[56] Corne JM, Holgate ST. Mechanisms of virus induced exacerbations of asthma.Thorax. 1997;52:380–389.

[57] Jackson D, Johnston S. The role of viruses in acute exacerbations of asthma.Journal of Allergy and Clinical Immunology. 2010; 125(6): 1178-1187.

[58] Papi A and Johnston SL. Rhinovirus Infection Induces Expression of Its Own Receptor Intercellular Adhesion Molecule 1 (ICAM-1) via Increased NF-kB-mediated Transcription. The Journal of Biological Chemistry. 1999; 274(14): 9707-9720.

[59] Papi A, Papadopulos NG, Stanciu LA, Pinamonti S, Degitz K, Holgate ST and Johnston SL. Reducing agents inhibit rhinovirus-induced upregulation of the rhinovirus receptor intercellular adhesion molecule-1 (ICAM-1) in respiratory epithelial cells. The FASEB Journal.2002; 16(14): 1934-1936.

[60] Wang X, Lau Ch, Pow A, Mazzulli T, Gutierrez, Proud D and Chow CW. Syk Is Downstream of Intercellular Adhesion Molecule-1 and Mediates Human Rhinovirus Activation of p38 MAPK in Airway Epithelial Cells.The Journal of Immunology. 2006; 17(10): 6859-6870.

[61] Zuñiga J, Torres M, Romo J, Torres D, Jiménez L, Ramírez G, et al. Immphamatory profiles in severe pneumonia associated with the pandemic influenza A(H1N1) virus isolated in Mexico city. Autoimmunity 2011; 44(7):562-570.

[62] Glezen WP, Taber LH, Frank AL, et al. Risk of primary infection and reinfection with respiratory syncytial virus. Am J Dis Child. 1986;140:543–6.

[63] Halls CB, Joyse M. Respiratory syncytial virus infections with families. J Med 1976; 294: 414- 419.

[64] Postma DS, Jones RO, Pillsbury HS. Severe hospitalized croup: treatment trends and prognosis. Laryngoscope 1984; 94: 1170-75.

[65] Glezen WP, Danny FW. Epidemiology of acute lower respiratory tract disease in children. N Engl J Med 1973; 288:498-505.

Chapter 2

Virology and Molecular Epidemiology of Respiratory Syncytial Virus (RSV)

Sameera Al Johani and Javed Akhter

Additional information is available at the end of the chapter

http://dx.doi.org/10.5772/53916

1. Introduction

Human respiratory syncytial virus (RSV) is a ubiquitous virus of worldwide distribution and is the leading cause of infant morbidity from respiratory infections. By the age of two years nearly all children have been infected and can cause severe bronchiolitis and pneumonia in this age group (Hall et al., 2009). Nearly 100% of children in the USA are infected with the virus by 2 to 3 years of age, several hundred infants may die directly from the infection, while the deaths of an additional several thousand may be attributed to RSV-related complications (Nair et al, 2010). The World Health Organization estimates that (RSV) is responsible for 64 million infections worldwide and 160,000 deaths per annum (Openshaw, 2002).

Although mostly young infants are affected, it is increasingly recognized as a significant cause of disease in the elderly population and can often be fatal for patients with impaired immune systems (Collins and Malero., 2011). The incubation period of RSV respiratory disease is estimated to be three to five days (Black, 2003). The virus can remain viable on hard surfaces (e.g., countertops) for up to 6hr, on rubber gloves for 90min, and on skin for 20min. (Hall et al., 1980). This prolonged survival highlights the need (and effectiveness) for hand washing and contact precautions in limiting the spread of RSV infection (Koetz et al, 2006). Viral shedding is significantly prolonged in immunocompromised individuals, and can continue for several months (Hall et al., 1981; Simoes, 2003).

2. Spectrum of respiratory disease

The spectrum of clinical manifestations ranges from mild upper tract illness, infection in middle ear which progresses to acute otitis media, croup, to apnoea in premature infants, pneumonia and bronchiolitis (Hall et al., 1975). At the beginning of the illness, the virus replicates in the nasopharynx. Common symptoms of an upper respiratory tract infection include a productive cough and mild to moderate nasal congestion with clear rhinorrhea.. A low-grade fever presents in the early stages of the infection and symptoms may persist for one to three weeks before complete recovery (Welliver, 2003).

Symptoms of lower respiratory tract disease include tachypnea (ie rapid breathing greater than 60 to 70 breaths/min), wheezing, and/or rales, that usually appear up to three days following onset of rhinorrhea. These symptoms are indicative of the virus spreading into the bronchi and bronchioles. A chest radiograph exhibits hyperinflation with flattened diaphragms. If the RSV further spreads to the alveoli, an interstitial pneumonia may develop, with middle and upper lobes affected. In such patients, tachypnea becomes severe respiratory distress, with deep retractions and grunting respirations. The risk for cardiovascular failure secondary to hypoxemia, acidosis, and dehydration increases significantly (Greenough, 2002). Immunocompromised and young infants, who have very narrow bronchioles, are at particularly high risk for complete bronchiolar obstruction. The risk for vomiting also increases, which is often related to respiratory distress and can increase the likelihood and of gastroesophogeal reflux. This may result in decreased oral intake with dehydration. Premature babies born at 30–35 weeks of gestation, HIV-infected patients, infants with cyanotic congenital heart disease,, and other immunosuppressive therapy such as bone marrow transplant are at increased risk for morbidity and mortality during RSV infection (Resch, 2011).

3. The structure of respiratory syncytial virus

RSV is a member of the subfamily *Pneumovirinae* in the family *Paramyxoviridae*, order *Mononegavirales*. RSV is closely related to several other RNA viruses, including measles, mumps, and parainfluenza types 1, 2, and 3. Respiratory syncytial virus is a medium-sized (120-200nm) enveloped virus that contains a lipoprotein coat and a linear minus-sense RNA genome. The entire genome of RSV is composed of approximately 15,000 nucleotides long (Dickens et al., 1984).

The genome contains 10 mRNAs, each coding for an individual protein (McIntosh,.1997). The structural proteins are divided into three functional groups, the nucleocapsid (N) protein, phosphoprotein (P) and viral polymerase (L). These proteins together, have been demonstrated to function as the RSV replicase. The outer envelope is lined internally with matrix (M) protein and is spiked externally with fusion (F) and attachment (G) glycoprotein projections, these are responsible for the initiation and propagation of an RSV infection (Empey et al., 2010). Another protein (M2) is also present in the viral envelope. The viral capsid is made up of a nucleoprotein, a phosphoprotein, and a polymerase protein (C). The F protein is a type 1 transmembrane glycoprotein with a Cleaved N-terminal signal sequence and a transmembrane anchor near the C terminus. It is cleaved into two subunits, F1 and F2 that are linked by disulfide bonds, after synthesis and modification by the addition of N-linked sugars. The G protein is of particular interest because variability in this protein is greater than that in the other proteins both between and within the major antigenic groups of RSV (Sullender, 2000).

4. Mechanism of infection

RSV does not normally replicate outside of the bronchopulmonary tree and is restricted to the respiratory mucosa (Othumganpat et al, 2009). The G protein initiates attachment of the virus to the epithelial cell. The virus fuses with the epithelial cell membrane and enters the cytoplasm after the F protein is cleaved by proteolytic enzymes of the infected cell. If the precursor is not cleaved it has no fusion activity, virion penetration will not occur and the virus particle is unable to initiate infection. Fusion by F1 occurs at the neutral PH of the extra cellular environment, allowing release of the viral nucleocapsid directly into the cell. This enables the virus to bypass internalization through endosomes. After replication the virus matures by budding from the cell surface. The new progeny nucleocapsids form in the cytoplasm and move to the cell surface. The M protein is essential for particle formation, probably serving to link the viral envelope to the nucleocapsid. During budding, most host proteins are excluded from the membrane. If appropriate host cell proteases are present, precursor proteins in the plasma membrane will be activated by cleavage. Activated fusion protein will then cause fusion of adjacent cell membranes, resulting in formation of large syncytia (Jawetz et al., 2004). The viral RNA can spread without forming complete viral particles. The infection results in the destruction of the epithelial cells of the upper respiratory tract. Exposure to RSV triggers humoral immune responses. Primary RSV infection results in only a weak antibody response with IgM, IgG, and IgA produced. This response is not sufficient to completely destroy the virus or to prevent upper respiratory tract replication of the virus, thus an upper respiratory tract illness develops (Smith et al., 2009).

Although, RSV mostly infects the nasal epithelial cells. However, development of extrapulmonary disease has been observed in certain T and B cell immunodeficiency states. The association of RSV with asthma and reversible reactive airway disease in early childhood has attracted significant attention (Mohapatra et al., 2008). Recurrent wheezing for up to 5 to 7 years of age and established airway disease has been observed in a significant number of children with a strong family history of allergy, after primary infection or reinfection with RSV (LeManske, 2004). Immune response to primary infection is relatively small but on reinfection, a significant booster effect with sustained immunologic reactivity is observed in serum and respiratory mucosa. Both CD4- and CD8-specific as well as Th1- and Th2-cell specific immune responses have been observed during human infection. In addition, proinflammatory as well as immunoregulatory cytokines and chemokines are induced in the respiratory tract after natural and induced (in vitro) infection. In vulnerable patients, the RSV infection will spread into the lower respiratory tract (Becker et al., 2006). In premature infants and immunocompromised hosts, the infection quickly progresses to the LRT. As the virus is destroyed within the lung by T cells, immunopathological responses cause further lung injury. Infected cells release proinflammatory cytokines and chemokines, including interlukins (IL-1, IL-6, and IL-8) and tumor necrosis factor-alpha (TNF-α). These actions result in activation of inflammatory cells, including macrophages, eosinophils, neutrophils, and T lymphocytes, into the airway lining and surrounding tissues.

5. Molecular epidemiology of RSV

Variability between RSV strains contributes to the ability of the virus to infect people repeatedly and cause annual outbreaks. Consistent shifts in RSV group dominance have been reported worldwide in which RSV group A viruses are more frequently detected. A new BA genotype was identified in Buenos Aires in 1999 that is characterized by a 60-nucleotide duplication starting after residue 791 of the G protein. Subsequently, strains with this duplication have been found in clinical specimens from distantly related places in the world, including Kenya in East

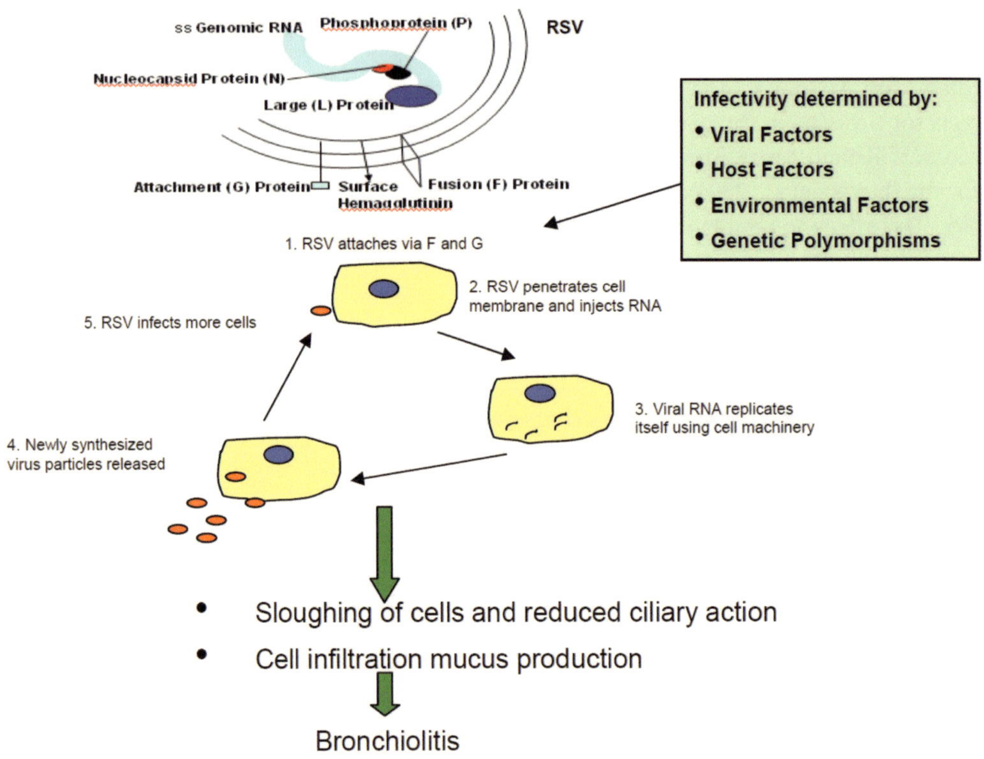

Figure 1. Mechanism of RSV Virus Entry and Replication in Respiratory Virus Infection

Africa. This BA genotype was first discovered in South Africa during the investigation of a nosocomial outbreak in Pretoria in 2006. (Niekerk and Venter, 2011). In Germany, RSV group A was dominant in seven out of nine epidemic seasons predominating between

http://dx.doi.org/10.5772/53916

1999 to 2007 seasons. During the same periods, mainly RSV group A dominated in several other countries.

The subgroup prevalence and genotype distribution patterns of RSV strains were investigated in a community in Belgium during 10 successive epidemic seasons (1996 to 2006). A regular 3-year cyclic pattern of subgroup dominance was observed, consisting of two predominant RSV-A seasons, followed by a single RSV-B-dominant year. RSV infections with both subgroups were more prevalent among children younger than 6 months and had a peak incidence in December. The most frequently detected genotypes were GA5 and GB13, the latter including strains with the 60-nucleotide duplication in the G gene (Zlateva et al, 2007). A study in India reported on RSV group A dominance for three consecutive epidemic seasons. RSV group B predominated for a single season in the countries investigated and at the same or similar time as observed in Germany. Thus, it can be concluded that RSV group A predominated within similar seasons, implicating that most RSV infections were caused by RSV group A worldwide at the same time.

The results of the first study to investigate the circulation and genetic diversity of RSV in Cambodia among different age ranges of population over 5 consecutive years (Arnott, et al., 2011). Circulation of RSV was seasonal, coinciding with the rainy season between July and November. The majority of RSV group B strains belonged to the BA genotype, with the exception of 10 strains classified as belonging to a novel RSV group B genotype,

In an Iranian study during the season 2009, samples were obtained from several provinces: Tehran, Hamadan, Isfahan, Kordestan, Zanjan, Lorestan and West Azarbayjan, and were tested for G protein gene of RSV by RT-PCR (Faghihloo et al., 2011). Of the respiratory samples tested, 22% were positive for RSV, of which 67% belonged to subgroup A and 33% to subgroup B. Phylogenetic analysis revealed that subgroup A strains fell in two genotypes GA1 and GA2, whereas subgroup B strains clustered in genotype BA. This study revealed that multiple genotypes of RSV cocirculate in Iran. Subgroup A strains are more prevalent than subgroup B strains, with genotype GA1 predominant.

There has been a distinct lack of data from the Middle East in terms of molecular typing of RSV. For example, In Saudi Arabia, only few reports have described the prevalence of RSV infection in sporadic districts of the kingdom including Riyadh, Al-Quassim and Abha (Jamjoom et al., 1993; Bakir et al., 1998; Al-Shehri et al., 2006; Meqdam and Subiah, 2006, Akhter and Johani., 2011). These reports covered short periods of time extending from 1991-1996, 2003-2004 and 2004-2010. Both virus subtypes in RSV infection of Saudi Arabia children are found to occur with a greater dominance of type A viruses in a three year cyclical pattern. However, a greater interest in RSV is needed for proper virus characterization. Molecular typing studies are required to elucidate the nature of RSV spread in these populations.

Similar viruses were first isolated around the same time in Europe, USA, The Gambia, Malaysia, Uruguay and Australia (Cane and Pringle, 1995). Further studies in North America (Peret et al., 2000), Europe (Lukic-Grlic et al., 1999), and Africa (Cane et al., 1999, Venter et al., 2002) have shown that similar strains of RSV appear simultaneously in indistinct geographic locations in these areas. It is clear that infections with very similar viruses may be occurring world-wide during the same season. Overall there appears to be very little geographic clustering of RSV strains and where this has been reported it may often be due to inadequate sampling or delayed reporting of strain variability, particularly from less developed parts of the world. As the virus is constantly accumulating genetic and antigenic change, this implies that when a new strain arises it is able to spread very rapidly around the world.

6. Vaccines

There have been exhaustive attempts to identify pharmacological therapies to improve the clinical course and outcomes of this disease. However, presently, there is no licensed vaccine against RSV. High-risk infants can be substantially protected by monthly intramuscular injections of a commercially available RSV-neutralizing antibody (palivizumab) administered during the RSV epidemic season (American Academy of Pediatrics, 2003). RSV is the focus of antiviral- and vaccine-development programmes because of the morbidity and mortality associated with bronchiolitis early in life. However, these goals are now being aided by an understanding of the virus genome architecture and the mechanisms by which it is expressed and replicated (Meisner and Long, 2003).

The reasons why an RSV vaccine is not yet available emanate from numerous problems with its development. First, is the possibility that vaccination will potentiate naturally occurring RSV disease, as observed with the formalin-inactivated vaccine (Domachowske and Rosenberg, 1996). Second, young infants exhibit relative immunologic immaturity or because of suppression of their immune response due to circulating maternally derived anti-RSV antibodies (Falsey and Walsh, 1996). Another important consideration is the need to provide protection against multiple antigenic strains of RSV in the two major groups, A and B. A number of strategies have been implemented recently to generate safe and effective subunit, inactivated, and live attenuated virus vaccines (Falsey and Walsh, 1997).

7. Inactivated and subunit respiratory syncytial virus vaccines

The first attempt at an RSV vaccine in the 1960s employed formalin-inactivated RSV particles (FIRSV). This vaccine failed to induce a protective immune response and led to enhanced disease upon natural infection with wild type (*wt*) RSV. As a result, 80% of the children vaccinated needed to be hospitalized following *wt* RSV infection, and two children died (Kim et al., 1969). Consequently, there was great apprehension to study any nonreplicating RSV vaccine in seronegative infants and children. Enhanced disease has never been observed with live attenuated vaccines and it is not seen in seropositive subjects, neither with inactivated nor with subunit RSV vaccines (Collins et al., 2001).

8. Sub unit vaccines

A large number of subunit vaccines have been studied in preclinical trials, and some have progressed into clinical trials. Most of these candidate vaccines consist of either or both of the RSV surface glycoproteins that mediate membrane fusion (F) and virus attachment (G). These vaccines were administered in various ways, such as using alum phosphate or alum hydroxide. Others were evaluated conjugated to bacterial toxins, as ISCOMs (immunostimulating complex), or with adjuvants such as CpGs (CpG-DNA), monophosphoryl lipid A, saponines, or oil-in-water emulsions (Piedra, 2003; Kneber and Kimpen, 2004). The use of inactivated and subunit vaccines seems safe in RSV seropositive individuals, however, two exceptions have been noted in seronegative infants: FI-RSV and subunit vaccines induced high RSV-binding antibody titers with low neutralizing activity and the enhanced disease seen with FI-RSV can be replicated in rodent models using subunit vaccines.(Openshaw et al., 2001; Johnson et al., 2004)

One of the more recent trials evaluated PFP-3 (purified F protein with aluminum phosphate) in seropositive children 1 to 12 years of age with cystic fibrosis. In this trial, PFP-3 was found to be safe and immunogenic but not protective. Similarly, in a trial of PFP-2 in healthy pregnant women and their offspring, PFP-2 was found to be safe but there was no significant increase in RSV neutralizing IgG titers following vaccination in the third trimester so that a protective effect in the offspring could not be expected (Munoz et al., 2003). A different subunit vaccine was tested consisting of copurified F, G, and M proteins from RSV subgroup A (sanofi-aventis, Bridgewater, NJ) in a phase 1 trial in healthy adult volunteers. Of those vaccinated, 80% developed a greater than fourfold increase in neutralizing antibody titers to RSV A and RSV B. However, these titers did not persist so that annual vaccination would be necessary to maintain potentially protective antibody titers with this candidate vaccine (Wright et al., 2000). BBG2Na (Pierre Fabre, Castres, France), a promising vaccine candidate that was developed by fusing the conserved central domain of the RSV G protein to the albumin-binding region of streptococcal protein G, was found to be safe and immunogenic in phase 1 and phase 2 studies. But in the phase 3 trial purpura / type III hypersensitivity resulted as an unexpected side-effect in a small number of vaccine recipients and so halted further development (Kneyber and Kimpen., 2003).

9. Live attenuated respiratory syncytial virus vaccines

Several live attenuated RSV vaccines have been identified by passage of RSV under different conditions such as lower temperatures, temperature- sensitive (*ts*), chemical mutagenesis and non-*ts* attenuating mutations. Several candidate vaccines went into clinical trials, but it was not possible to find an appropriate balance between immunogenicity and attenuation, particularly in young infants.

The development of a method to generate infectious virus from a cDNA copy of the negative-sense single-stranded virus genome initiated the era of rational RSV vaccine design. It allowed the use of site-directed mutagenesis to introduce desired mutations into the RSV genome and to evaluate the contribution of each mutation to the attenuation phenotype by introducing individual mutations or sets of mutations into the RSV genome. Reverse genetics has also been used to generate attenuated deletion mutants that are useful as live attenuated RSV vaccines. Deletion of the genes for the interferon antagonists NS1 or xlink, the small hydrophobic gene SH, or the M2–2 regulator of transcription and replication produced viable viruses that displayed restricted replication in nonhuman primates. Candidate vaccines bearing these deletions with or without additional attenuating point mutations were identified as suitable for clinical development (Collins and Murphy, 2005).

A promising candidate vaccine is an RSV subgroup A mutant designated *cp*248/404/1030ΔSH. This mutated virus has 11 mutations identified in the biologically derived *cpts*248/ 404RSV, a further mutation in the large polymerase protein L (the 1030 mutation), and a deletion of the SH protein. It was was evaluated in a phase 1 trial in 1- to 2-month-old infants, replication was highly restricted in seronegative infants and the vaccine was well tolerated (Karron et al., 2005). Although neither systemic nor mucosal antibody responses were repeatedly observed in the youngest vaccinated infants, but complete restriction of a second dose of vaccine given 4 weeks after the first dose indicated that protective immunity could be induced.

10. Future strategies

One of the most promising current strategies for protection against respiratory tract infection is intranasal treatment with vectors capable of generating RNAs that block viral replication. RNA interference (RNAi) is a natural defense of the innate immune system against viruses (Dallas and Vlassov, 2006). Following viral replication, double-stranded viral RNA is recognized by the host RNAi system which cuts it into short oligoribonucleotides, 20–30 bases long. These short sequences activate the cell's RNA cleavage machinery (the RNA interference silencing complex, or RISC) to destroy the viral RNA. By introducing siRNAs complementary to specific viral mRNAs, double-stranded activating RNA can be generated that activates the RISC cleavage system and destroys the viral message. This approach using antiviral siRNA has been reviewed by Manjunath et al, 2009. The use of siRNA as an antiviral agent involves a relatively straightforward attack on one or more key viral genes and should be effective against many human pathogens. The use of non-integrating plasmid vectors removes the risk of mutagenesis caused by some viral vectors.

11. Summary

The burden of acute respiratory infections (ARIs) caused by viral pathogens is impressive and leaves no doubt that effective and affordable vaccines are urgently needed. The impact of respiratory viral infection is greatest in the very young, the elderly, and people with an impaired immune system or other chronic conditions. LRIs are a common cause of hospital admission and excess mortality. RSV infection is the most frequent etiology of a child's first LRI. Presently, passive protection against RSV is achieved successfully through monthly intramuscular injection of the humanized monoclonal anti-RSV antibody palivizumab However, immunoglobulin products are expensive to administer

Attempts to develop a vaccine against RSV have been unsuccessful to date. A formalin-inactivated RSV vaccine was developed in the 1960s. Although initial serological responses to this vaccine appeared promising, children who received this vaccine developed more severe disease, with a number of deaths, when exposed to natural RSV infection. The development of a successful RSV vaccine must address this issue and achieve protection of very young children if it is to have an impact on severe RSV disease. Recent progress in this area has included development of stable, live-attenuated RSV vaccines that can be administered as nasal spray. Despite progress in this area, a vaccine that is ready for use in clinical practice is still many years away.

Another approach is the development of an RSV vaccine that involves use of cloned RSV surface proteins as potential subunit vaccines. RSV fusion (F) and glycoprotein (G) can induce neutralizing and protective antibodies and are the components in development. Phase 1 trials of Fusion (F) protein nanoparticle RSV vaccine candidates have shown that they are generally well-tolerated, highly immunogenic and produce functional antibodies that neutralize RSV. These are being evaluated for potential immunization of young children and also for administration to pregnant women during the last trimester to boost anti-RSV antibody levels transferred to the infant (Schmidt, 2007).

Author details

Sameera Al Johani[1,2] and Javed Akhter[1]

1 Microbiology Section, Department of Pathology and Laboratory Medicine, King AbdulAziz Medical City, Riyadh, Saudi Arabia

2 Microbiology, College of Medicine, King Saud Bin AbdulAziz University for Health Sciences, Riyadh, Saudi Arabia

References

[1] Akhter J, Johani S. Epidemiology and diagnosis of human respiratory syncytial virus infections. In Human Respiratory syncytial virus infection edited by Resch B. 2011, Part 2, Chapter 8: 161-176 Intech open access publishers

[2] Al-Shehri, M.A., A. Sadeq, and K. Quli, 2006. Bronchiolitis in Abha, Southwest Saudi Arabia: Viral etiology and predictors for hospital admission. West. Afr. J. Med., 24: 299-304.

[3] American Academy of Pediatrics, C. O. I. D. A. C. O. F. A. N. Revised indications for theuse of palivizumab and respiratory syncytial virus immune globulin intravenous for theprevention of respiratory syncytial virus infections. Pediatrics 2003; 112: 1442.

[4] Arnott A, Vong S, Mardy S, Chu S, Naughtin M, Sovann L, Buecher C, Beauté J, Rith S, Borand L, Asgari N, Frutos R, Guillard B, Touch S, Deubel V, Buchy P.

[5] A study of the genetic variability of human respiratory syncytial virus (HRSV) in Cambodia reveals the existence of a new HRSV group B genotype. J Clin Microbiol. 2011, 49(10):3504-13.

[6] Becker Y. Respiratory syncytial virus (RSV) evades the human adaptive immune system by skewing the Th1/Th2 cytokine balance toward increased levels of Th2 cytokines and IgE, markers of allergy--a review. Virus Genes. 2006 33(2):235-52.

[7] Black CP. Systematic review of the biology and medical management of respiratory syncytial virus infection. Respir Care 2003;48:209-231.

[8] Cane, P. A., and C. R. Pringle. Molecular epidemiology of respiratory syncytial virus: a review of the use of reverse transcription-polymerase chain reaction in the analysis of genetic variability. Electrophoresis 1995. 16:329-333.

[9] Cane PA, Weber M, Sanneh M, Dackour R, Pringle CR, Whittle H. Molecular epidemiology of respiratory syncytial virus in The Gambia. Epidemiol Infect 1999; 122: 155-60.

[10] Collins PL, Chanock RM, Murphy BR. Respiratory syncytial virus. In: Knipe DM, Howley PM, Griffin DE, et al, eds. Fields Virology. Vol 1. 4th ed. Philadelphia: Lippincott Williams & Wilkins; 2001:1443–1486

[11] Collins PL, Melero JA: Progress in understanding and controlling respiratory syncytial virus: still crazy after all these years. Virus Res 2011, 162:80-99.

[12] Collins PL, Murphy BR. New generation live vaccines against human respiratory syncytial virus designed by reverse genetics. Proc Am Thorac Soc 2005;2:166–173

[13] Dallas A, Vlassov AV. RNAi: A novel antisense technology and its therapeutic potential. Med Sci Monit. 2006;12:RA67–74.

[14] Dickens, L.E., Collins,P.L.,and Wertz,G.W.(1984).Transcriptional Mapping Of Human Respiratory Syncytial Virus. Journal Of Virology 52:364-369.

[15] Domachowske J.B., Rosenberg H.F. (1999). Respiratory Syncytial virus infection. Immune Response, Immunopathogenesis and Treatment. Clinical Microbiology Review 12:298 - 309.

[16] Empey, KM., Peebles Jr, RS, Kolls JK. Pharmacologic Advances in the Treatment and Prevention of Respiratory Syncytial Virus *Clin Infect Dis. (2010) 50 (9): 1258-1267. doi: 10.1086/651603*

[17] Faghihloo, E.; Salimi, V.; Rezaei, F.; Naseri, M.; Mamishi, S.; Mahmoodi, M.; Mokhtari-Azad, T.Genetic diversity in the G protein gene of human respiratory syncytial virus among Iranian children with acute respiratory symptoms. Iranian Journal of Pediatrics 2011 21 (1): 58-64

[18] Falsey,A.R.,andWalsh,E.E.(1996).Safety And Immunogenicity OF A Respiratory Syncytial Virus Subunit Vaccine (PFP- 2) In Ambulatory Adults Over Age 60. Vaccine 14: 1214- 1218.

[19] Falsey,A.R.,and Walsh,E.E.(1997).Safety and Immunogenicity of a Respiratory Syncytial Virus Subunit Vaccine (PFP-2) In The Institutionalized Elderly. Vaccine 15: 1130-1132.

[20] Greenough A. Respiratory syncytial virus infection: Clinical features, management, and prophylaxis. Curr Opin Pulm Med 2002;8:214-217.

[21] Hall CB. Respiratory syncytial virus and parainfluenza virus. N Engl J Med 2001;344:1917-1928.

[22] Hall CB, Douglas RG, Jr., Geiman JM. Quantitative shedding patterns of respiratory syncytial virus in infants. J Infect Dis 1975;132:151–156.

[23] Hall CB, Douglas RG, Jr., Geiman JM. Possible transmission by fomites of respiratory syncytial virus. J Infect Dis 1980;141:98102.

[24] Hall CB, Douglas RG, Jr. Modes of transmission of respiratory syncytial virus. J Pediatr 1981;99:100–103.

[25] Hall CB, Douglas RG, Jr., Schnabel KC, Geiman JM. Infectivity of respiratory syncytial virus by various routes of inoculation. Infect Immune 1981;33:779–783.

[26] Hall CB, Weinberg G, Iwane M, Blumkin A,Ewards K, Staat M. The burden of Respiratory Syncytial Virus infection in young children. N Engl J Med 2009; 360: 588-98.

[27] Jamjoom, G.A., A.M. Al-Semrani, A. Board, A.R. Al-Frayh, F. Artz and K.F. Al-Mobaireek, 1993. Respiratory syncytial virus infection in young children hospitalized with respiratory illness in Riyadh. J. Trop. Pediatr., 39: 346-349.

[28] Jawetz, Melnick and Adelbergs (2004). Paramyxo viruses and Rubella viruses. In C.F. Brooks, J.S. Butes, S.A. Morse (ed), Medical microbiology 23rd ed, Pp 558-560.

[29] Johnson TR, Graham BS. Contribution of respiratory syncytial virus G antigenicity to vaccine-enhanced illness and the implications for severe disease during primary respiratory syncytial virus infection. Pediatr Infect Dis J 2004;23(Suppl 1):S46–S57

[30] Karron RA, Wright PF, Belshe RB, et al. Identification of a recombinant live attenuated respiratory syncytial virus vaccine candidate that is highly attenuated in infants. J Infect Dis 2005;191:1093–1104

[31] Kim HW, Canchola JG, Brandt CD, et al. Respiratory syncytial virus disease in infants despite prior administration of antigenic inactivated vaccine. Am J Epidemiol 1969;89: 422–434

[32] Kneyber MC, Kimpen JL. Advances in respiratory syncytial virus vaccine development. Curr Opin Investig Drugs 2004; 5:163–170

[33] Koetz A, Nilsson P, Linden M, van derHoek L, Ripa T. Detection of human coronavirus NL63, human metapneumovirus and respiratory syncytial virus in children with respiratory tract infections in south-west Sweden. Clin Microbiol Infect 2006; 12:1089–1096.

[34] Lemanske RF. J Allergy Clin Immunol. 2004 Nov;114(5):1023-6. Viral infections and asthma inception.

[35] Lukic-Grlic A, Bace A, Lokar-Kolbas R, et al. Clinical and epidemiological aspects of respiratory syncytial virus lower respiratory tract infections. Eur J Epidemiol 1999; 15: 361-5.

[36] Manjunath N, Wu H, Subramanya S, Shankar P. Lentiviral delivery of short hairpin RNAs. *Adv Drug Deliv Rev* 2009, 61(9):732-45,.

[37] McIntosh,K. (1997). Respiratory Syncytial Virus. In: Evans, A., Kaslow. R., (Ed). Viral Infections in Humans: Epidemiology and control. 4th edition. New York: plenum; Pp 691-705.

[38] Meissner HC, Long , SS. Revised Indications for the Use of Palivizumab and Respiratory Syncytial Virus Immune Globulin Intravenous for the Prevention of Respiratory Syncytial Virus Infections. Pediatrics Vol. 112 No. 6 December 1, 2003 pp. 1447 -1452

[39] Meqdam, M.M. and S.H. Subaih, 2006. Rapid detectionand clinical features of infants and young children with acute lower respiratory tract infection due to respiratory syncytial virus. FEMS Immunol. Med. Microbiol., 47: 129-133.

[40] Mohapatra SS, Boyapalle S.Epidemiologic, Experimental, and Clinical Links between Respiratory Syncytial Virus Infection and Asthma. *Clin. Microbiol. Rev.* 2008 (21)3: 495-504

[41] Munoz FM, Piedra PA, Glezen WP. Safety and immunogenicity of respiratory syncytial virus purified fusion protein-2 vaccine in pregnant women. Vaccine 2003;21:3465–3467

[42] Nair H, Nokes DJ, Gessner BD, Dherani M, Madhi SA, Singleton RJ, et al. Global burden of acute lower respiratory infections due to respiratory syncytial virus in young children: a systematic review and meta-analysis. Lancet. 2010;375:1545–55. doi: 10.1016/S0140-6736(10)60206-1

[43] Niekerk SV, Venter M. Replacement of Previously Circulating Respiratory Syncytial Virus Subtype B Strains with the BA Genotype in South Africa *J. Virol.* September 2011 85(17) 8789-8797

[44] Openshaw PJ, Culley FJ, Olszewska W. Immunopathogenesis of vaccine-enhanced RSV disease. Vaccine 2001; 20(Suppl 1):S27–S31

[45] Openshaw, PJM. Potential therapeutic implications of new insights into respiratory syncytial virus disease. Respir Res 2002, 3 (suppl 1):S15-S20

[46] Othumpangat S, Gibson L, Samsell L, Piedimonte G. NGF is an essential survival factor for bronchial epithelial cells during respiratory syncytial virus infection. PLoS ONE 2009;4:e6444

[47] Piedra PA. Clinical experience with respiratory syncytial virus vaccines. Pediatr Infect Dis J 2003;22(Suppl 2):S94–S99

[48] Peret TC, Hall CB, Hammond GW, et al. Circulation patterns of group A and B human respiratory syncytial virus genotypes in 5 communities in North America. J Infect Dis 2000; 181: 1891-6.

[49] Resch B. Respiratory Syncytial Virus Infection in High-Risk Infants *The Open Microbiology Journal,* 2011, *5,* (Suppl 2-M1) 127

[50] Schmidt., AC.Progress in Respiratory Virus Vaccine Development. Semin Respir Crit Care Med. 2007;28(2):243-252.

[51] Simões EA. Environmental and demographic risk factors for respiratory syncytial virus lower respiratory tract disease. *J Pediatr.* 2003;143(5 suppl):S118-S126.

[52] Smith EC, Popa A, Chang A, Masante C, Dutch RE. Viral entry mechanisms: the increasing diversity of paramyxovirus entry. FEBS J. 2009; 276(24): 7217–7227.

[53] Stensballe LG, Devasundaram JK., Simoes, EAF. Pediatr Infect Dis J, 2003; 22(2): 22:S21–32. Respiratory syncytial virus epidemics: the ups and downs of a seasonal virus

[54] Sullender WM.. Respiratory Syncytial Virus Genetic and Antigenic Diversity. Clinical Microbiology Reviews, Jan. 2000, p. 1–15

[55] Trento A, Viegas M, Galiano M, Videla C, Carballal G, Mistchenko AS., Melero JA. Natural History of Human Respiratory Syncytial Virus Inferred from Phylogenetic Analysis of the Attachment (G) Glycoprotein with a 60-Nucleotide Duplication J. Virol. 2006 80(2) 975-984

[56] Venter M, Collinson M, Schoub BD. Molecular epidemiological analysis of community circulating respiratory syncytial virus in rural South Africa: comparison of viruses and genotypes responsible for different disease manifestations. J Med Virol 2002; 68: 452-61

[57] Welliver RC. Respiratory syncytial virus and other respiratory viruses. Pediatr Infect Dis J 2003;22:S6-S10.

[58] Wright PF, Karron RA, Belshe RB, et al. Evaluation of a live, cold-passaged, temperature-sensitive, respiratory syncytial virus vaccine candidate in infancy. J Infect Dis 2000; 182:1331–1342

[59] Wright PF, Karron RA, Madhi SA, et al. The interferon antagonist xlink protein of respiratory syncytial virus is an important virulence determinant for humans. J Infect Dis 2006;193:573–581

[60] Zlateva KT, Vijgen L, Dekeersmaeker N, Naranjo C, Van Ranst M. Subgroup prevalence and genotype circulation patterns of human respiratory syncytial virus in Belgium during ten successive epidemic seasons. J Clin Microbiol. 2007 45(9):3022-30.

Chapter 3

Structural and Functional Aspects of Viroporins in Human Respiratory Viruses: Respiratory Syncytial Virus and Coronaviruses

Wahyu Surya, Montserrat Samsó and Jaume Torres

Additional information is available at the end of the chapter

http://dx.doi.org/10.5772/53957

1. Introduction

Viroporins are an increasingly recognized class of small viral membrane proteins (~60-120 amino acids) which oligomerize to produce hydrophilic pores at the membranes of virus-infected cells [1]. The existence of 'viroporins' was proposed more than 30 years ago after observing enhanced membrane permeability in infected cells [2]. These proteins form oligomers of defined size, and can act as proton or ion channels, and in general enhancing membrane permeability in the host [3]. Even though viroporins are not essential for the replication of viruses, their absence results in attenuated or weakened viruses or changes in tropism (organ localization) and therefore diminished pathological effects [4, 5].

In addition to having one – sometimes two – α-helical transmembrane (TM) domain(s), viroporins usually contain additional extramembrane regions that are able to make contacts with viral or host proteins. Indeed, the network of interactions of viroporins with other viral or cellular proteins is key to understand the regulation of viral protein trafficking through the vesicle system, viral morphogenesis and pathogenicity.

In general, viroporins participate in the entry or release of viral particles into or out of cells, and membrane permeabilization may be a desirable functionality for the virus. Indeed, several viral proteins that are not viroporins are known to affect membrane permeabilization, e.g., A38L protein of vaccinia virus, a 33-kDa glycoprotein that allows Ca^{2+} influx and induces necrosis in infected cells [6]. In viruses that lack typical viroporins, their function may be replaced by such pore-forming glycoproteins. For example, HIV-2 lacks typical viroporins, and ROD10 Env is an envelope glycoprotein that enhances viral particle release. In HIV-1, this function is attributed to the viroporin Vpu [7].

An important point that needs to be established, in view of the observed channel activity of viroporins, is whether the channels they form are selective, with a controlled gating mechanism, or whether permeabilization is non selective, like in some antimicrobial peptides [8]. Viroporins have also been found to modulate endogenous cellular channels [9-12] and this activity may also have an important regulatory role during the life cycle of the virus.

Viroporins can be found in all kinds of viruses, RNA, DNA, enveloped and non-enveloped. Examples of viroporins are picornavirus 2B [13], alphavirus 6K [14-16], HIV-1 Vpu [17, 18], influenza virus A M2, (also called AM2) [19], RSV SH protein [20], p10 protein of avian reovirus [21], Human hepatitis C virus (HCV) and bovine viral diarrhea virus (BVDV) p7 [22, 23], Paramecium bursaria chlorella virus (PBCV-1) Kcv [24], and coronavirus envelope proteins, e.g., SARS-CoV E [25, 26]. Recent reviews [27, 28] provide more examples and possible functional roles.

The most extensively studied viroporin to date is probably the M2 protein from influenza A virus (AM2). AM2 protein is 97-residue long, with one transmembrane (TM) domain and a C-terminal cytoplasmic amphiphilic helix. AM2 forms homotetramers and is located in the viral envelope, where it enables protons from the endosome to enter the viral particle (virion). This lowers the pH inside the viral particle, causing dissociation of the viral matrix protein M1 from the ribonucleoprotein RNP, uncoating of the virus and exposure of the content to the cytoplasm of the host cell. AM2 also delays acidification of the late Golgi in some strains [29, 30].

The proton channel activity of AM2 can be inhibited by antiviral drugs amantadine and rimantadine, which block the virus from taking over the host cell. Two different high-resolution structures of truncated forms of AM2 have been reported: the structure of a mutated form of its TM region (residues 22-46) [31], and a slightly longer form (residues 18-60) containing the TM region and a segment of the C-terminal domain [32, 33]. These studies suggest that the known AM2 adamantane inhibitors, amantadine and rimantadine, act by either blocking the pore [31, 34] or by an allosteric mechanism [32]. New AM2 inhibitors have been reported [35], but their effectiveness against adamantane-resistant viruses remains to be established. The use of these drugs presents a classical example of targeting viral channels to treat viral infection infection [31, 32, 36].

The case of AM2 protein in influenza A represents a link between viroporin activity and structure to viral pathogenesis. Unfortunately, for many viroporins even rudimentary structural models are lacking due to high hydrophobicity, conformational flexibility and tendency to aggregate. For some viroporins however, increasing degrees of structural information can be obtained due to availability of high quality purified protein. Examples of these are the viroporins present in coronaviruses (CoV) and in the respiratory syncytial virus (RSV), envelope (E) protein and the small hydrophobic (SH) protein, respectively. Both types of virus infect the upper and lower respiratory tract of humans, and their viroporins are the subject of this chapter.

2. Envelope (E) and Small Hydrophobic (SH) proteins in respiratory viruses

2.1. SH protein in hRSV

Medical impact of the human respiratory syncytial virus (hRSV) infection. hRSV is a member of the *Paramyxoviridae* family, and is the leading cause of bronchiolitis and pneumonia in infants and the elderly worldwide [37]. hRSV infection is the most frequent cause of hospitalization of infants and young children in industrialized countries. In the USA alone, around 100,000 infants with hRSV infection are hospitalized annually. hRSV also is a significant problem in the elderly, patients with cardiopulmonary diseases and in immunocompromised individuals. hRSV accounts for approximately 10,000 deaths per year in the group of >64 years of age in the US. Globally, hRSV infection results in 64 million cases and 160,000 deaths every year (http://www.who.int/vaccine_research/diseases/ari/en/index2.html).

There is currently no effective vaccine available to prevent hRSV infection. Development of vaccines has been complicated by the fact that host immune responses appear to play a significant role in the pathogenesis of the disease [38]. Naturally acquired immunity to hRSV is neither complete nor durable, and recurrent infections occur frequently during the first three years of life. Palivizumab, a humanized monoclonal antibody directed against hRSV surface fusion F protein (Synagis, by MedImmune), is moderately effective but very expensive. It is currently available as prophylactic drug for infants at high risk. Cost of prevention limits its use in many parts of the world. The only licensed drug for use in infected people is ribavirin, but its efficacy is limited. Antibodies against both F (fusion) and G (attachment) proteins have been found in the serum of hRSV infected patients, but only provide temporary protection. Therefore, low immunoprotection and lack of suitable antivirals leads towards the search and characterization of new drug targets for the effective treatments of hRSV infection. A possible suitable target is the SH protein as will be elaborated below.

The viral particle formation in RSV. Based on the reactive patterns to monoclonal antibodies, there are two hRSV strains that co-circulate in human populations, subtypes A and B. The hRSV genome comprises a nonsegmented negative-stranded RNA of ~15 kb that transcribes 11 proteins, including the three membrane proteins fusion (F), attachment (G), and small hydrophobic (SH) [39, 40]. The F protein is sufficient for mediating viral entry into cells *in vitro*, and the G protein plays a role in viral attachment [41, 42]. In contrast, the precise role of SH protein is still unclear.

hRSV also contains six internal structural proteins: the matrix (M) protein, which provides structure for the virus particle, nucleoprotein (N), phosphoprotein (P) and large (L) polymerase protein form the ribonucleoprotein (RNP) complex, which encapsidates the RSV genome and functions as the RNA-dependent RNA polymerase. Lastly, two isoforms of matrix protein 2 (M2-1 and M2-2) are accessory proteins that control transcription and replication [43]. Viral proteins traffic to the apical surface of polarized epithelial cells, where they assemble into virus filaments at the plasma membrane [44], although the mechanisms that drive assembly into filaments and budding are not well understood.

Generation of nascent hRSV genomic RNA appears to occur in discrete cytoplasmic inclusion bodies that contain the hRSV N, P, L, M2-1 and M2-2 proteins but not the F, G, or SH proteins [45]. It is suspected that the RNP complexes form in the inclusions and then traffic to the apical membrane, where they meet with the surface glycoproteins F, G, and SH arriving from the Golgi apparatus through the secretory pathway [46]. hRSV proteins and viral RNA assemble into virus filaments at the cell surface. These filaments are thought to contribute to cell-cell spread of the virus and morphologically resemble the filamentous form of virions seen in electron microscopy (EM) studies of virus produced in polarized cells [47].

The small hydrophobic (SH) protein. The SH protein is 65 or 64 amino acids long, in subtype A or B, respectively. SH protein has a single membrane-spanning hydrophobic region [48], and a C-terminal extramembrane tail, oriented extracellularly/lumenally [48]. The sequence of SH protein is highly conserved, especially at the TM domain [49, 50]. hRSV that lacks SH protein, hRSVΔSH, is still viable, and still forms syncytia [51-53]. However, hRSVΔSH was attenuated in *in vivo* mouse and chimpanzee models [4, 5], which indicates that SH protein is important for hRSV pathogenesis. SH protein has been suggested to play an ancillary role in virus-mediated cell fusion [54, 55]. Also, the presence of SH protein has been shown to reduce cytopathic effect (CPE) and apoptosis in L929 and A549 (lung epithelial cell line) infected cells, at least in part by inhibiting tumor necrosis factor α (TNF-α) production [56], similarly to parainfluenza virus 5 (PIV5).

Interaction of SH protein with viral and host proteins. Extensive protein-protein interactions have been observed between the three membrane proteins on the hRSV envelope, F, G, and SH [51, 57, 58] and these interactions have an effect on fusion activity of hRSV on the host [51, 54]. In cells transiently expressing hRSV membrane proteins, the presence of G and SH proteins enhanced fusion activity mediated by F protein [54, 55]. Thus, SH protein has been suggested to play an ancillary role in virus-mediated cell fusion. However, using virus-infected cells the presence of G protein alone enhanced F-mediated fusion activity [51], whereas SH protein in the absence of G protein inhibited it, suggesting a possible interaction between SH and G [51]. Viruses where the SH protein gene was deleted grew better in HEp-2 cells [55], leading to the suggestion of a negative regulatory effect of SH protein on virus-induced membrane fusion, although direct interaction between SH protein and fusion-responsible F protein has not been observed [58], whereas complexes F-G and G-SH have been detected on the surface of infected cells using immunoprecipitation [58] and heparin agarose affinity chromatography [57]. These three proteins not only form hetero-oligomers, but also homo-oligomers: F forms trimers [59], G forms tetramers [60], and SH forms pentamers [48, 61, 62]. Thus, a complicated regulatory network of interactions may exist which probably includes both homo- and hetero-oligomeric forms.

In addition to interactions with viral proteins, the fact that SH proteins of hRSV and parainfluenza virus 5 (PIV5) are necessary for the inhibition of tumor necrosis factor alpha (TNF-α)-induced apoptosis [56, 63] also suggests a possible interaction with host proteins, although this has not been confirmed experimentally. However, in another study, deletion of SH protein gene from RSV did not result in increased apoptosis in infected H441 cells [11].

Localization and post-translational modifications of SH protein during viral infection. In infected cells, some SH protein is found in plasma membrane and cytoplasm, but most of the SH protein accumulates at the membranes of the Golgi complex and only very low amounts are found in the viral envelope [64]. Several forms of the SH protein, glycosylated and non-glycosylated, are present during infection [65], but the non-glycosylated form appears to be the most abundant [66]. SH protein is also modified by tyrosine phosphorylation [61], and increased accumulation of SH in the Golgi complex was observed in the presence of a kinase inhibitor. Thus, SH protein is modified by a MAPK p38-dependent tyrosine kinase activity and this modification influences its cellular distribution. Although SH contains one cysteine residue, no palmitoylation has been detected in SH protein in conditions where F and G were palmitoylated [48].

Structural determination of SH protein. An important step towards the understanding of viroporin function at the molecular level is the availability of these proteins in a highly pure form. This has been so far difficult due to their high hydrophobicity, toxicity to expression hosts, and tendency to aggregate. However, recently we have been able to obtain the full length SH protein [67] that allows structural and biophysical studies (Fig. 1A).

SH protein after cross-linking has been shown to form multiple oligomers of increasing size in SDS [66, 68]. Later, we showed that the TM domain of SH protein forms only homopentamers in perfluoro-octanoic acid (PFO) gels [69]. Reports using purified full-length SH protein have confirmed the pentameric nature of the oligomer formed by this protein. For example, a bundle formation of a tagged SH protein construct was visualized under electron microscopy and was interpreted as a pentameric or a hexameric structure [70]. Using a purified tag-free SH protein, we have unequivocally demonstrated the homo-pentameric nature of these oligomers in a variety of detergents using analytical ultracentrifugation and electrophoresis (Fig. 1) [71]. Indeed, in the presence of PFO (Fig. 1B) and a variety of other detergents under Blue-native gel electrophoresis (Fig. 1C), the full-length SH protein migrates as a single band with a molecular weight ~40 kDa, consistent with a pentameric oligomer. The pentameric form of SH has been further confirmed by analytical ultracentrifugation sedimentation equilibrium in detergents DPC, C14SB and C8E5 micelles. In these detergents, the species distribution profiles show a best fit to a monomer-pentamer self-association model (Fig. 1 D-E).

Secondary structure of SH protein. The SH protein is predicted to have an α-helical region spanning residues 16-46, which includes its predicted TM region (residues ~20-40, Fig. 1A). Fourier Transform infrared (FTIR) data for the full-length SH protein reconstituted in model lipid bilayers shows the presence of ~60% α-helical structure, whereas the rest is β-structure [71]. The availability of purified, isotopically labeled protein allowed us to obtain a model for this pentameric oligomer where SH protein was reconstituted in DPC micelles using NMR (Fig. 2). The model shows the lumen of the hypothetic channel, sufficient for the passage of ions.

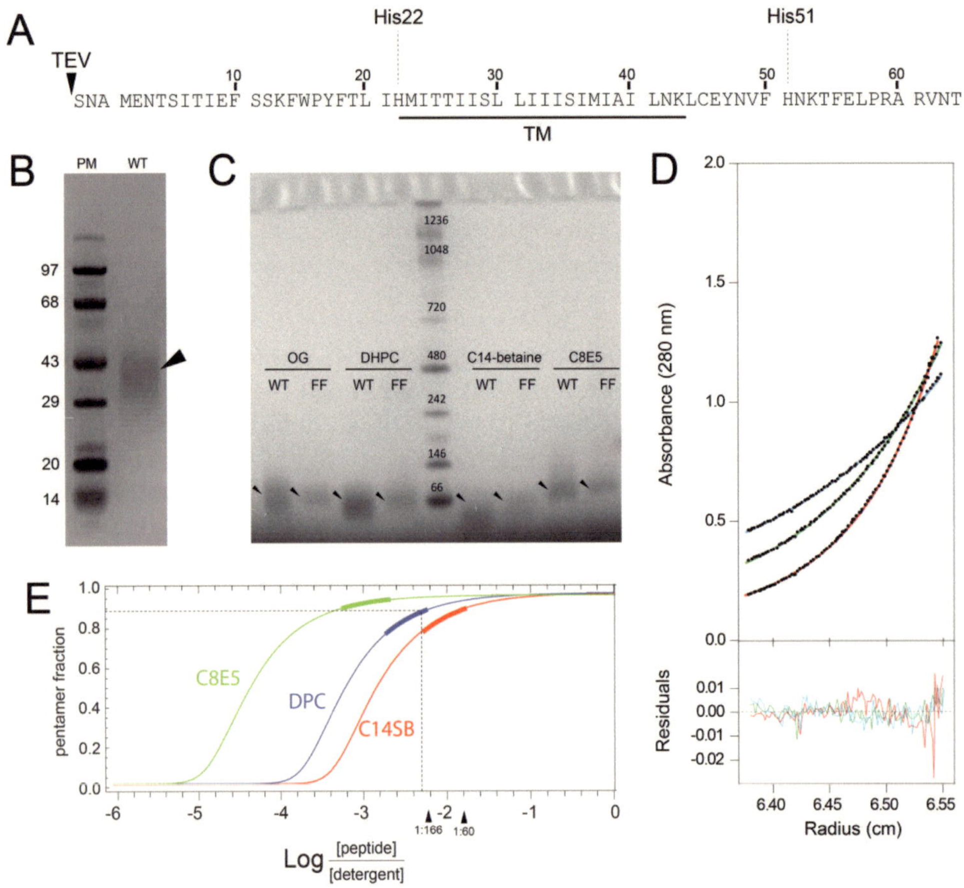

Figure 1. Sequence and oligomerization of SH protein from hRSV subtype A. (A) Amino acid sequence of full-length SH protein, with three additional N-terminal residues, SNA, as a result of tobacco etch virus (TEV) protease cleavage to remove the expression tag [71]; (B) Gel electrophoresis analysis of SH protein in PFO shows a band consistent with pentamers (arrow); (C) Blue-native gel electrophoresis of wild type SH protein (WT) and double mutant H22F/H51F (FF) presolubilized in a variety of detergents show one band migrating consistent with pentamers (arrows); (D) Analytical ultracentrifugation sedimentation equilibrium data for 50 μM SH (WT) protein collected at three different speeds: 16,000 (blue), 19,500 (green), and 24,000 (red) rpm. Sedimentation profile was globally best-fitted to a monomer-pentamer equilibrium model. The graph shows both data points (black filled circles) and fitted function (in color). Lower panels represent fit residuals; (E) SH (WT) oligomeric species distribution in C14SB, C8E5 and DPC detergents, where the thick bar on the curve represents the range of protein:detergent molar ratios used in the AUC experiment. The dotted line indicates the protein:DPC molar ratio (1:200) used in the NMR experiments [71] and its corresponding pentamer fraction (~90%). C14SB, DPC and C8E5 detergent concentrations were 5, 15 and 33 mM, respectively.

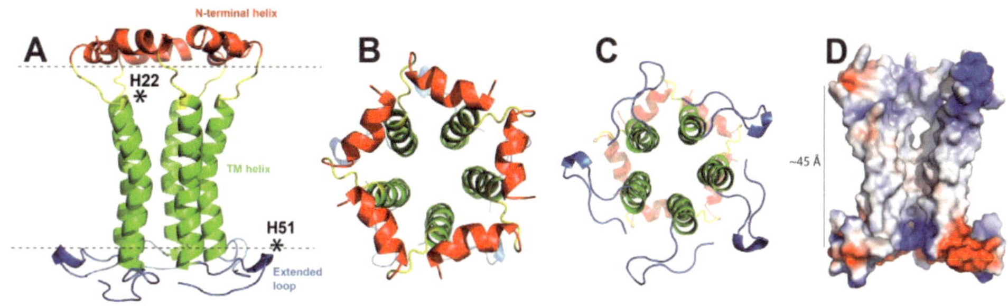

Figure 2. NMR-based pentameric model of RSV SH protein in detergent DPC micelles [71]. (A) Side view; (B) N-terminal (cytoplasmic) view; (C) C-terminal (extracellular or lumenal) view; (D) Electrostatic surface of the assembly showing the mostly hydrophobic central lumen. The SH protein assembly spans the entire bilayer with an overall length of about 45 Å.

Ion channel activity of SH protein. The presence of SH protein at the plasma membrane of HEK293 transfected cells allowed the study of SH protein channel activity [71], which was reported to be pH sensitive. Mutants where both histidines, H22 and H51 (Fig. 1A), were changed to phenylalanine (FF mutant, Fig. 1C), were found to be channel inactive. In a Blue-native gel electrophoresis, this FF mutant showed similar electrophoretic mobility (Fig. 1C) and similar plasma membrane localization to the wild type [71], which suggests that the observed channel activity is not mediated by direct or indirect interaction of SH protein with host-endogenous channels.

One of the two histidines, His22, was suggested to face the lumen of the pentameric oligomer using site-specific infrared dichroism of the isotopically labeled TM domain reconstituted in model lipid bilayers [69]. In the NMR based model of the full length protein (Fig. 2), although His22 adopts a lumenal orientation, the second histidine, His51, appears in an extra-membrane location, at the tip of the C-terminal extended loop (Fig. 2A), which is difficult to reconcile with an activation role based on His protonation. Thus, it is possible that the structure of this C-terminal domain in detergent micelles, used for the NMR experiment, does not represent accurately the structure of SH protein in lipid bilayers, where we obtained the patch clamp data. Nevertheless, the pH-activated channel activity observed, and the histidine-less inactive mutant strongly suggests that protonation of histidines may be involved in channel activity. Indeed, the presence of a lumenal histidine sidechain is reminiscent of the one found in the TM domain of the influenza A AM2 proton channel, which is also activated at low pH via histidine protonation [33].

Despite the similarities between AM2 and SH protein, we have been unable to observe strong proton channel activity of SH protein *in vitro* (unpublished observations). In addition, the different life cycle of hRSV and influenza virus A does not provide a rationale for this hypothetic proton channel activity. Equally, no obvious rationale can be assigned to pH mediated activation. The use of specific channel inhibitors for SH protein could contribute to clarify the precise role of channel activity in this protein, disentangled from other effects.

2.2. E protein in coronaviruses

Medical impact of coronaviruses. Coronaviruses (family *Coronaviridae*, genus *Coronavirus* [72]) are enveloped viruses that cause common cold in humans and a variety of lethal diseases in birds and mammals [73]. The species in the genus *Coronavirus* have been organized into 3 groups with genetic and antigenic criteria [74]: α-coronaviruses include the porcine *Transmissible gastroenteritis virus* (TGEV) and *Human coronaviruses 229E* (HCoV-229E) or NL63 (HCoV-NL63). β-coronaviruses include *Murine hepatitis virus* (MHV) and *Human coronavirus OC43* (HCoV-OC43). γ-coronaviruses include the avian *Infectious bronchitis virus* (IBV) and the Turkey coronavirus (TCoV). The virus responsible for the severe acute respiratory syndrome (SARS-CoV), a respiratory disease in humans, is close to the β-coronaviruses, formerly group 2 [75].

SARS produced a near pandemic in 2003, with 8,096 infected cases and 774 deaths worldwide (fatality rate of 9.6%). Mortality was 6% for those aged 25-44, 15 % for the 45-64 group and >50% for those over 65 (*http://www.who.int/csr/sarsarchive/2003_05_07a/en/*). For comparison, the case fatality rate for influenza A is usually around 0.6% (primarily among the elderly) and 33% in locally severe epidemics of new strains. SARS-CoV was enzootic in an unknown animal or bird species, probably a bat [76], before suddenly emerging as a virulent virus in humans. A similar crossing of the animal-human species barrier is thought to have occurred between the bovine coronavirus (BCoV) and human coronavirus OC43 (HCoV-OC43) more than 100 years ago [77]. Such interspecies jumps, from animal hosts to humans, are likely to reoccur.

Protective efficacy of candidate vaccines against coronaviruses in humans has been mainly studied in animals so far, and only few vaccines have entered Phase 1 human trials [78]. Ribavirin [79], interferons [80], unconventional agents [81-83] and non-steroidal anti-inflammatory agents [84] have shown activity against SARS-CoV and HCoV-229E, but there is no data from animal studies or clinical trials [85]. Studies of antiviral therapy against coronaviruses other than SARS-CoV have been scarce; *in vitro* data show that several chemicals may have inhibitory activities on HCoV-NL63 and HCoV-229E [86, 87].

In addition to the genes involved in viral RNA replication and transcription, other essential genes in coronaviruses encode the common viral structural proteins, S (spike), E (envelope), M (membrane) and N (nucleocapsid). Of these, S, E, and M are incorporated into the virion lipidic envelope, and S protein is involved in fusion with host membranes during entry into cells. The M protein is the most abundant constituent of coronaviruses and gives the virion envelopes their shape; the E protein is only a minor constituent of the virion but is abundantly expressed inside the infected cell [88-90].

The E protein in SARS-CoV is the shortest, with only 76 amino acids, whereas that of IBV E is one of the longest (109 amino acids). E protein sequences are extremely divergent in their sequence, but the same general architecture is found in all of them: a short hydrophilic N-terminus (8–12 residues), an N-terminal TM domain (21–29 residues) followed by a cluster of 2-3 cysteines which are likely to be palmitoylated, and finally a less hydrophobic C-terminal tail (39–76 residues). Prediction of TM domains of representatives of coronavirus E proteins from several species using a hidden Markov model (e.g., http://phobius.sbc.su.se/) [91] shows that they have at least one α-helical TM domain. In some cases a second TM domain is also predicted, e.g., in IBV E and MHV E (Fig 3). However, in none of these coronavirus E proteins this second putative TM has a predicted α-helical conformation. Instead, a β-coil-β motif appears to predominate in that part of the sequence, with a totally conserved Pro residue in a central position ('P' in Fig. 3).

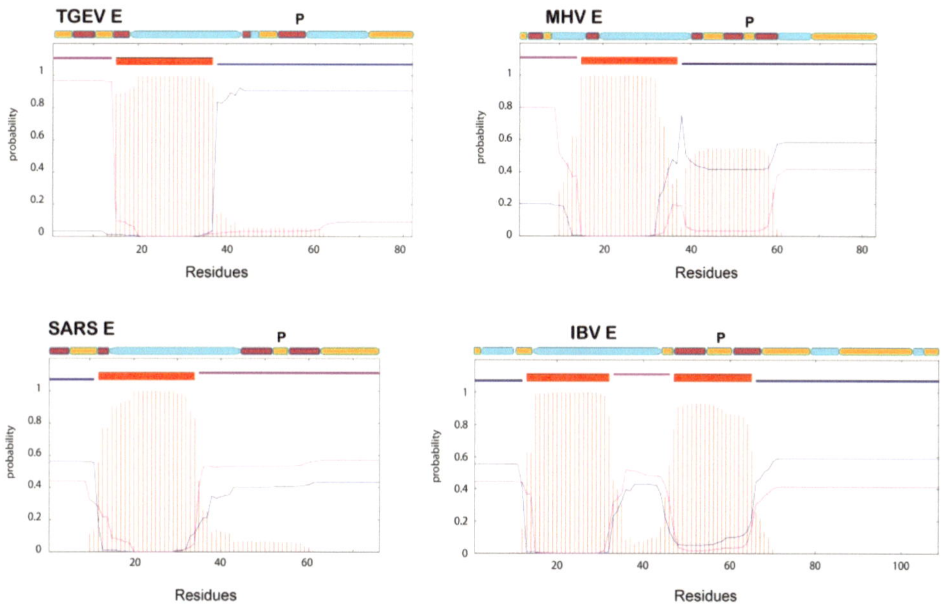

Figure 3. Secondary structure and TM prediction of E proteins of coronaviruses. E proteins from four representatives of coronavirus are presented: TGEV, MHV, SARS-CoV and IBV E proteins. Regions predicted to be α-helical, β-sheet, or random coil are marked in blue, red, and yellow, respectively. Red bars show the probability of a region being a TM domain. The location of the conserved Pro residue in each protein is indicated by a 'P'.

Topology of E proteins. The topology of coronavirus envelope proteins is an issue still under debate. Experimental determination of E protein orientation in infected cells [88, 92, 93] has shown that in TGEV E, the N-terminus is exposed to the cytoplasm, with the C-terminus facing the Golgi lumen ($N_{cyto}C_{exo}$). In MHV E, both N and C-terminal ends were found to face the cytoplasm ($N_{cyto}C_{cyto}$). For SARS-CoV E, an $N_{cyto}C_{cyto}$ topology, similar to MHV E, was reported in transfected cells [94], consistent with two TM domains ($N_{cyto}C_{cyto}$), although a small fraction of the population (~10%) was found to be glycosylated at residue N66. As glycosylation must have occurred in the Golgi lumen, the authors suggested the existence of a minor fraction of E protein in an $N_{cyto}C_{exo}$ topology. However, a study in infected cells detected the C terminus oriented cytoplasmically and the N-terminus lumenally [95], consistent with a single TM domain. Lastly, in IBV E, the C-terminus was found exposed to the cytoplasm, but not the N-terminus, suggesting a topology $N_{exo}C_{cyto}$, with the N-terminus facing the lumen of the Golgi [96].

The results of these experiments should be interpreted with caution, especially comparing data from transfected cells and infected cells. Equally, the possible lack of accessibility to antibodies of parts of the protein plays a part. Indeed, as discussed elsewhere [97], in the case of IBV E, if the entire N-terminal region of IBV E protein was buried within the intracellular membrane, it would have remained inaccessible to the antibodies used. Several coexisting forms may exist for E proteins, which would have different roles in the life cycle of the virus.

The factors that would favour one topology over another are unknown, but one possible candidate is palmitoylation. Indeed, E proteins of SARS [26], IBV [98] and MHV [99] are palmitoylated at one or more cysteines. This modification is likely to have structural and functional consequences, because removal of the cysteines in MHV E resulted in deformed viruses [100, 101]. Experimental determination of the topology of these E protein homologs – with or without palmitoylation – in model membranes or membrane-like detergents is critical to understand the function of the envelope protein in coronavirus biology. Unfortunately, these detailed structural studies are still not available.

The importance of the correct topology in E proteins may be highlighted by a recent study [102] that showed that E protein in MHV could be replaced by some heterologous E proteins. The MHV virus became viable when the replacement was from groups 2, i.e., β-coronaviruses (SARS-CoV E) and 3, i.e., γ-coronaviruses (IBV E), but not when TGEV E (group 1, or α-coronaviruses) was used. This discrimination may have to do with topology considerations, because the contribution of E proteins to the formation of viral particles in coronaviruses could be provided by a broad range of sequences, and not by specific interactions.

Localization of E protein during viral infection. E protein can be found between the ER and Golgi compartments inside the cell [103-105]. However, only a small amount ends up in the virion [88-90], suggesting that its main role is inside the cell [95]. In transfected HeLa cells, SARS-CoV E protein is targeted to the Golgi complex, and this localization has been attributed, at least in part, to the β-hairpin motif in its C-terminus [106] (see Fig. 3). In infected Vero E6 cells, SARS-CoV E protein accumulates in the ER-Golgi intermediate compartment (ERGIC) [95]; the latter study could not detect any SARS-CoV E protein in the plasma membrane.

Effect of coronavirus E gene deletion. While the absence of S and M protein are clearly deleterious to the virus because of their abundance and key role in envelope formation, the E protein is not essential for *in vitro* or *in vivo* coronavirus replication. However, the absence of E protein results in an attenuated virus, as shown for SARS-CoV [107] and other coronaviruses (see below). Recently, it has been shown that SARS viruses lacking gene E, in addition to being attenuated, did not grow in the central nervous system, in contrast to the wild type virus [108]. This suggests a role of the SARS-CoV E gene as a virulence factor influencing tissue tropism and pathogenicity. Recently, SARS-CoV lacking E gene has been suggested as vaccine candidate [109]. Studies using the E deleted SARS-CoV E have shown that E protein affects stress and inflammation responses [110], which probably contribute to the attenuation of the virus observed in the absence of this protein [107].

In other coronaviruses, it has been found that E protein is involved in viral morphogenesis, e.g., co-expression of M and E is sufficient for formation and release of virus-like particles (VLP) in the host cell [93, 111-115]. Also, mutations in the extramembrane domain of E protein were shown to impair viral assembly and maturation in MHV [116], probably due to a defective interaction with M protein. In TGEV, the absence of E protein resulted in a blockade of virus trafficking in the secretory pathway, and the prevention of virus maturation [117, 118].

Interaction partners of E proteins. The interaction of E protein with M in IBV has already been reported by two different labs [96, 119] and involves at least the C-terminal tail of these two proteins, which therefore should be on the same side of the lipid bilayer. Additionally, the extramembrane cytoplasmic tail of SARS-CoV E has also been reported to bind Bcl-X_L [120] and the N-terminal domain of non-structural protein 3 (nsp3) [121]. Similar studies have shown that SARS-CoV E via its four last C-terminal amino-acids, interacts with the host protein, PALS1, a tight junction-associated protein. Intercellular tight junctions are a physical barrier that protects underlying tissues from pathogen invasions. In SARS-CoV–infected Vero E6 cells, PALS1 redistributes to the ERGIC/Golgi region, where E accumulates. Hijacking PALS1 by SARS-CoV E may play a determinant role in the disruption of the lung epithelium in SARS patients [122]. SARS-CoV E has also been found to interact with Na^+/K^+ ATPase α-1 subunit and stomatin [95].

Channel activity in coronavirus E proteins. Enhanced permeability has been observed in bacterial and mammalian cells expressing MHV E [123] or SARS-CoV E [26]. In addition, E proteins of SARS, human coronavirus 229E, MHV, and IBV, have shown *in vitro* ion channel activity in planar lipid bilayers [124, 125], which in some cases was inhibited by the drug hexamethylene amiloride (HMA) [125]. In a patch clamp study, channel activity was observed in cells transfected with SARS-CoV E [25], although another study could not detect SARS-CoV E protein in the plasma membrane of transfected or infected cells [95]. Nevertheless, channel activity has been shown in black lipid membranes for purified synthetic TM domains and full length SARS-CoV [67, 126, 127], and inactivating mutations located in the TM domain, N15A and V25F [126], have been confirmed recently in a separate study [128]. In the latter, a significant contribution of lipid composition was observed, and a protein-lipid complex forming pore was proposed. These mutants may help elucidate the contribution of channel activity to SARS-CoV E protein function.

Structural determination of E protein. At present, detailed structures of coronavirus envelope proteins are lacking. This is due difficulties in both expression and purification, and to their high tendency to aggregate which makes crystallization and NMR studies extremely challenging. Recently, we have successfully utilized a modified β-barrel fusion protein construct to express and subsequently purify full-length SARS-CoV E and IBV E proteins [67].

We showed that both full length proteins form homopentamers, confirming previous results obtained only with the synthetic TM domain [25].

Previous reports have studied the oligomerization of coronavirus E proteins. However, results were not conclusive, partly because these experiments were performed in SDS, a harsh detergent that leads to monomers or to non-specific aggregates. For example, SARS-CoV E oligomerization has been studied in Western Blots after SDS-PAGE and labeling with polyclonal antibodies [99], antibodies against a hemagglutinin-derived C-terminal tag [100], or using non purified or truncated synthetic E proteins [124, 125]. In the latter approach, a predominanly monomeric form was observed in SDS. In our hands, synthetic SARS-CoV E also produced in SDS mostly monomers, and a minor fraction of dimers (unpublished observations), but several oligomers were observed for the recombinant form (Fig. 4, lane WT). The differences between synthetic and recombinant E protein may be due to unwanted side reactions that take place during synthesis. Addition of DTT (Fig. 4B) produces bands compatible with monomers and trimers, whereas cysteine-less mutants only produced monomers. Thus, the three cysteines in SARS-CoV E seem to participate in some inter-monomeric contacts. Indeed, sedimentation data for SARS-CoV E could only be fitted after addition of reductant [67] in the case of SARS-CoV E. Differences between absence and presence of reductant were observed even when only one cysteine was available (Fig. 4B), therefore these disulfide bonds may not be specific. Changes in hydrophobicity and local secondary structure seem to play a major role in the results observed. Further, disulfide bonds are not necessary to form pentamers; sedimentation equilibrium of full-length SARS-CoV E or IBV E in C14SB detergent and in the presence of reducing agent produced best fit to a monomer-pentamer equilibrium model [67], similar to what has been observed for the TM region alone [127].

The likely orientation of these cysteine residues relative the pentameric bundle can be determined on the basis of the available structure formed by synthetic TM_{8-38} [25]. That structure did not include any of the three cysteines of SARS-CoV E, but if the structural model is prolonged by two turns (Fig. 5), the three cysteines are seen oriented either towards the lumen of the channel or inter-helically.

The juxtamembrane cysteines in coronavirus envelope proteins are well conserved, and have been found to be crucial in the coronavirus cycle. For example, in MHV E, removal of the cysteines resulted in deformed viruses [99-101]. Using the full length infectious clone [99], double- and triple-mutants to alanine produced smaller plaques and decreased virus yields. Single-substitution mutants, in contrast, did not produce anomalous growth, whereas replacement of all three cysteines resulted in crippled virus with significantly reduced yields. In these reports, these effects were attributed to the absence of palmitoylation sites, which may direct E proteins towards lipid rafts [129]. E proteins of SARS [26], IBV [98] and MHV [99] have been shown to be palmitoylated at one or more cysteines. It is possible that an additional role of palmitoylation is to drag the C-terminal tail of E proteins towards the membrane and trigger a conformational change.

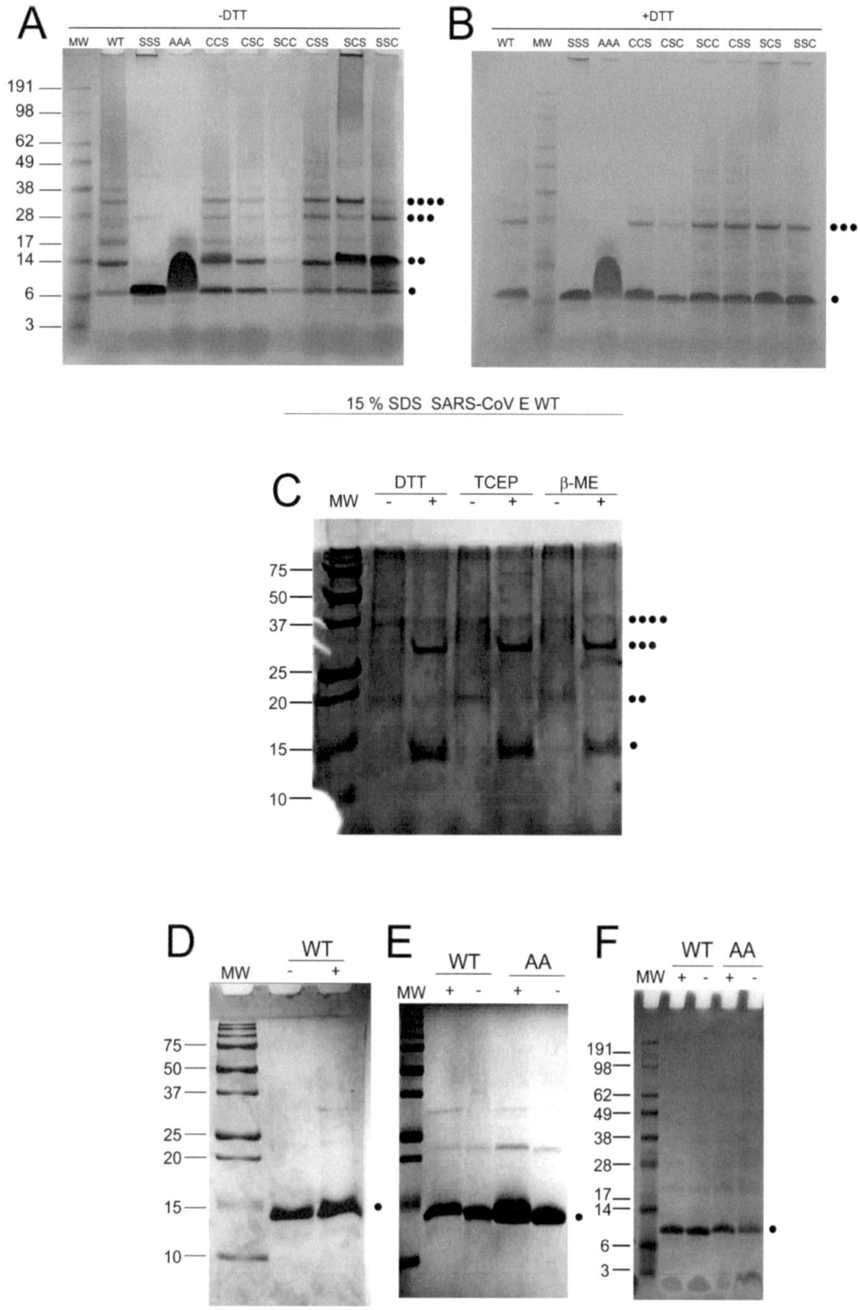

Figure 4. SDS-PAGE electrophoresis of SARS-CoV E and IBV E. (A) SARS-CoV E wild type (WT) and cysteine mutants in the absence of DTT in gel 4-12 % Nu-PAGE in MES/SDS buffer; (B) same as A in presence of DTT. The lane containing the molecular weight markers (MW) is indicated. The oligomeric size is indicated by black circles (●); (C) Effect of three reductants (DTT, TCEP and β-mercaptoethanol (β-ME) on the electrophoretic mobility SARS-CoV E WT in 15% SDS PAGE gel.

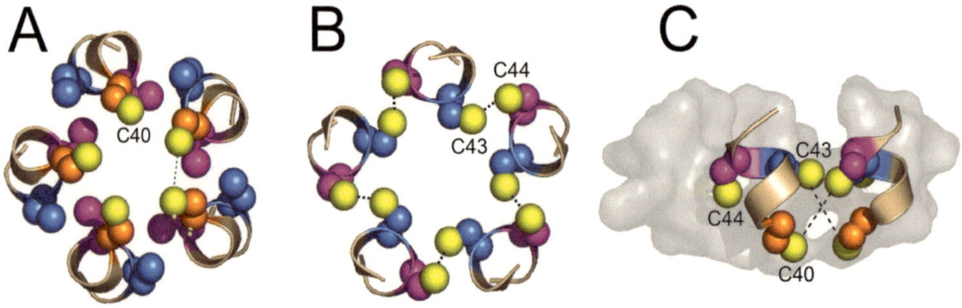

Figure 5. Cysteine location in the pentameric arrangement of the TM domain of SARS-CoV E. The scheme is arranged according to previous published models [25, 130] after prolonging the helices 2 turns at the C-terminal end, and shows the position of the three cysteines in SARS-CoV E, C40, C43 and C44; A and B, views from the N-terminus of the pentamer, with C40 (A) and C43 and C44 (B); C, Side view, showing only two helices for clarity, and possible inter-helical disulfide bonds C43-C40 and C44-C40.

Dissection of the domains of SARS-CoV E. The four representatives of CoV E proteins have a predicted α-helical TM domain (Fig. 6a) and a C-terminal region predicted to have β-structure. Synthetic peptide 36-76 encompasses the C-terminal extramembrane domain and was analyzed in the presence of DMPC lipid membranes using FTIR. This peptide presented limited solubility both in water and in organic solvents. The amide I spectrum of this peptide (Fig. 6b) shows bands assigned to antiparallel β-sheet, because of the splitting of the amide I band caused by strong inter- and intra-strand transition dipole coupling (TDC) [131-133], resulting in a weak band at high frequency (1675–1690 cm^{-1}) and a strong band at lower frequency (1625–1640 cm^{-1}). The band at 1666 cm^{-1} can be assigned to disordered structure [134, 135]. The amide A frequency was blue-shifted from that observed for the TM domain alone [130] (3,305 cm^{-1}) or full length SARS-CoV E (3294 cm^{-1}, not shown) to 3281 cm^{-1}, again consistent with the presence of β-structure. The intensity of the amide II band decreased upon exposure to D_2O (dotted line, Fig. 6b) by about 30 ± 5%, i.e., ~28 residues are resistant to exchange in this peptide. The fast-exchanging fraction is likely due to the region predicted to have random coil conformation. Thus, the 36-76 fragment has an intrinsic tendency to fold as β-sheet, and presents both β-structure and random coil, in agreement with the secondary structure prediction (Fig. 6a). In fact, the spectrum resulting from the addition of TM α-helix (8-38) [130] and C-terminal tail (36-76), shown in Fig. 6b, is very similar to the spectrum obtained for full length SARS-CoV E (Fig. 6e, dotted line) reconstituted in the same conditions.

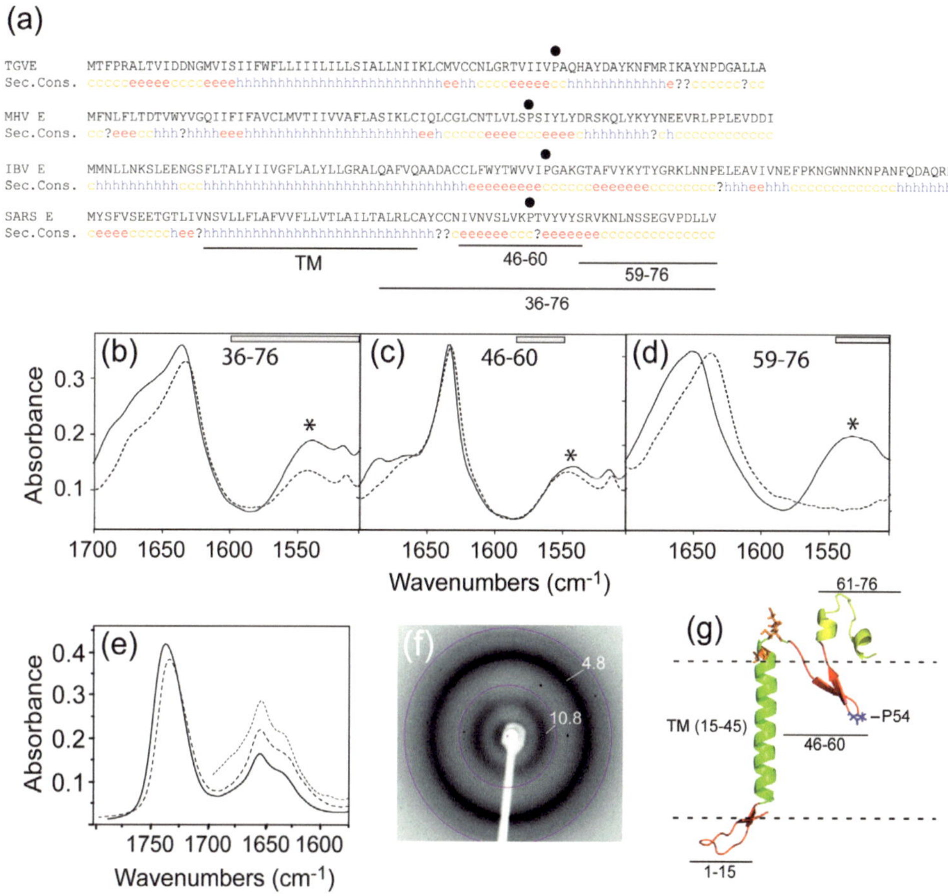

Figure 6. Secondary structure prediction of coronavirus envelope proteins and correspondence with results obtained for synthetic peptides of SARS-CoV E. (a) Sequences corresponding to E proteins representative of coronavirus groups 1 (TGEV E), 2 (MHV E), 3 (IBV E) and SARS CoV E, and their predicted secondary structure (consensus)[136]. The position of the conserved proline is indicated with a black dot; (b-d) amide I and II bands of the synthetic SARS-CoV E peptides indicated when incorporated in DMPC bilayers in H_2O (solid) or after D_2O (dash) hydration. The position of amide II band is indicated by a star; (e) ATR-FTIR spectra corresponding to SARS-CoV E (solid line), and IBV E (broken line) reconstituted in DMPC bilayers, in the lipid ester region (1740 cm^{-1}) and amide I region (C=O stretching, 1650 cm^{-1}). The dotted line resulted from the addition of the spectra corresponding to the TM [130] and fragment 36-76 (panel b); (f) X-ray diffraction pattern for peptides (36-76) or (46-60) after drying from acetonitrile. The inter-sheet spacing is 10.8 Å (inner ring) whereas the hydrogen bond spacing is represented by the outer ring at 4.8 Å, characteristic of amyloid fibrils. Due to poor alignment, the reflection at distance 4.8 Å appeared as a ring; (g) schematic model of full length SARS-CoV E build using prediction tools and experimental data obtained using infrared spectroscopy.

Similar experiments with fragments 46-60 and 59-76 (Fig. 6, c-d) showed that 46-60 forms β-sheets resistant to H/D exchange. Indeed, this latter peptide showed limited solubility, similar to the 'parent' peptide 36-76. Further, its amide I spectrum in DMPC displayed the features of antiparallel β-sheet, with bands at 1635 cm^{-1} and 1685 cm^{-1} (Fig. 6c) and showed no H/D exchange in the amide II region (Fig. 6c, star). In contrast, fragment 61-76 is predicted to form random coil (Fig. 6a), and should show complete H/D exchange. Indeed, the hydrophilic fragment 59–76 dissolved readily in water (>5 mg/ml), produced an amide I spectrum in DMPC consistent with random structure (Fig. 6d), with a broad amide I band at 1645 cm^{-1}, and showed complete H/D exchange at the amide II region (star).

The two folding domains observed in the C-terminal domain of SARS-CoV E are reminiscent of the two separate domains reported for the amyloid peptide [137], where fragment 34–42 has limited solubility and adopts antiparallel β-sheet structure, and fragment 26–33 is more soluble in water, and has a disordered conformation. Thus, we tested if peptide (36-76) can form amyloid-like fibrils. The aggregate obtained after drying this peptide from acetonitrile showed intense X-ray reflections at ~4.8 Å and ~10.8 Å (Fig. 6f), which correspond to the distances between hydrogen bonded peptide backbones and β–pleated sheets, respectively, characteristically found in Alzheimer disease amyloid plaque cores [137]. This peptide was monomeric in SDS. Based on the above results, a topological model for SARS-CoV E can be proposed, with one α-helical TM domain and a C-terminal β-hairpin (Fig. 6g). We have reported previously that SARS-CoV E secondary structure in lipid bilayers is predominantly α-helical [67], in contrast with the results shown in Fig. 6e. However, we have found that the secondary structure of E protein is strongly dependent on the reconstitution conditions. In our previous report [67], the protein was presolubilized in hexafluoroisopropanol, an α-helix inducer, whereas in Fig. 6e pre-solubilization was done in methanol. Thus, the β-hairpin prediction for the residues around the highly conserved residue P54, may be correct only in certain experimental conditions. The dual conformation, α-helical and β-hairpin, conformation proposed here is reminiscent of the proposed dual topology of a similar β-hairpin with central conserved Pro residue found in stomatin. In that case, secondary structure changed to α-helix when Pro was mutated to Ser [138].

Examination of the peptide (36-76) precipitate by electron microscopy (Fig. 7A) revealed a protofibrillar morphology [139-141]. These structures were not observed in the control specimen prepared in the absence of peptide (Fig. 7B). The fibrils form an ordered mesh structure characterized by straight sections intervened by bends. The fibril width was 7, 8 and 10 nm, consistent with reports of other filaments derived from β-sheet structures [141-143]. The length of the straight sections was rather homogenous, with most measurements falling between 20-40 nm and with an average value of 32 nm.

The formation of fibrils is anticipated by the residue composition in the region around the conserved proline (P54). For example, from the 17 residues in the stretch I46 to V62, 9 residues are either V, I or Y. Amino acids with β-branched side chains, e.g. valine and isoleucine, or bulky residues, have been shown previously to disfavor α-helical conformation, and to pack efficiently along the surface of a β-sheet [144, 145]. Accordingly, a series of hexapeptides containing similar motifs (e.g., VxVx) have been shown to be good amyloid-forming peptides [146]. We speculate that changing some of these residues to non-branched, for example from V to L, would abolish the ability of SARS-CoV E to form fibers, and possibly attenuate the observed cytopathological effects of SARS-CoV E in cells. Indeed, a similar strategy led to disruption of Golgi targeting in SARS-CoV E [106].

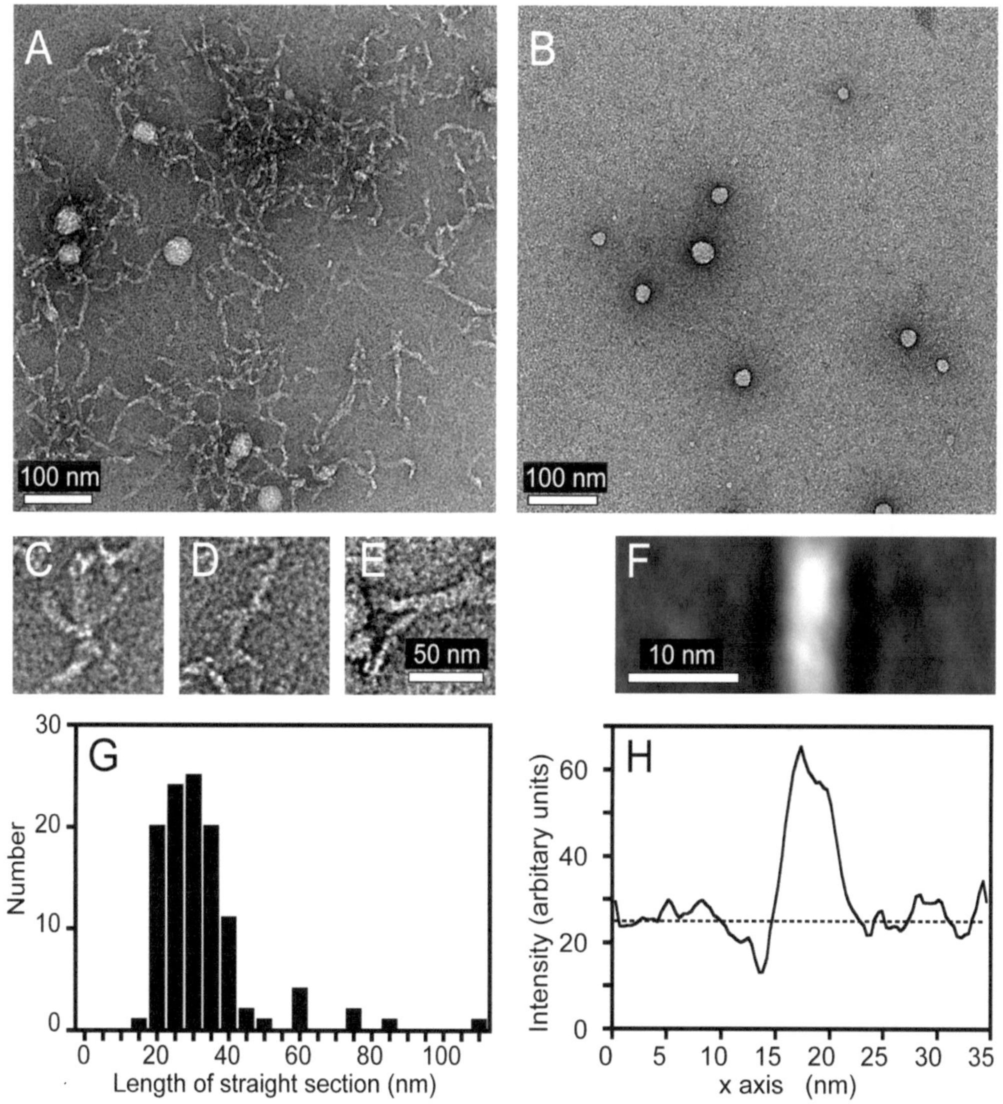

Figure 7. Electron microscopy and image processing; (A) Micrograph of a negatively stained sample of peptide 36-76 dissolved in acetonitrile. The ordered mesh is formed by 7-10 nm wide fibrils with 20-40 nm long straight sections. Globular structures of 10-50 nm diameter are also present; (B) Control specimen without peptide showing similar globular structures; (C, D) Magnified views of fibril branching points; (E) Two thin fibrils merging into a thicker one; (F) Class average of the 8 nm fibril; (G) Histogram of the lengths of the fibril straight sections. (H) Intensity profile along the x-axis of panel (F). The width of the peak above background level indicates filament thickness. The scale bar is shown in each panel.

In addition, a sequence of ordered fragments (α-helices or strands) flanking a disordered or turn loop, with Pro at its center, has been described for several fusion peptides, e.g., in EnvA of the Avian sarcoma/leukosis virus subtype A (ASLV-A) [147], Ebola virus GP [148] and mouse or macaque fertilin α (ADAM 1) [149], which suggests that this part of SARS-CoV E is analogous to an internal fusion peptide. This motif has also been observed in a cis-proline turn [150] linking two β-hairpin strands in the structure of an HIV-1_{III}B V3 peptide. It was found by mutagenesis of the fusion peptide of Env in ASLV-A, that proline, or a residue of similar intermediate hydrophobicity, are part of an accessible loop and was needed for initial interactions of fusion peptides with target membranes.

Amyloid fiber formation has been reported for fragments of many non pathogenic proteins [151], and they have been found in a variety of proteins which are not associated with disease [152, 153]. Therefore, this finding may not have relevance for the toxicity of the virus. Nevertheless, this possibility cannot be discarded in view of other roles of similar semen-derived fibers in HIV viral entry which dramatically enhance HIV infection [154]. A more likely possibility, however, is that this conformational plasticity is needed during membrane fusion; a transition form a α-helical conformation to an antiparallel β-structure, with Pro as a hinge, could drive membrane fusion by pulling the two membranes in close apposition.

NMR studies: towards the high-resolution structure of SARS-CoV E. Full-length SARS-CoV E protein shows a high tendency to aggregate when solubilized in detergents, making it difficult to find a suitable condition for structural determination. While the TM region could be studied in DPC [25], 2D-HSQC spectra of full-length SARS-CoV E protein show poor quality in DPC-solubilized samples, even when SDS is included to improve spectral quality (Fig. 8A). Some degree of improvement can be observed with a truncated version of SARS-CoV E, which is lacking ~10 amino acids at both termini (Fig. 8B). We have also obtained a good, well-dispersed spectrum for this construct in SDS (Fig. 8C), allowing us to begin the structural determination of the extramembrane regions of SARS-CoV E.

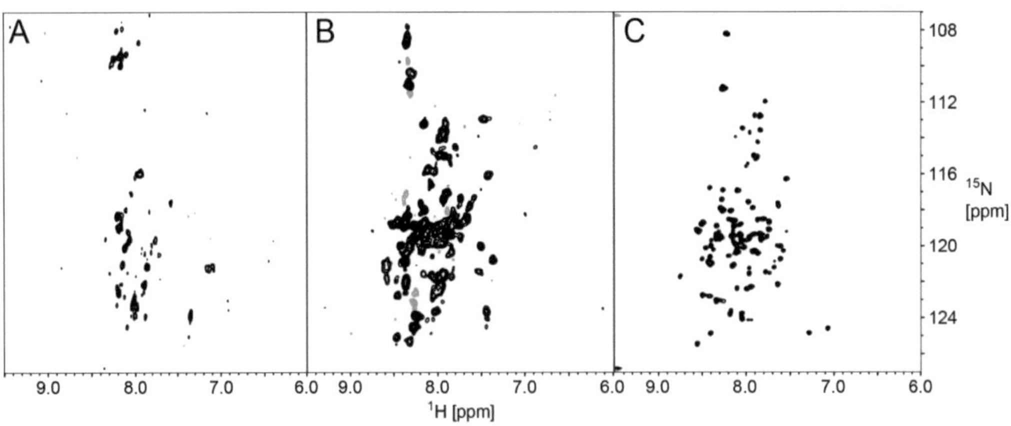

Figure 8. TROSY-HSQC of SARS-CoV E protein in various detergent micelles. (A) full-length SARS-CoV E in a mixture of DPC and SDS, (B) truncated SARS-CoV E in DPC and (C) in SDS.

http://dx.doi.org/10.5772/53957

3. Conclusion

Viroporins constitute important components of viruses, and we are just beginning to understand what is their biological role during the viral life cycle. One of the main problems in their *in vitro* structural and functional study is high hydrophobicity and strong tendency to aggregate. This may reflect their likely multifunctional role in the cell, interacting with several viral and host partners. This multifunctionality seems dictated by genetic minimalism observed in viruses, in turn forced by the need to rapidly produce new progeny inside an alien environment. Viroporins such as those presented here, SH protein and CoV E proteins, form complexes that are still not well characterized that are critical for viral eggress. In this context, the biological function of channel activity is still unknown. More data is becoming available with more purified proteins, and inevitably extrapolations will have to be made from easier to handle proteins. For example, we could obtain a reasonably detailed SH protein NMR spectrum in detergents, but that is still not possible for E proteins. Even when structural data can be obtained, efforts will be directed towards environments that best mimic the conditions of natural lipid bilayers, as protein conformation is likely to change. With multidisciplinary action, the key roles of viroporins will be elucidated in the near future.

Acknowledgements

J.T. acknowledges the funding of the National Research Foundation grant NRF-CRP4-2008-02.

Author details

Wahyu Surya[1], Montserrat Samsó[2] and Jaume Torres[1*]

*Address all correspondence to: jtorres@ntu.edu.sg

1 School of Biological Sciences, Nanyang Technological University, Singapore

2 School of Medicine, Virginia Commonwealth University, Richmond, VA, USA

References

[1] Gonzalez, M.E. and L. Carrasco, Viroporins. FEBS Lett., 2003. 552(1): p. 28-34.

[2] Carrasco, L., *Membrane leakiness after viral infection and a new approach to the development of antiviral agents.* Nature, 1978. 272(5655): p. 694-699.

[3] Carrasco, L., *Modification of Membrane Permeability by Animal Viruses*, in *Advances in Virus Research*, F.A.M. Karl Maramorosch and J.S. Aaron, Editors. 1995, Academic Press. p. 61-112.

[4] Bukreyev, A., et al., *Recombinant respiratory syncytial virus from which the entire SH gene has been deleted grows efficiently in cell culture and exhibits site-specific attenuation in the respiratory tract of the mouse.* J Virol, 1997. 71(12): p. 8973-82.

[5] Whitehead, S.S., et al., *Recombinant respiratory syncytial virus bearing a deletion of either the xlink or SH gene is attenuated in chimpanzees.* J Virol, 1999. 73(4): p. 3438-42.

[6] Sanderson, C.M., et al., *Overexpression of the vaccinia virus A38L integral membrane protein promotes Ca2+ influx into infected cells.* J. Virol., 1996. 70(2): p. 905-914.

[7] Bour, S. and K. Strebel, *The human immunodeficiency virus (HIV) type 2 envelope protein is a functional complement to HIV type 1 Vpu that enhances particle release of heterologous retroviruses.* J. Virol., 1996. 70(12): p. 8285-8300.

[8] Shai, Y., *Mechanism of the binding, insertion and destabilization of phospholipid bilayer membranes by alpha-helical antimicrobial and cell non-selective membrane-lytic peptides.* Biochim. Biophys. Acta - Biomem., 1999. 1462(1-2): p. 55-70.

[9] Shimbo, K., et al., *Viral and cellular small integral membrane proteins can modify ion channels endogenous to Xenopus oocytes.* Biophys. J., 1995. 69(5): p. 1819-29.

[10] Hsu, K., et al., *Mutual functional destruction of HIV-1 Vpu and host TASK-1 channel.* Mol. Cell, 2004. 14(2): p. 259-267.

[11] Song, W.F., et al., *Respiratory Syncytial Virus Inhibits Lung Epithelial Na(+) Channels by Up-regulating Inducible Nitric-oxide Synthase.* J. Biol. Chem., 2009. 284(11): p. 7294-7306.

[12] Lazrak, A., et al., *Influenza virus M2 protein inhibits epithelial sodium channels by increasing reactive oxygen species.* FASEB J., 2009. 23(11): p. 3829-3842.

[13] Cuconati, A., et al., *A protein linkage map of the P2 nonstructural proteins of poliovirus.* J. Virol., 1998. 72(2): p. 1297-1307.

[14] Strauss, J.H. and E.G. Strauss, *The alphaviruses: Gene expression, replication, and evolution.* Microbiological Reviews, 1994. 58(3): p. 491-562.

[15] Sanz, M.A., L. Pel̀rez, and L. Carrasco, *Semliki forest virus 6K protein modifies membrane permeability after inducible expression in Escherichia coli cells.* J. Biol. Chem., 1994. 269(16): p. 12106-12110.

[16] Melton, J.V., et al., *Alphavirus 6K proteins form ion channels.* J. Biol. Chem., 2002. 277(49): p. 46923-31.

[17] Schubert, U., et al., *Identification of an ion channel activity of the Vpu transmembrane domain and its involvement in the regulation of virus release from HIV-1-infected cells.* FEBS Lett., 1996. 398(1): p. 12-18.

[18] Chen, M.Y., et al., *Human immunodeficiency virus type 1 Vpu protein induces degradation of CD4 in vitro: The cytoplasmic domain of CD4 contributes to Vpu sensitivity.* J. Virol., 1993. 67(7): p. 3877-3884.

[19] Lamb, R.A., L.J. Holsinger, and L.H. Pinto, *The influenza A virus M2 ion channel protein and its role in the influenza virus life cycle.* Receptor-Mediated Virus Entry into Cells, 1994: p. 303-321.

[20] Perez, M., et al., *Membrane permeability changes induced in Escherichia coli by the SH protein of human respiratory syncytial virus.* Virology, 1997. 235(2): p. 342-51.

[21] Bodelon, G., et al., *Modification of late membrane permeability in avian reovirus-infected cells: viroporin activity of the S1-encoded nonstructural p10 protein.* J. Biol. Chem., 2002. 277(20): p. 17789-96.

[22] Penin, F., et al., *Structural biology of hepatitis C virus.* Hepatology (Baltimore, Md, 2004. 39(1): p. 5-19.

[23] Harada, T., N. Tautz, and H.J. Thiel, *E2-p7 region of the bovine viral diarrhea virus polyprotein: Processing and functional studies.* J. Virol., 2000. 74(20): p. 9498-9506.

[24] Plugge, B., et al., *A potassium channel protein encoded by chlorella virus PBCV-1.* Science, 2000. 287(5458): p. 1641-1644.

[25] Pervushin, K., et al., *Structure and inhibition of the SARS coronavirus envelope protein ion channel.* PLoS Path., 2009. 5(7).

[26] Liao, Y., et al., *Biochemical and functional characterization of the membrane association and membrane permeabilizing activity of the severe acute respiratory syndrome coronavirus envelope protein.* Virology, 2006. 349(2): p. 264-275.

[27] Nieva, J.L., V. Madan, and L. Carrasco, *Viroporins: structure and biological functions.* Nature Reviews Microbiology, 2012. 10(8): p. 563-574.

[28] Wang, K., S. Xie, and B. Sun, *Viral proteins function as ion channels.* Biochim. Biophys. Acta, 2011. 1808(2): p. 510-5.

[29] Grambas, S. and A.J. Hay, *Maturation of Influenza-a Virus Hemagglutinin - Estimates of the Ph Encountered during Transport and Its Regulation by the M2 Protein.* Virology, 1992. 190(1): p. 11-18.

[30] Sakaguchi, T., G.P. Leser, and R.A. Lamb, *The ion channel activity of the influenza virus M2 protein affects transport through the Golgi apparatus.* J. Cell Biol., 1996. 133(4): p. 733-747.

[31] Stouffer, A.L., et al., *Structural basis for the function and inhibition of an influenza virus proton channel.* Nature, 2008. 451(7178): p. 596-9.

[32] Schnell, J.R. and J.J. Chou, *Structure and mechanism of the M2 proton channel of influenza A virus.* Nature, 2008. 451(7178): p. 591-5.

[33] Pielak, R.M., J.R. Schnell, and J.J. Chou, *Mechanism of drug inhibition and drug resistance of influenza A M2 channel.* Proc. Nat. Acad. Sci. USA, 2009. 106(18): p. 7379-7384.

[34] Cady, S.D., T.V. Mishanina, and M. Hong, *Structure of Amantadine-Bound M2 Transmembrane Peptide of Influenza A in Lipid Bilayers from Magic-Angle-Spinning Solid-State NMR: The Role of Ser31 in Amantadine Binding.* J. Mol. Biol., 2009. 385(4): p. 1127-1141.

[35] Wang, J., et al., *Discovery of spiro-piperidine inhibitors and their modulation of the dynamics of the M2 proton channel from influenza A virus.* J. Am. Chem. Soc., 2009. 131(23): p. 8066-8076.

[36] Skehel, J.J., A.J. Hay, and J.A. Armstrong, *On the mechanism of inhibition of influenza virus replication by amantadine hydrochloride.* J Gen Virol, 1978. 38(1): p. 97-110.

[37] Dowell, S.F., et al., *Respiratory syncytial virus is an important cause of community-acquired lower respiratory infection among hospitalized adults.* J Infect Dis, 1996. 174(3): p. 456-62.

[38] Delgado, M.F., et al., *Lack of antibody affinity maturation due to poor Toll-like receptor stimulation leads to enhanced respiratory syncytial virus disease.* Nat. Med., 2009. 15(1): p. 34-41.

[39] Collins, P.L. and J.A. Melero, *Progress in understanding and controlling respiratory syncytial virus: Still crazy after all these years.* Virus Res., 2011. 162(1-2): p. 80-99.

[40] Melero, J.A., *Molecular Biology of Human Respiratory Syncytial Virus*, in *Respiratory Syncytial Virus*, P. Cane, Editor 2007, Elsevier B.V. p. 1-41.

[41] Krusat, T. and H.J. Streckert, *Heparin-dependent attachment of respiratory syncytial virus (RSV) to host cells.* Arch Virol, 1997. 142(6): p. 1247-54.

[42] Lamb, R.A., *Paramyxovirus fusion: a hypothesis for changes.* Virology, 1993. 197(1): p. 1-11.

[43] Fields, B.N., D.M. Knipe, and P.M. Howley, Fields Virology, 1996.

[44] Roberts, S.R., R.W. Compans, and G.W. Wertz, *Respiratory syncytial virus matures at the apical surfaces of polarized epithelial cells.* J. Virol., 1995. 69(4): p. 2667-2673.

[45] Lindquist, M.E., et al., *Respiratory syncytial virus induces host RNA stress granules to facilitate viral replication.* J. Virol., 2010. 84(23): p. 12274-12284.

[46] Brock, S.C., et al., *The transmembrane domain of the respiratory syncytial virus F protein is an orientation-independent apical plasma membrane sorting sequence.* J. Virol., 2005. 79(19): p. 12528-12535.

[47] Utley, T.J., et al., *Respiratory syncytial virus uses a Vps4-independent budding mechanism controlled by Rab11-FIP2.* Proceedings of the National Academy of Sciences of the United States of America, 2008. 105(29): p. 10209-10214.

[48] Collins, P.L. and G. Mottet, *Membrane orientation and oligomerization of the small hydrophobic protein of human respiratory syncytial virus.* J Gen Virol, 1993. 74: p. 1445-1450.

[49] Chen, M.D., et al., *Conservation of the respiratory syncytial virus SH gene.* J Infect Dis, 2000. 182(4): p. 1228-33.

[50] Collins, P.L., R.A. Olmsted, and P.R. Johnson, *The small hydrophobic protein of human respiratory syncytial virus: comparison between antigenic subgroups A and B.* J Gen Virol, 1990. 71 (Pt 7): p. 1571-6.

[51] Techaarpornkul, S., N. Barretto, and M.E. Peeples, *Functional analysis of recombinant respiratory syncytial virus deletion mutants lacking the small hydrophobic and/or attachment glycoprotein gene.* J. Virol., 2001. 75(15): p. 6825-34.

[52] Bukreyev, A., et al., *Recombinant respiratory syncytial virus from which the entire SH gene has been deleted grows efficiently in cell culture and exhibits site-specific attenuation in the respiratory tract of the mouse.* J. Virol., 1997. 71(12): p. 8973-82.

[53] Karron, R.A., et al., *Respiratory syncytial virus (RSV) SH and G proteins are not essential for viral replication in vitro: clinical evaluation and molecular characterization of a cold-passaged, attenuated RSV subgroup B mutant.* Proc. Nat. Acad. Sci. USA, 1997. 94(25): p. 13961-6.

[54] Heminway, B.R., et al., *Analysis of respiratory syncytial virus F, G, and SH proteins in cell fusion.* Virology, 1994. 200(2): p. 801-5.

[55] Techaarpornkul, S., N. Barretto, and M.E. Peeples, *Functional analysis of recombinant respiratory syncytial virus deletion mutants lacking the small hydrophobic and/or attachment glycoprotein gene.* J Virol, 2001. 75(15): p. 6825-34.

[56] Fuentes, S., et al., *Function of the respiratory syncytial virus small hydrophobic protein.* Journal of Virology, 2007. 81(15): p. 8361-6.

[57] Feldman, S.A., et al., *Human respiratory syncytial virus surface glycoproteins F, G and SH form an oligomeric complex.* Arch Virol, 2001. 146(12): p. 2369-83.

[58] Low, K.W., et al., *The RSV F and G glycoproteins interact to form a complex on the surface of infected cells.* Biochem Biophys Res Commun, 2008. 366(2): p. 308-13.

[59] Calder, L.J., et al., *Electron microscopy of the human respiratory syncytial virus fusion protein and complexes that it forms with monoclonal antibodies.* Virology, 2000. 271(1): p. 122-31.

[60] Escribano-Romero, E., et al., *The soluble form of human respiratory syncytial virus attachment protein differs from the membrane-bound form in its oligomeric state but is still capable of binding to cell surface proteoglycans.* J Virol, 2004. 78(7): p. 3524-32.

[61] Rixon, H.W.M., et al., *The respiratory syncytial virus small hydrophobic protein is phosphorylated via a mitogen-activated protein kinase p38-dependent tyrosine kinase activity during virus infection.* J Gen Virol, 2005. 86(2): p. 375-384.

[62] Gan, S.W., et al., *Structure and ion channel activity of the human respiratory syncytial virus (hRSV) small hydrophobic protein transmembrane domain.* Protein Sci, 2008. 17(5): p. 813-20.

[63] Lin, Y., et al., *Induction of apoptosis by paramyxovirus simian virus 5 lacking a small hydrophobic gene.* J Virol, 2003. 77(6): p. 3371-83.

[64] Rixon, H.W., et al., *The small hydrophobic (SH) protein accumulates within lipid-raft structures of the Golgi complex during respiratory syncytial virus infection.* J Gen Virol, 2004. 85(Pt 5): p. 1153-65.

[65] Olmsted, R.A. and P.L. Collins, *The 1A protein of respiratory syncytial virus is an integral membrane protein present as multiple, structurally distinct species.* J Virol, 1989. 63(5): p. 2019-29.

[66] Collins, P.L. and G. Mottet, *Membrane orientation and oligomerization of the small hydrophobic protein of human respiratory syncytial virus.* J Gen Virol, 1993. 74 (Pt 7): p. 1445-50.

[67] Parthasarathy, K., et al., *Expression and purification of coronavirus envelope proteins using a modified β-barrel construct.* Protein Expression and Purification, 2012. 85(1): p. 133-141.

[68] Rixon, H.W., et al., *The respiratory syncytial virus small hydrophobic protein is phosphorylated via a mitogen-activated protein kinase p38-dependent tyrosine kinase activity during virus infection.* J Gen Virol, 2005. 86(Pt 2): p. 375-84.

[69] Gan, S.W., et al., *Structure and ion channel activity of the human respiratory syncytial virus (hRSV) small hydrophobic protein transmembrane domain.* Protein Sci., 2008. 17: p. 813-820.

[70] Carter, S.D., et al., *Direct visualization of the small hydrophobic protein of human respiratory syncytial virus reveals the structural basis for membrane permeability.* FEBS Letters, 2010. 584(13): p. 2786-2790.

[71] Gan, S.-W., et al., *The Small Hydrophobic Protein of the Human Respiratory Syncytial Virus Forms Pentameric Ion Channels.* Journal of Biological Chemistry, 2012. 287(29): p. 24671-24689.

[72] Gonzalez, J.M., et al., *A comparative sequence analysis to revise the current taxonomy of the family Coronaviridae.* Arch Virol, 2003. 148(11): p. 2207-2235.

[73] Siddell, S.G., *The Coronaviridae; an introduction*1995: Plenum Press, New York, N.Y.

[74] Enjuanes, L., et al., *Coronaviridae,* in *Virus taxonomy. Classification and nomenclature of viruses.,* M.H.V. van Regenmortel, et al., Editors. 2000, Academic Press: San Diego. p. 835-849.

[75] Gorbalenya, A.E., E.J. Snijder, and W.J. Spaan, *Severe acute respiratory syndrome coronavirus phylogeny: toward consensus.* J. Virol., 2004. 78(15): p. 7863-6.

[76] Hon, C.C., et al., *Evidence of the recombinant origin of a bat severe acute respiratory syndrome (SARS)-like coronavirus and its implications on the direct ancestor of SARS coronavirus.* J. Virol., 2008. 82(4): p. 1819-26.

[77] Vijgen, L., et al., *Complete genomic sequence of human coronavirus OC43: molecular clock analysis suggests a relatively recent zoonotic coronavirus transmission event.* J. Virol., 2005. 79(3): p. 1595-604.

[78] Lin, J.T., et al., *Safety and immunogenicity from a phase I trial of inactivated severe acute respiratory syndrome coronavirus vaccine.* Antivir Ther, 2007. 12(7): p. 1107-13.

[79] Barnard, D.L., et al., *Enhancement of the infectivity of SARS-CoV in BALB/c mice by IMP dehydrogenase inhibitors, including ribavirin.* Antiviral Res, 2006. 71(1): p. 53-63.

[80] Loutfy, M.R., et al., *Interferon alfacon-1 plus corticosteroids in severe acute respiratory syndrome: a preliminary study.* JAMA, 2003. 290(24): p. 3222-8.

[81] Keyaerts, E., et al., *In vitro inhibition of severe acute respiratory syndrome coronavirus by chloroquine.* Biochem Biophys Res Commun, 2004. 323(1): p. 264-8.

[82] Wu, C.J., et al., *Inhibition of severe acute respiratory syndrome coronavirus replication by niclosamide.* Antimicrob Agents Chemother, 2004. 48(7): p. 2693-6.

[83] Chen, F., et al., *In vitro susceptibility of 10 clinical isolates of SARS coronavirus to selected antiviral compounds.* J Clin Virol, 2004. 31(1): p. 69-75.

[84] Amici, C., et al., *Indomethacin has a potent antiviral activity against SARS coronavirus.* Antivir Ther, 2006. 11(8): p. 1021-30.

[85] Stockman, L.J., R. Bellamy, and P. Garner, *SARS: systematic review of treatment effects.* PLoS medicine, 2006. 3(9): p. e343.

[86] Cheng, P.W., et al., *Antiviral effects of saikosaponins on human coronavirus 229E in vitro.* Clin. Exp. Pharmacol. Physiol., 2006. 33(7): p. 612-6.

[87] Pyrc, K., et al., *Inhibition of human coronavirus NL63 infection at early stages of the replication cycle.* Antimicrob Agents Chemother, 2006. 50(6): p. 2000-8.

[88] Godet, M., et al., *TGEV corona virus ORF4 encodes a membrane protein that is incorporated into virions.* Virology, 1992. 188(2): p. 666-75.

[89] Liu, D.X. and S.C. Inglis, *Association of the infectious-bronchitis virus-3c protein with the virion envelope.* Virology, 1991. 185(2): p. 911-917.

[90] Yu, X., et al., *Mouse hepatitis-virus gene 5b protein is a new virion envelope protein.* Virology, 1994. 202(2): p. 1018-1023.

[91] Kall, L., A. Krogh, and E.L. Sonnhammer, *Advantages of combined transmembrane topology and signal peptide prediction--the Phobius web server.* Nucleic Acids Res., 2007. 35(Web Server issue): p. W429-32.

[92] Maeda, J., et al., *Membrane topology of coronavirus E protein.* Virology, 2001. 281(2): p. 163-169.

[93] Corse, E. and C.E. Machamer, *Infectious bronchitis virus E protein is targeted to the Golgi complex and directs release of virus-like particles.* J. Virol., 2000. 74(9): p. 4319-4326.

[94] Yuan, Q., et al., *Biochemical evidence for the presence of mixed membrane topologies of the Severe Acute Respiratory Syndrome coronavirus envelope protein expressed in mammalian cells.* FEBS Lett., 2006. 580: p. 3192-3200.

[95] Nieto-Torres, J.L., et al., *Subcellular location and topology of severe acute respiratory syndrome coronavirus envelope protein.* Virology, 2011. 415(2): p. 69-82.

[96] Corse, E. and C.E. Machamer, *Infectious bronchitis virus E protein is targeted to the Golgi complex and directs release of virus-like particles.* J Virol, 2000. 74(9): p. 4319-26.

[97] Maeda, J., et al., *Membrane topology of coronavirus E protein.* Virology, 2001. 281(2): p. 163-9.

[98] Corse, E. and C.E. Machamer, *The cytoplasmic tail of infectious bronchitis virus E protein directs Golgi targeting.* J. Virol., 2002. 76(3): p. 1273-1284.

[99] Lopez, L.A., et al., *Importance of conserved cysteine residues in the coronavirus envelope protein.* J. Virol., 2008. 82(6): p. 3000-3010.

[100] Boscarino, J.A., et al., *Envelope protein palmitoylations are crucial for murine coronavirus assembly.* J. Virol., 2008. 82(6): p. 2989-99.

[101] Thorp, E.B., et al., *Palmitoylations on murine coronavirus spike proteins are essential for virion assembly and infectivity.* J. Virol., 2006. 80(3): p. 1280-9.

[102] Kuo, L., K.R. Hurst, and P.S. Masters, *Exceptional flexibility in the sequence requirements for coronavirus small envelope protein function.* J. Virol., 2007. 81(5): p. 2249-62.

[103] Lim, K.P. and D.X. Liu, *The missing link in coronavirus assembly - Retention of the avian coronavirus infectious bronchitis virus envelope protein in the pre-Golgi compartments and physical interaction between the envelope and membrane proteins.* Journal of Biological Chemistry, 2001. 276(20): p. 17515-17523.

[104] Nal, B., et al., *Differential maturation and subcellular localization of severe acute respiratory syndrome coronavirus surface proteins S, M and E.* Journal of General Virology, 2005. 86: p. 1423-1434.

[105] Raamsman, M.J.B., et al., *Characterization of the coronavirus mouse hepatitis virus strain A59 small membrane protein E.* Journal of Virology, 2000. 74(5): p. 2333-2342.

[106] Cohen, J.R., L.D. Lin, and C.E. Machamer, *Identification of a Golgi Complex-Targeting Signal in the Cytoplasmic Tail of the Severe Acute Respiratory Syndrome Coronavirus Envelope Protein.* Journal of Virology, 2011. 85(12): p. 5794-5803.

[107] DeDiego, M.L., et al., *A severe acute respiratory syndrome coronavirus that lacks the E gene is attenuated in vitro and in vivo.* J. Virol., 2007. 81(4): p. 1701-13.

[108] Dediego, M.L., et al., *Pathogenicity of severe acute respiratory coronavirus deletion mutants in hACE-2 transgenic mice.* Virology, 2008. 376(2): p. 379-89.

[109] Netland, J., et al., *Immunization with an attenuated severe acute respiratory syndrome coronavirus deleted in E protein protects against lethal respiratory disease.* Virology, 2010. 399(1): p. 120-128.

[110] DeDiego, M.L., et al., *Severe acute respiratory syndrome coronavirus envelope protein regulates cell stress response and apoptosis.* PLoS Path., 2011. 7(10): p. e1002315.

[111] Bos, E.C., et al., *The production of recombinant infectious DI-particles of a murine coronavirus in the absence of helper virus.* Virology, 1996. 218(1): p. 52-60.

[112] Vennema, H., et al., *Nucleocapsid-independent assembly of coronavirus-like particles by co-expression of viral envelope protein genes.* EMBO Journal., 1996. 15(8): p. 2020-2028.

[113] Baudoux, P., et al., *Coronavirus pseudoparticles formed with recombinant M and E proteins induce alpha interferon synthesis by leukocytes.* J. Virol., 1998. 72(11): p. 8636-8643.

[114] Corse, E. and C.E. Machamer, *The cytoplasmic tails of infectious bronchitis virus E and M proteins mediate their interaction.* Virology, 2003. 312(1): p. 25-34.

[115] Mortola, E. and P. Roy, *Efficient assembly and release of SARS coronavirus-like particles by a heterologous expression system.* FEBS Lett., 2004. 576(1-2): p. 174-8.

[116] Fischer, F., et al., *Analysis of constructed E gene mutants of mouse hepatitis virus confirms a pivotal role for E protein in coronavirus assembly.* J. Virol., 1998. 72(10): p. 7885-7894.

[117] Curtis, K.M., B. Yount, and R.S. Baric, *Heterologous gene expression from transmissible gastroenteritis virus replicon particles.* J. Virol., 2002. 76(3): p. 1422-34.

[118] Ortego, J., et al., *Generation of a replication-competent, propagation-deficient virus vector based on the transmissible gastroenteritis coronavirus genome.* J. Virol., 2002. 76(22): p. 11518-29.

[119] Lim, K.P. and D.X. Liu, *The missing link in coronavirus assembly. Retention of the avian coronavirus infectious bronchitis virus envelope protein in the pre-Golgi compartments and physical interaction between the envelope and membrane proteins.* J. Biol. Chem., 2001. 276(20): p. 17515-17523.

[120] Yang, Y., et al., *Bcl-xL inhibits T-cell apoptosis induced by expression of SARS coronavirus E protein in the absence of growth factors.* Biochem. J., 2005. 392(1): p. 135-143.

[121] Alvarez, E., et al., *The envelope protein of severe acute respiratory syndrome coronavirus interacts with the non-structural protein 3 and is ubiquitinated.* Virology, 2010. 402(2): p. 281-91.

[122] Yoshikawa, T., et al., *Severe acute respiratory syndrome (SARS) coronavirus-induced lung epithelial cytokines exacerbate SARS pathogenesis by modulating intrinsic functions of monocyte-derived macrophages and dendritic cells.* J. Virol., 2009. 83(7): p. 3039-48.

[123] Madan, V., et al., *Viroporin activity of murine hepatitis virus E protein.* FEBS Lett., 2005. 579(17): p. 3607-12.

[124] Wilson, L., et al., *SARS coronavirus E protein forms cation-selective ion channels.* Virology, 2004. 330(1): p. 322-31.

[125] Wilson, L., P. Gage, and G. Ewart, *Hexamethylene amiloride blocks E protein ion channels and inhibits coronavirus replication.* Virology, 2006. 353(2): p. 294-306.

[126] Torres, J., et al., *Conductance and amantadine binding of a pore formed by a lysine-flanked transmembrane domain of SARS coronavirus envelope protein.* Protein Sci., 2007. 16(9): p. 2065-2071.

[127] Parthasarathy, K., et al., *Structural flexibility of the pentameric SARS coronavirus envelope protein ion channel.* Biophys. J., 2008. 95(6): p. L39-41.

[128] Verdia-Baguena, C., et al., *Coronavirus E protein forms ion channels with functionally and structurally-involved membrane lipids.* Virology, 2012. 432(2): p. 485-94.

[129] McBride, C.E. and C.E. Machamer, *Palmitoylation of SARS-CoV S protein is necessary for partitioning into detergent-resistant membranes and cell-cell fusion but not interaction with M protein.* Virology. 405(1): p. 139-48.

[130] Torres, J., et al., *Model of a putative pore: the pentameric α-helical bundle of SARS coronavirus E protein in lipid bilayers.* Biophys. J., 2006. 91: p. 938-947.

[131] Moore, W.H. and S. Krimm, *Vibrational analysis of peptides, polypeptides, and proteins. II. beta-poly(L-alanine) and beta-poly(L-anaylglycine).* Biopolymers, 1976. 15(12NA-NA-770103-770104): p. 2465-83.

[132] Moore, W.H. and S. Krimm, *Transition dipole coupling in Amide I modes of betapolypeptides.* Proc. Nat. Acad. Sci. USA, 1975. 72(12): p. 4933-4935.

[133] Krimm, S. and J. Bandekar, *Vibrational spectroscopy and conformation of peptides, polypeptides, and proteins.* Adv.Protein Chem., 1986. 38: p. 181-364.

[134] Byler, D.M. and H. Susi, *Examination of the secondary structure of proteins by deconvolved FTIR spectra.* Biopolymers, 1986. 25(3): p. 469-487.

[135] Torii, H. and M. Tasumi, *Model-Calculations on the Amide-I Infrared Bands of Globular-Proteins.* J. Chem. Phys., 1992. 96(5): p. 3379-3387.

[136] Combet, C., et al., *NPS@: network protein sequence analysis.* Trends Biochem Sci, 2000. 25(3): p. 147-50.

[137] Halverson, K., et al., *Molecular determinants of amyloid deposition in Alzheimer's disease: conformational studies of synthetic beta-protein fragments.* Biochemistry, 1990. 29(11): p. 2639-44.

[138] Kadurin, I., S. Huber, and S. Grunder, *A single conserved proline residue determines the membrane topology of stomatin.* Biochem. J., 2009. 418: p. 587-594.

[139] Kheterpal, I. and R. Wetzel, *Hydrogen/deuterium exchange mass spectrometry--a window into amyloid structure.* Acc Chem Res, 2006. 39(9): p. 584-93.

[140] Williams, A.D., et al., *Structural properties of Abeta protofibrils stabilized by a small molecule.* Proc. Nat. Acad. Sci. USA, 2005. 102(20): p. 7115-20.

[141] Nguyen, J.T., et al., *X-ray diffraction of scrapie prion rods and PrP peptides.* J. Mol. Biol., 1995. 252(4): p. 412-22.

[142] Geisler, N., et al., *Peptides from the conserved ends of the rod domain of desmin disassemble intermediate filaments and reveal unexpected structural features: a circular dichroism, Fourier transform infrared, and electron microscopic study.* J. Struct. Biol., 1993. 110(3): p. 205-14.

[143] Kreplak, L. and U. Aebi, *From the polymorphism of amyloid fibrils to their assembly mechanism and cytotoxicity.* Adv Protein Chem, 2006. 73: p. 217-33.

[144] Arfmann, H.A., R. Labitzke, and K.G. Wagner, *Conformational properties of L-leucine, L-isoleucine, and L-norleucine side chains in L-lysine copolymers.* Biopolymers, 1977. 16(8): p. 1815-26.

[145] Mutter, M., et al., *Sequence-dependence of secondary structure formation: conformational studies of host-guest peptides in alpha-helix and beta-structure supporting media.* Biopolymers, 1985. 24(6): p. 1057-74.

[146] Lopez de la Paz, M. and L. Serrano, *Sequence determinants of amyloid fibril formation.* Proc. Nat. Acad. Sci. USA, 2004. 101(1): p. 87-92.

[147] Hernandez, L.D. and J.M. White, *Mutational analysis of the candidate internal fusion peptide of the avian leukosis and sarcoma virus subgroup a envelope glycoprotein.* J. Virol., 1998. 72(4): p. 3259-3267.

[148] Ito, H., et al., *Mutational analysis of the putative fusion domain of Ebola virus glycoprotein.* J. Virol., 1999. 73(10): p. 8907-12.

[149] Wolfsberg, T.G., et al., *ADAM, a widely distributed and developmentally regulated gene family encoding membrane proteins with a disintegrin and metalloprotease domain.* Dev. Biol., 1995. 169(1): p. 378-83.

[150] Tugarinov, V., et al., *A cis proline turn linking two beta-hairpin strands in the solution structure of an antibody-bound HIV-1IIIB V3 peptide.* Nat Struct Biol, 1999. 6(4): p. 331-5.

[151] Pedersen, J.S. and D.E. Otzen, *Amyloid-a state in many guises: survival of the fittest fibril fold.* Protein Sci., 2008. 17(1): p. 2-10.

[152] Fandrich, M., M.A. Fletcher, and C.M. Dobson, *Amyloid fibrils from muscle myoglobin.* Nature, 2001. 410(6825): p. 165-6.

[153] Guijarro, J.I., et al., *Amyloid fibril formation by an SH3 domain.* Proceedings of the National Academy of Sciences of the United States of America, 1998. 95(8): p. 4224-8.

[154] Munch, J., et al., *Semen-derived amyloid fibrils drastically enhance HIV infection.* Cell, 2007. 131(6): p. 1059-71.

Section 2

Bacterial Infections

Chapter 4

Biophysical Effects on Chronic Rhinosinusitis Bacterial Biofilms

Mohammed Al-Haddad, Ahmed Al-Jumaily,
John Brooks and Jim Bartley

Additional information is available at the end of the chapter

http://dx.doi.org/10.5772/53860

1. Introduction

Chronic rhinosinusitis (CRS) is a common debilitating condition. In the United States alone according to recent data from the National Health Interview Survey CRS affects approximately 31 million people [1] resulting in an estimated annual cost of $6 billion. Bacterial biofilms have been implicated in the pathogenesis of CRS [2-4].

This literature review focuses on the effect of physical excitation by ultrasound and/or electric fields on bacterial biofilms. The associated research is based on the hypothesis that *external forces applied by ultrasound and electric fields can alter the attachment forces of biofilms and possibly help patients with chronic infective diseases such as chronic rhinosinusitis.*

Firstly, the role of bacterial biofilms in CRS is discussed identifying the major bacterial species involved in CRS (section 2). Secondly, the importance of the cyclic process of biofilm formation is reviewed focusing on the nature of the attachment and detachment process (section 3). Thirdly, treatments are categorized into medication and physical methods (section 4), with a major emphasis on ultrasound and the bioelectric effect. Finally, future directions on the use of ultrasound and electric fields, and their potential effects on biofilms are discussed (section 5).

2. Chronic rhinosinusitis

The respiratory system is divided into the upper and the lower airways. In the upper airways, the air is filtered, warmed and moistened by the nasal cavity, which is surrounded by a ring of air-filled cavities called the paranasal sinuses. These consist of the maxillary, sphenoid, frontal and ethmoid sinuses (Fig. 1). The proposed functions of the sinuses include moisturizing and humidifying ambient air, acting as resonators for speech, lightening the weight of the skull bones, providing protection to the brain from trauma, and producing nitric oxide.

Rhinosinusitis is defined as a group of disorders characterized by inflammation of the nose and paranasal sinuses. Based on the duration of inflammation, rhinosinusitis is classified as acute (< 4 weeks), subacute (4-12 weeks) or chronic (>12 weeks). CRS symptoms have been classified as major, which includes facial pain or pressure, nasal obstruction or blockage, discolored postnasal drainage, hyposmia (a reduced ability to smell) and purulence in nasal cavity, or minor, which includes headache, fever, dental pain and ear pain [5].

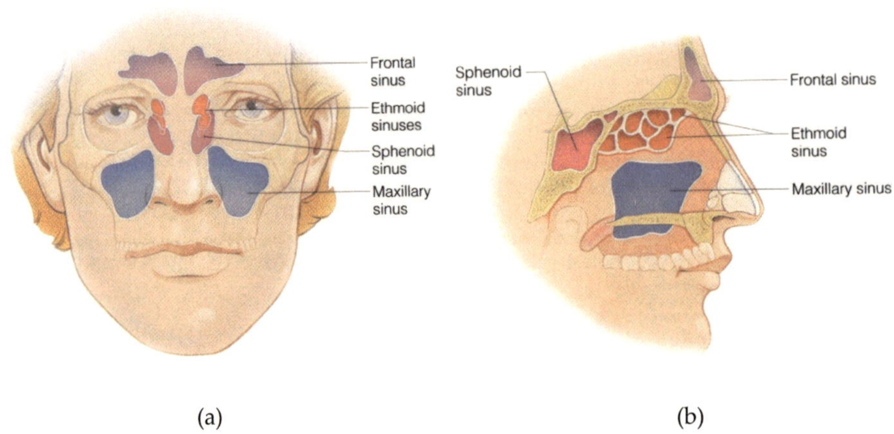

Figure 1. The paranasal sinuses from (a) front and (b) side view [6]

While the pathology of CRS remains unclear and is described as multifactorial, bacterial biofilms have been implicated as a major contributing factor [2-4]. Bacteria are now recognized as existing in two forms: free floating (planktonic) or in sophisticated communities called biofilms. They have been defined as "a structured community of bacterial cells enclosed in a self-produced polymeric matrix adherent to an inert or living surface" [7].

2.1. Biofilms

Biofilms are composed of two major components: microorganism cells that account for less than 10% and a matrix of extracellular polymer substances (EPS) that account for more than 90% of biofilms [8-10]. The characteristics of the cells in biofilms differ from their planktonic counterparts [11]. EPS is considered the primary matrix material of biofilms and is comprised of 50-90% organic carbon [10]. The biofilm matrix is composed of secreted polymers (polysaccharides), lipids, proteins, DNA and RNA [12]. Normally biofilms protect their inhabitants against environmental and biological threats [13].

Bacteria in a biofilm communicate chemically by using molecular chemical signals, a phenomenon called quorum sensing. It plays a major role in structuring complex communities and regulates a variety of physiological functions in both Gram-negative and Gram-positive bacteria [14]. Physical signals may also be involved in bacterial communication [15], but this communication is not well understood.

The knowledge relating to the structure, function and mechanisms of quorum sensing is limited. It has been proposed that quorum sensing generates and responds to physical signals including sound waves, electric current and electromagnetic radiation [15]. Production of sound waves has been observed with *Bacillus subtilis* [16], however, measurable data have not been reported in the literature. Intensity limitations and time scale requirements are challenges in acquiring physical quantitative data from biofilms.

Generally, bacteria are described as negatively charged under most physiological conditions [17]. However, the net charge varies from species to species and is most likely influenced by culture conditions [18], age of the culture [19], ionic strength [20] and pH [21]. During the formation of biofilms, the net negative charge of the bacteria is reduced in order to modify their cellular surface charge [22]. This phenomenon has been observed with *Staphylococcus aureus* [23, 24]. Similarly, the measurement of surface charge of *Staphylococcus epidermidis* shows a variation in the net charge suggesting that different regions of the cell on the surface have different surface charges although the overall net charge may be negative [25]. The net charge has been decreased by increasing pH [21].

In addition to the biological and physical attributes of bacterial biofilms, they have a resistance to antibiotics 10-1000 times higher than planktonic bacteria of the same species [26]. A simple description of the biofilm resistance is the formation of a physical barrier to prevent antibiotics from penetrating biofilms [27]. Specifically, it has been reported that mechanisms include restricted penetration, enzymatic destruction of antimicrobial, gene transfer, quorum sensing, altered growth rate (persister cells), stress response to hostile environmental conditions and over-expression of genes [28]. Multiple mechanisms may work together to increase bacterial biofilm resistance to antibiotics.

Several studies have investigated the relationship between biofilms and CRS [2, 3, 29, 30]. The most common bacterial biofilms in CRS are *S. aureus*, *Pseudomonas aeruginosa*, coagulase-negative staphylococci, *Streptococcus pneumoniae*, *Moraxella catarrhalis* and *Haemophilus influenzae*. Using scanning electron microscopy, Cryer et al. obtained the first evidence of biofilms in CRS showing the presence of *P. aeruginosa* biofilm in specimens taken from maxillary and ethmoid sinus mucosa [31]. Healy et al. investigated the presence of bioflms in CRS by using microscopic fluorescent *in situ* hybridization and showed that *H. influenzae* was most frequently present (80%) among the species identified, which included *S. aureus*, *P. aeruginosa*, *S. pneumoniae* and fungi [32]. However, confocal scanning microscopy and transmission electron microscopy studies have shown that *S. aureus* and *P. aeruginosa* respectively are the most common biofilm bacteria in CRS [33, 34]. Despite the uncertainty with respect to the dominant bacterial species of biofilms in CRS, they have been reported as the major cause of CRS. In addition, biofilms are found attached to sinus surfaces and/or aggregated with a surrounding mucus layer or fluid [35-37]. However, regarding the aggregation, it is not well known whether they detach from surfaces, or whether aggregated biofilms form in the fluids themselves [38].

3. Biofilm formation

Before biofilms form, microorganisms move or are moved to a surface. Planktonic cells conventionally are thought to initiate contact with surfaces. However, this phenomenon and the mechanism behind it are not well understood. It is hypothesized to include random contact caused by several factors. These include Brownian motion, sedimentation owing to differences in specific gravity between the bacteria and the bulk liquid, convective mass transport in which cells are physically transported towards the surface, and active transport owing to the activity of the filamentous cell appendages such as flagella, in which chemotaxis may or may not be included [39].

The formation of a biofilm is divided into attachment, growth and detachment. Although the growth is a part of the cyclical process of biofilm formation, the focus will be on the physical mechanisms influencing the attachment and detachment of biofilms to surfaces.

3.1. Attachment

Several experimental and theoretical approaches have been used to investigate the attachment process. The process of attachment is generally divided into two stages, reversible and irreversible, or similarly named as docking and locking [13]. Numbers of environmental, physical, chemical and biological variables initiate the attachment, including extracellular DNA (eDNA), temperature, electrostatic charges and acid base interaction forces. The role of eDNA in the initial cell attachment is not fully understood, despite its role in the growth and development of *P. aeruginosa* biofilm [40, 41]. However, eDNA enhances the adhesion of Gram-positive bacteria [42].

Temperature effects appear to be different depending on the microorganisms. *P. aeruginosa* has been observed to adhere better to hydrophilic contact lenses at 37 °C than at 26 °C [43]. On the other hand, *S. pneumoniae* adhere better at 24° C than at 10 °C [44]. The temperature may cause an increase in nutrient intake by increasing the activity of enzymes in the production of EPS [45]. It has been observed that the temperature has an impact on the presence of bacterial surface appendages and a decrease in temperature may initiate adhesion [46]. The temperature may also change the environmental conditions surrounding the bacteria by changing the ionic strength of the polysaccharides [47].

A number of physical and chemical forces, including van der Waals, electrostatic charges and acid base interactions, initiate the attachment during the reversible stage [48]. Generally, van der Waals forces are described as an attractive force, while electrostatic forces are a repulsive force [49]. If the repulsive forces are greater than the attractive forces, small shear forces can detach bacteria from surfaces, unless a conditioning film on the substrate is formed by the presence of EPS [49, 50].

http://dx.doi.org/10.5772/53860

The transition from weak interactions (forces) of the cell with the substratum to a permanent bonding is mediated by the presence of EPS [51], which increases the strength of attachment [13]. In this transition, a process of attachment transfers from the reversible to the irreversible stage. Several forces, including covalent and hydrogen bonding as well as hydrophobic interactions, are generated [52]. In addition, electron transfer has been suggested as an extra step involved, by either donating electrons to, or accepting electrons from the substratum [53]. This might explain why the production of EPS is suggested to be mediated by electrostatic charges [54]. Electrostatic interaction forces contribute to the cross-linkers of the biofilm matrix [55]. Aggregated interaction (forces) between positive and negative charges are shown between exo-polysaccharide alginate of *P. aeruginosa* and extracellular enzymes [56]. Electrostatic interaction and hydrogen bonding forces are suggested to be the dominant forces in biofilm formation [57].

Bacterial adhesion forces change depending on the distance between the cells and the substratum. Force-distance relations are proposed to consist of three steps: van der Waals forces at a distance greater than 50 nm, van der Waals and electrostatic interaction between 10 and 20 nm and van der Waals, electrostatic interaction and other interactions at a distance less than 1.5 nm [58]. However, these physical forces have been further classified as long and short range interaction forces [59]. Long range occurs at a distance greater than 50 nm while short range occurs at less than 5 nm. Long and short range physical forces are related forces and highly dependent on the distance between the biofilm and a surface.

Adhesion forces have recently been measured using an atomic force microscope and optical tweezers [60-62]. However, a clear quantitative measurement of the bacterial forces has not yet been defined. Although all microscopic techniques including scanning electron microscopy, optical microscopy, and confocal laser microscopy do not quantitatively measure the adhesion forces, they qualitatively do observe the morphology of biofilms. Hence, a new technique is needed for accurately quantifying bacterial forces.

Although most of the above techniques were based on the experimental approaches, the theoretical analysis of bacterial adhesion is determined by three approaches: the Derjaguin-Landau-Verwey-Overbeek (DLVO) model, the thermodynamic approach and the extended DLVO theory. The DLVO model calculates the net energy of interaction between a cell and a surface [50]:

$$net\ energy\ of\ interaction = van\ der\ Waals\ energy + electrostatic\ energy \tag{1}$$

However, this approach does not consider molecular and acid-base interactions. The thermodynamic approach calculates the surface free energies, assuming that the process is reversible only while it is described as distance dependent in the DLVO model. In addition, the thermodynamic system is assumed to be a closed system without any external input energy. Furthermore, electrostatic interactions are not taken into account in the surface free energies [63]. Neither the DLVO model nor the thermodynamic approach explain clearly the bacterial adhesion. Extended DLVO theory has been proposed recently by calculating the total adhesion energy in which the acid base interactions are included and given by:

$$\Delta G^{adh} = \Delta G^{vdW} + \Delta G^{dl} + \Delta G^{AB} \tag{2}$$

Where ΔG^{adh} : Total adhesion energy

ΔG^{vdW} :van der Waals interactionΔG^{dl} :Electric double layer interactionΔG^{AB} :Acid-base interactions

Although extended DLVO seems to be a promising theoretical approach, further investigation is needed to explain the exact mechanism of bacterial adhesion.

3.2. Detachment

The detachment of biofilms is influenced by several physical, chemical and biological conditions. This may lead to changes in the biofilm cells. Physical conditions play a major role in the bulk liquid surrounding biofilms and physical forces have been reported to change the structure of biofilms [64]. In addition, high shear forces have been shown to change the strength and weakness of biofilms [65]. Increasing the velocity and particle concentration of the liquid normally increases the detachment rate [66]. Shear forces influence biofilm thicknesses [51]; however variations in these forces depend on the biofilm formation [67, 68]. It has been observed that under steady shear forces that biofilms roll along surfaces [69].

A direct electric current was reported to enhance the detachment of *S. epidermidis* biofilm from surgical stainless steel [70]. However, a variation in the detachment rate was observed when the direction of the current was changed between electrodes at the same magnitude [71]. Direct current appears to cause a disruption of the electrical bi-layer on the substrate [72].

In addition to the above physical factors, the detachment of a biofilm can be attributed to changes in the chemical properties of the biofilm or surrounding media. pH has been shown to influence the structure of biofilms in a form of expansion and contraction [73]. The effect of nutrients on biofilm detachment is not well understood. Limitation of nutrients at the biofilm-liquid interface increases the detachment rate [74]; however, another study has shown that the increased availability of nutrients also increases the detachment rate [75].

Apart from the above physical and chemical changes, there are biological factors influencing the detachment process. These include polysaccharide, enzymes, genes and quorum sensing. While these factors have shown a marginal effect, surface-protein-releasing-enzyme produced by *Streptococcus mutans* has caused the release of biofilms from tooth surfaces at rates 20% higher than control samples [76].

Physical and biological parameters appear to be more significant than chemical ones despite the fact that the latter have an important role in the detachment process. The significance of the physical detachment is attributed to attachment forces; however, quorum sensing is biologically significant in structuring the biofilm community. A question worth raising is would a change in the physical parameters, such as frequency, break down and disrupt biofilm attachment to surfaces? Would these changes block quorum sensing in biofilms?

4. Methods of disrupting biofilms

Available methods of treatment for CRS bacterial biofilms are classified into two categories; conventional medication (biochemical) and biophysical.

4.1. Medication

Medication is the current recommended treatment method for CRS. However, they do not seem to improve long-term outcomes [77]. In addition, there are side effects [78] and there is a possibility of changing pathogens and resistance patterns that result in the persistence of CRS [79]. A problem of CRS antibiotic treatment is that these treatments are not able to eradicate bacteria in a biofilm state.

Alternative natural substances similar to antibiotics have been proposed such as honey and garlic. Manuka honey has been reported to be an effective treatment for CRS without damaging respiratory epithelium [80]. However, it does not block biofilm quorum sensing; in contrast, garlic has been shown to be effective in blocking quorum sensing [81]. Both conventional antibiotics and alternative natural substances are often ineffective against biofilms [82].

Vitamin D recently has been proposed as a treatment for CRS and to decrease the viability of *P. aeroginosa* biofilms [83]. However, the mechanism of action is unclear. As another treatment, baby shampoo as simple chemotherapy has been proposed for treating CRS [84]. However, side effects were observed in more than 10% of the patients who could not continue in the study.

4.2. Biophysical approach

Physical methods are classified into two categories: ultrasound and bioelectric effect.

4.2.1. Ultrasound

Ultrasound is a cyclic sound pressure utilizing frequencies higher than 20 kHz. It has been employed in a variety of medical applications ranging from diagnostic imaging to physical therapy [85]. Variables in ultrasound therapy include the type of ultrasound (continuous or pulsed), frequency, intensity, duty cycle, individual treatment duration and overall treatment length. Recently, it has been suggested that ultrasound could be a promising alternative method for treating biofilms [86].

In vitro [87] and *in vivo* research [88] has shown that ultrasound has a role in disrupting bacterial biofilms. It disrupts *Escherichia coli* [89], *S. epidermidis* [88], *P. aerginosa* [90], coagulase-negative Staphylococci [87] and *S. aureus* [87] bacterial biofilms. Bacterial viability is further reduced when ultrasound is combined with antibiotics [91, 92]. The susceptibility of biofilms from different bacterial species to ultrasound appears to vary. Under identical conditions, ultrasound at 67 kHz was effective against Gram-negative *E. coli* and *P. aeruginosa* cultures but not against Gram-positive *S. aureus* and *S. epidermidis* cultures [92]. However, *S. epider-*

midis responded favourably at a lower frequency (28.48 kHz) and a longer treatment time [88]. A variety of frequencies ranging from 28.48 kHz to 10 MHz has been utilised on bacterial biofilms [91, 93, 94]. A comparison between frequencies (70 kHz, 500 kHz, 2.25 MHz and 10 MHz) shows that lower frequencies appear more effective than higher ones [93, 95]. In both continuous and pulse ultrasound modes, high power intensities (200 mW/cm^2) appear more efficacious than low power intensities (2 and 20 mW/cm^2) [95, 96].

Most studies describe the effect of ultrasound on bacterial viability in terms of the changes in colony forming unit (CFU) per unit area. Although this provides an indication as to changes in the number of bacterial biofilm cells, it cannot measure physical changes in biofilms. Using ultrasound, one study suggests that bioacoustical affect biofilms [97], while another suggests it affects planktonic bacteria rather than biofilms [92]. It has also been suggested that ultrasound also enhances the transport of antimicrobial agents to bacteria [98], increases the transport of oxygen and nutrient to the cell and waste product away from the cell increasing bacterial growth rate [99], disturbs the cations in biofilms [100], and increases the permeability of the cell membrane [101-103].

Continuous [104] and pulsed [105] ultrasound at a frequency of 1 MHz with power intensities of 1 and 0.5 W/cm^2 for maxillary and frontal sinuses respectively have been evaluated in CRS treatment. Continuous ultrasound is more likely to cause a thermal effect [105], however, no thermal effect has been observed with pulsed ultrasound. In acute rhinosinusitis the efficacy of ultrasound is comparable to antibiotics and when compared to antibiotics was also the preferred treatment option [106]. Therapeutic ultrasound is also effective in treating CRS [86, 104, 105, 107, 108].

4.2.2. *Bioelectric effect*

In the last decade the influence of high and low intensity electric fields and current densities on biofilms has been studied. High intensity electric fields influence the organization of biological membranes [109], membrane analogues [110], the shape of the cell [111], cell behaviour [112] and the dimensions of the bacterial glycocalyx [113]. However, low electrical current has been shown to enhance the efficacy of antimicrobial agents against *P. aeruginosa* [114], *S. epidermidis* [114], *Streptocoocus gordonii* [115], *E. coli* [116] and *S. aureus* [114] biofilms. This phenomenon has been referred to as the bioelectric effect.

Several methodologies of bioelectric effect on bacterial biofilms have been investigated, including direct current [117-119], radio frequency [116] and electromagnetic pulses [120]. The mechanism(s) of bioelectric actions on bacterial biofilms is not understood yet. A number of hypotheses have been proposed to explain the action(s) on biofilms [121]. These include increased bacterial growth due to electrolytic oxygen generation [122, 123], increased connective transport due to expansion and contraction of the biofilms [73], electrochemical generation of oxygen [119], and increased membrane permeability [124]. Most of the bioelectric studies on biofilms have analyzed the effects in terms of the changes in the number of CFU. Although this provides an indication of the effects on the number of biofilm cells, it does not measure chemical changes in biofilms including chemical bonds from covalent and hydrogen bonds, hydrophobic interactions, pH and EPS matrix. In addition, this analysis does not explain physical changes in biofilms on either the nature of biofilms or attachment processes. Hence, it does not explain electrostatic charges, van der Waals forces, electron transportation or electromagnetic radiation.

The effects of application of a variety of currents ranging from 1 to 2000 mA and 15 $\mu A/cm^2$ to 9 mA/cm^2 have been investigated on biofilms [121]. The main variables in the use of bioelectric effects are electric field and current density. Although these variables have been thoroughly investigated on biofilms, their significance has not yet been established. In contrast, in the laboratory, the electric field is probably not the variable that breaks down the biofilms; however, it has been suggested that the current drives charged molecules and ions into the biofilm matrix [119]. Applying electric current alone has been reported as not killing biofilms [122, 124]; however, other studies have reported some electric current effects [123, 125].

Results have been analyzed in terms of changes in CFU with respect to time. Application of electric fields alone, have reduced the number of CFU of biofilms for a certain period of time, but they return to the original number of bacteria at the end of the treatment period [118, 119]. Time of treatment has been evaluated at 12, 24 and 48 hours [114, 124, 126]. When time was increased from 12 to 48 hours, electric current showed a slight increase in the viable count of biofilms compared with the absence of electric current [122]. A dual treatment by bioelectric effect and antibiotics showed a further reduction in biofilms beyond the use antibiotics alone. The reduction is varied by a difference in magnitude ranging from 1-2 to 6-8 log [121]. However, variation in action on biofilms has shown different reactions according to type and concentration of antibiotics at the same level of electric field on the same species [114]. The morphology of biofilms could show the exact changes due to bioelectric effects if the bacterial biofilms behaviour were analysed by the changes of CFU in real time rather at a discrete point of time.

5. Summary

Ultrasound and bioelectric effect are new strategies for breaking down biofilms. However, their mechanisms are not well understood. Ultrasound frequencies that disturb bacterial biofilms need further investigation. The roles of time in the treatment and overall time of treatment have not been investigated and its effect with ultrasound has gained little attention. Bioelectric effect may disrupt bi-layer; however, the mechanisms through which electric currents or applied voltages cause a reduction in the number of viable biofilm cells is not conclusively understood. Evidence suggests that the biophysical approach could prevent the formation of biofilms and thus be clinically applicable to treat many chronic infectious diseases including chronic rhinosinusitis.

Several questions need to be answered. Are attachment bonds broken by ultrasound or does ultrasound disturb the biofilm structures? Is this caused by stretching the biofilm beyond the attachment forces or does the frequency affect the structural resonance of biofilms?

Author details

Mohammed Al-Haddad[1], Ahmed Al-Jumaily[1*], John Brooks[2] and Jim Bartley[1,3]

*Address all correspondence to: ahmed.al-jumaily@aut.ac.nz, mohammed.alhaddad@aut.ac.nz

1 Institute of Biomedical Technologies (IBTec), Auckland University of Technology, Auckland, New Zealand

2 Biotechnology Research Institute, Auckland University of Technology, Auckland, New Zealand

3 Department of Surgery, University of Auckland, Auckland, New Zealand

References

[1] Meltzer E, Hamilos D, Hadley J, Lanza D, Marple B, Nicklas R, et al. Rhinosinusitis: Establishing Definitions for Clinical Research and Patient Care. Journal of Allergy and Clinical Immunology. 2004 December;114(6):155-212.

[2] Hunsaker DH, Leid JG. The Relationship of Biofilms to Chronic Rhinosinusitis. Current Opinion in Otolaryngology & Head & Neck Surgery. 2008;16(3):237-41.

[3] Ramadan HH. Chronic Rhinosinusitis and Bacterial Biofilms. Current Opinion in Otolaryngology & Head & Neck Surgery. 2006;14(3):183-6.

[4] Macassey E, Dawes P. Biofilms and their Role in Otorhinolaryngological Disease. The Journal of Laryngology and Otology. 2008;122(12):1273-8.

[5] Benninger MS, Ferguson BJ, Hadley JA, Hamilos DL, Jacobs M, Kennedy DW, et al. Adult chronic Rhinosinusitis: Definitions, Diagnosis, Epidemiology, and Pathophysiology. Otolaryngology - Head and Neck Surgery. 2003;129(3, Supplement 1):S1-S32.

[6] Marieb EN. Human anatomy & physiology. 4th ed. ed. Menlo Park, Calif.: Addison Wesley Longman; 1998.

[7] Costerton JW, Stewart PS, Greenberg EP. Bacterial Biofilms: A Common Cause of Persistent Infections. . Science. 1999;284(5418):1318.

[8] De Beer D, Stoodley P, Lewandowski Z. Liquid Flow and Mass Transport in Heterogeneous Biofilms. Water Research. 1996;30(11):2761-5.

[9] Christensen B, Characklis WG. Physical and chemical properties of biofilms. In: Characklis WG, Marshall KC, editors. Biofilms: Wiley; 1990. p. 93-130.

[10] Nielsen PH, Jahn A, Palmgren R. Conceptual Model for Production and Composition of Exopolymers in Biofilms. Water Sci Technol. 1997;36(1):11-9.

[11] Costerton W, Veeh R, Shirtliff M, Pasmore M, Post C, Ehrlich G. The Application of Biofilm Science to the Study and Control of Chronic Bacterial Infections. Journal of Clinical Investigation. 2003;112(10):1466-77.

[12] Sutherland IW. The Biofilm Matrix - an Immobilized but Dynamic Microbial Environment. Trends in Microbiology. 2001;9(5):222-7.

[13] Dunne WM. Bacterial Adhesion: Seen any Good Biofilms Lately? Clinical Microbiological Review. 2002;15(2):155-66.

[14] Waters CM, Bassler BL. Quorum Sensing: Cell-to-Cell Communication in Bacteria. Annual Review Of Cell and Developmental Biology. 2005;21:319-46.

[15] Reguera G. When Microbial Conversations Get Physical. Trends in Microbiology. 2011;19(3):105-13.

[16] Matsuhashi M, Pankrushina AN, Takeuchi S, Ohshima H, Miyoi H, Endoh K, et al. Production of Sound Waves by Bacterial Cells and the Response of Bacterial Cells to Sound. Journal of General and Applied Microbiology. 1998 Feb;44(1):49-55.

[17] Rijnaarts HHM, Norde W, Lyklema J, Zehnder AJB. DLVO and Steric Contributions to Bacterial Deposition in Media of Different Ionic Strengths. Colloids and Surfaces B: Biointerfaces. 1999;14(1-4):179-95.

[18] Gilbert P, Evans DJ, Evans E, Duguid IG, Brown MR. Surface Characteristics and Adhesion of Escherichia coli and Staphylococcus epidermidis. The Journal of Applied Bacteriology. 1991;71(1):72-7.

[19] Walker SL, Hill JE, Redman JA, Elimelech M. Influence of Growth Phase on Adhesion Kinetics of Escherichia coil D21g. Applied and Environmental Microbiology 2005;71(6):3093-9.

[20] Dan N. The Effect of Charge Regulation on Cell Adhesion to Substrates: Salt-induced Repulsion. Colloids and Surfaces B: Biointerfaces. 2003;27(1):41-7.

[21] Palmer JS, Flint SH, Schmid J, Brooks JD. The Role of Surface Charge and Hydrophobicity in the Attachment of Anoxybacillus Flavithermus Isolated from Milk Powder. Journal Of Industrial Microbiology & Biotechnology. 2010;37(11):1111-9.

[22] Peschel A. How do Bacteria Resist Human Antimicrobial Peptides? Trends in Microbiology. 2002 Apr;10(4):179-86.

[23] Peschel A, Otto M, Jack RW, Kalbacher H, Jung G, Gotz F. Inactivation of the dlt operon in Staphylococcus aureus confers sensitivity to defensins, protegrins, and other antimicrobial peptides. J Biol Chem. 1999 Mar;274(13):8405-10.

[24] Peschel A, Collins LV. Staphylococcal Resistance to Antimicrobial Peptides of Mammalian and Bacterial Origin. Peptides. 2001 Oct;22(10):1651-9.

[25] Jones DS, Adair CG, Mawhinney WM, Gorman SP. Standardisation and Comparison of Methods Employed for Microbial Cell Surface Hydrophobicity and Charge Determination. International Journal of Pharmaceutics. 1996;131(1):83-9.

[26] Costerton JW, Montanaro L, Arciola CR. Biofilm in Implant Infections: Its Production and Regulation. International Journal of Artificial Organs. 2005;28(11):1062-8.

[27] Stewart PS, William Costerton J. Antibiotic Resistance of Bacteria in Biofilms. The Lancet. 2001;358(9276):135-8.

[28] del Pozo JL, Patel R. The Challenge of Treating Biofilm-associated Bacterial Infection. Clinical Pharmacology and Therapeutics. 2007 Aug;82(2):204-9.

[29] Suh JD, Cohen NA, Palmer JN. Biofilms in Chronic Rhinosinusitis. Current Opinion in Otolaryngology & Head & Neck Surgery. 2010;18(1):27-30.

[30] Cohen M, Kofonow J, Nayak JV, Palmer JN, Chiu AG, Leid JG, et al. Biofilms in Chronic Rhinosinusitis: A Review. American Journal of Rhinology & Allergy. 2009;23:255-60.

[31] Cryer J, Schipor I, Perloff JR, Palmer JN. Evidence of Bacterial Biofilms in Human Chronic Sinusitis. ORL: Journal for Oto-Rhino-Laryngology and its Related Specialties. 2004;66(3):155-8.

[32] Healy DY, Leid JG, Sanderson AR, Hunsaker DH. Biofilms with Fungi in Chronic Rhinosinusitis. Otolaryngology - Head and Neck Surgery. 2008;138(5):641-7.

[33] Psaltis AJ, Ha KR, Beule AG, Tan LW, Wormald P-J. Confocal Scanning Laser Microscopy Evidence of Biofilms in Patients with Chronic Rhinosinusitis. The Laryngoscope. 2007;117:1302-6.

[34] Ferguson BJ, Stolz DB. Demonstration of Biofilm in Human Bacterial Chronic Rhinosinusitis. American Journal of Rhinology & Allergy. 2005;19(5):452-7.

[35] Prince AA, Steiger JD, Khalid AN, Dogrhamji L, Reger C, Chiu AG, et al. Prevalence of Biofilm-forming Bacteria in Chronic Rhinosinusitis. American Journal of Rhinology & Allergy. 2008;22(3):239-45.

[36] Psaltis AJ, Ha KR, Beule AG, Tan LW, Wormald P-J. Confocal scanning laser microscopy evidence of biofilms in patients with chronic rhinosinusitis. The Laryngoscope. 2007;117(7):1302-6.

[37] Stoodley P, Nistico L, Johnson S, Lasko LA, Baratz M, Gahlot V, et al. Direct Demonstration of Viable Staphylococcus aureus Biofilms in an Infected Total Joint Arthroplasty: a Case Report. The Journal of Bone and Joint Surgery American volume. 2008;90(8):1751.

[38] Hall-Stoodley L, Stoodley P. Evolving Concepts in Biofilm Infections. Cellular Microbiology. 2009;11(7):1034-43.

[39] van Loosdrecht MC, Lyklema J, Norde W, Zehnder AJ. Influence of Interfaces on Microbial Activity. Microbiological Reviews. 1990;54(1):75-87.

[40] Whitchurch CB, Tolker-Nielsen T, Ragas PC, Mattick JS. Extracellular DNA Required for Bacterial Biofilm Formation. Science. 2002;295(5559):1487-.

[41] Molin S, Tolker-Nielsen T. Gene Transfer Occurs with Enhanced Efficiency in Biofilms and Induces Enhanced Stabilisation of the Biofilm Structure. Current Opinion in Biotechnology. 2003;14(3):255-61.

[42] Das T, Sharma PK, Busscher HJ, van der Mei HC, Krom BP. Role of Extracellular DNA in Initial Bacterial Adhesion and Surface Aggregation. Applied and Environmental Microbiology 2010;76(10):3405-8.

[43] Klotz SA, Butrus SI, Misra RP, Osato MS. The Contribution of Bacterial Surface Hydrophobicity to the Process of Adherence of Pseudomonas aeruginosa to Hydrophilic Contact Lenses. Current Eye Research. 1989;8(2):195-202.

[44] Oztuna F, Ozlü T, Bülbül Y, Buruk K, Topbaş M. Does Cold Environment Affect Streptococcus pneumoniae Adherence to Rat Buccal Epithelium? Respiration; International Review of Thoracic Diseases. 2006;73(4):546-51.

[45] Stepanović S, Ćirković I, Mijač V, Švabić-Vlahović M. Influence of the Incubation Temperature, Atmosphere and Dynamic Conditions on Biofilm Formation by Salmonella spp. Food Microbiology. 2003;20(3):339-43.

[46] Herald PJ, Zottola EA. Attachment of Listeria Monocytogenes to Stainless Steel Surfaces at Various Temperatures and pH values. Journal of Food Science. 1988;53(5): 1549-62.

[47] Nisbet BA, Sutherland IW, Bradshaw IJ, Kerr M, Morris ER, Shepperson WA. XM-6: A New Gel-forming Bacterial Polysaccharide. Carbohydrate Polymers. 1984;4(5): 377-94.

[48] Van Oss CJ. The Forces Involved in Bioadhesion to Flat Surfaces and Particles -- their Determination and Relative Roles. Biofouling. 1991;4:25-35.

[49] Carpentier B, Cerf O. Biofilms and Their Consequences, with Particular Reference to Hygiene in the Food Industry. Journal of Applied Bacteriology. 1993;75(499-511).

[50] Marshall KC, Stout R, Mitchell R. Mechanism of the Initial Events in the Sorption of Marine Bacteria to Surfaces. J Gen Microbiol. 1971;68(NOV):337-48.

[51] Characklis WG. Biofilm Process. In: Characklis WG, Marshall KC, editors. Biofilms. New York: Wiley; 1990. p. 195-231.

[52] Kumar CG, Anand SK. Significance of Microbial Biofilms in Food Industry: a Review. International Journal of Food Microbiology. 1998;42(1-2):9-27.

[53] Poortinga AT, Bos R, Busscher HJ. Charge Transfer During Staphylococcal Adhesion to TiNOX® Coatings with Different Specific Resistivity. Biophysical Chemistry. 2001;91(3):273-9.

[54] Otto M. Bacterial Evasion of Antimicrobial Peptides by Biofilm Formation. Current Topics in Microbiology and Immunology. 2006;306:251-8.

[55] Chen X, Stewart PS. Role of Electrostatic Interactions in Cohesion of Bacterial Biofilms. Applied Microbiology and Biotechnology. 2002;59(6):718-20.

[56] Flemming H-C, Wingender J. The Biofilm Matrix. Nature Reviews Microbiology. 2010;8(9):623-33.

[57] Mayer C, Moritz R, Kirschner C, Borchard W, Maibaum R, Wingender J, et al. The Role of Intermolecular Interactions: Studies on Model Systems for Bacterial Biofilms. International Journal of Biological Macromolecules. 1999;26(1):3-16.

[58] Busscher HJ, Weerkamp AH. Specific and Non-specific Interactions in Bacterial Adhesion to Solid Substrata. FEMS Microbiology Letters. 1987;46(2):165-73.

[59] Gottenbos B, Busscher HJ, van der Mei HC, Nieuwenhuis P. Pathogenesis and Prevention of Biomaterial Centered Infections. Journal of Materials Science: Materials in Medicine. 2002;13(8):717-22.

[60] Wright CJ, Shah MK, Powell LC, Armstrong I. Application of AFM from Microbial Cell to Biofilm. Scanning. 2010;32(3):134-49.

[61] Fang HH, Chan KY, Xu LC. Quantification of Bacterial Adhesion Forces Using Atomic Force Microscopy (AFM). Journal of Microbiological Methods. 2000;40(1):89-97.

[62] Otto K. Biophysical Approaches to Study the Dynamic Process of Bacterial Adhesion. Research in Microbiology. 2008;159(6):415-22.

[63] Vernhet A, Bellon-Fontaine MN. Role of Bentonites in the Prevention of Saccharomyces Cerevisiae Adhesion to Solid Surfaces. Colloids and Surfaces B: Biointerfaces. 1995;3(5):255-62.

[64] Stoodley P, Lewandowski Z, Boyle JD, Lappin-Scott HM. Structural Deformation of Bacterial Biofilms Caused by Short-term Fluctuations in Fluid Shear: An in situ Investigation of Biofilm Rheology. Biotechnology and Bioengineering. 1999;65(1):83-92.

[65] Stoodley P, Cargo R, Rupp CJ, Wilson S, Klapper I. Biofilm Material Properties as Related to Shear-induced Deformation and Detachment Phenomena. Journal of Industrial Microbiology and Biotechnology 2002;29(6):361-7.

[66] Chang HT, Rittmann BE, Amar D, Heim R, Ehlinger O, Lesty Y. Biofilm Detachment Mechanisms in a Liquid-fluidized Bed. Biotechnology and Bioengineering. 1991;38(5):499-506.

[67] Horn H, Reiff H, Morgenroth E. Simulation of Growth and Detachment in Biofilm Systems Under Defined Hydrodynamic Conditions. Biotechnology and Bioengineering. 2003;81(5):607-17.

[68] Choi YC, Morgenroth E. Monitoring Biofilm Detachment under Dynamic Changes in Shear Stress Using Laser-based Particle Size Analysis and Mass Fractionation. Water Sci Technol. 2003;47(5):69-76.

[69] Rupp CJ, Fux CA, Stoodley P. Viscoelasticity of Staphylococcus aureus Biofilms in Response to Fluid Shear Allows Resistance to Detachment and Facilitates Rolling Migration. Applied and Environmental Microbiology 2005;71(4):2175-8.

[70] van der Borden AJ, van der Werf H, van der Mei HC, Busscher HJ. Electric Current-induced Detachment of Staphylococcus Epidermidis Biofilms from Surgical Stainless Steel. Applied and Environmental Microbiology 2004 Nov;70(11):6871-4.

[71] Hong SH, Jeong J, Shim S, Kang H, Kwon S, Ahn KH, et al. Effect of Electric Currents on Bacterial Detachment and Inactivation. Biotechnology and Bioengineering. 2008;100(2):379-86.

[72] Brooks JD, Flint SH. Biofilms in the Food Industry: Problems and Potential Solutions. International Journal of Food Science & Technology. 2008;43(12):2163-76.

[73] Stoodley P, DeBeer D, Lappin-Scott HM. Influence of Electric Fields and pH on Biofilm Structure as Related to the Bioelectric Effect. Antimicrobial Agents and Chemotherapy 1997;41(9):1876-9.

[74] Sawyer LK, Hermanowicz SW. Detachment of Biofilm Bacteria due to Variations in Nutrient Supply. Water Sci Technol. 1998;37(4-5):211-4.

[75] Characklis WG, Mcfeters GA, Marshall KC. Physiological ecology in biofilm systems. In: Characklis WG, Marshall KC, editors. Biofilms. New York: Wiley; 1990. p. 341-94.

[76] Vats N, Lee SF. Active Detachment of Streptococcus mutans Cells Adhered to Epon-hydroxylapatite Surfaces Coated with Salivary Proteins in vitro. Archives of Oral Biology. 2000;45(4):305-14.

[77] Ponikau JU, Sherris DA, Kita H, Kern EB, Rochester M. Intranasal Antifungal Treatment in 51 Patients with Chronic Rhinosinusitis. Journal of Allergy and Clinical Immunology. 2002 December 110(06):862-6.

[78] Vaughan WC, Carvalho G. Use of Nebulized Antibiotics for Acute Infections in Chronic Sinusitis. Otolaryngology - Head and Neck Surgery. 2002 December;127(06): 558-68.

[79] Chan KH, Abzug MJ, Coffinet L, Simoes EAF, Cool C, Liu AH. Chronic Rhinosinusitis in Young Children Differs from Adults: a Histopathology Study. The Journal of Pediatrics. 2004 February;144 (2):206-12.

[80] Kilty SJ, AlMutari D, Duval M, Groleau MA, Nanassy JD, Gomes MM. Manuka Honey: Histological Effect on Respiratory Mucosa. American Journal of Rhinology & Allergy. 2010;24(2):63.

[81] Rasmussen TB, Bjarnsholt T, Skindersoe ME, Hentzer M, Kristoffersen P, Köte M, et al. Screening for Quorum-sensing Inhibitors (QSI) by Use of a Novel Genetic System, the QSI Selector. Journal of Bacteriology. 2005;187(5):1799-814.

[82] Smith A, Buchinsky FJ, Post JC. Eradicating Chronic Ear, Nose, and Throat Infections: a Systematically Conducted Literature Review of Advances in Biofilm Treatment. Otolaryngology - Head and Neck Surgery. 2011;144(3):338-47.

[83] Bartley J. Vitamin D, Innate Immunity and Upper Respiratory Tract Infection. The Journal of Laryngology and Otology. 2010;124(5):465.

[84] Chiu AG, Palmer JN, Woodworth BA, Doghramji L, Cohen MB, Prince A, et al. Baby Shampoo Nasal Irrigations for the Symptomatic Post-functional Endoscopic Sinus Surgery Patient. American Journal of Rhinology & Allergy. 2008;22(1):34.

[85] Sahlstrand-Johnson P, Jönsson P, Persson HW, Holmer N-G, Jannert M, Jansson T. In Vitro Studies and Safety Assessment of Doppler Ultrasound as a Diagnostic Tool in Rhinosinusitis. Ultrasound in Medicine & Biology. 2010;36(12):2123-31.

[86] Bartley J, Young D. Ultrasound as a Treatment for Chronic Rhinosinusitis. Medical Hypotheses. 2009;73(1):15-7.

[87] Ensing GT, Neut D, van Horn JR, van der Mei HC, Busscher HJ. The Combination of Ultrasound with Antibiotics Released from Bone Cement Decreases the Viability of Planktonic and Biofilm Bacteria: an in vitro Study with Clinical Strains. J Antimicrob Chemother. 2006 Dec;58(6):1287-90.

[88] Carmen JC, Roeder BL, Nelson JL, Beckstead BL, Runyan CM, Schaalje GB, et al. Ultrasonically Enhanced vancomycin Activity against Staphylococcus epidermidis Biofilms in vivo. J Biomater Appl. 2004 Apr;18(4):237-45.

[89] Hedges M, Lewis M, Lunec J, Cramp WA. The Effect of Ultrasound at 1.5 MHz on Escherichia coli. International Journal of Radiation Biology and Related Studies in Physics, Chemistry and Medicine. 1980;37(1):103-8.

[90] Huang C-T, James G, Pitt WG, Stewart PS. Effects of Ultrasonic Treatment on the Efficacy of Gentamicin against Established Pseudomonas aeruginosa Biofilms. Colloids and Surfaces B: Biointerfaces. 1996;6(4-5):235-42.

[91] Rediske AM, Roeder BL, Brown MK, Nelson JL, Robison RL, Draper DO, et al. Ultrasonic Enhancement of Antibiotic Action on Escherichia coli Biofilms: an in vivo Model. Antimicrobial Agents and Chemotherapy 1999 May;43(5):1211-4.

[92] Pitt WG, McBride MO, Lunceford JK, Roper RJ, Sagers RD. Ultrasonic Enhancement of Antibiotic Action on gram-negative Bacteria. Antimicrobial Agents and Chemotherapy 1994 Nov;38(11):2577-82.

[93] Qian Z, Sagers RD, Pitt WG. The Effect of Ultrasonic Frequency upon Enhanced killing of P. aeruginosa biofilms. Ann Biomed Eng. 1997 Jan-Feb;25(1):69-76.

[94] Nishikawa T, Yoshida A, Khanal A, Habu M, Yoshioka I, Toyoshima K, et al. A study of the Efficacy of Ultrasonic Waves in Removing Biofilms. Gerodontology. 2010;27(3): 199-206.

[95] Peterson RV, Pitt WG. The Effect of Frequency and Power Density on the Ultrasonically-enhanced Killing of Biofilm-sequestered Escherichia coli. Colloids and Surfaces B: Biointerfaces. 2000;17(4):219-27.

[96] Qian Z, Sagers RD, Pitt WG. The role of Insonation Intensity in Acoustic-enhanced Antibiotic Treatment of Bacterial Biofilms. Colloids and Surfaces B: Biointerfaces. 1997;9(5):239-45.

[97] Qian Z, Sagers RD, Pitt WG. Investigation of the Mechanism of the Bioacoustic Effect. Journal of Biomedical Materials Research. 1999;44(2):198-205.

[98] Rapoport N, Smirnov AI, Pitt WG, Timoshin AA. Bioreduction of Tempone and Spin-Labeled Gentamicin by Gram-Negative Bacteria: Kinetics and Effect of Ultrasound. Archives of Biochemistry and Biophysics. 1999;362(2):233-41.

[99] Pitt WG, Ross SA. Ultrasound Increases the Rate of Bacterial Cell Growth. Biotechnology Progress. 2003;19(3):1038-44.

[100] Broekman S, Pohlmann O, Beardwood ES, de Meulenaer EC. Ultrasonic Treatment for Microbiological Control of Water Systems. Ultrasonics Sonochemistry. 2010;17(6): 1041-8.

[101] Rapoport N, Smirnov AI, Timoshin A, Pratt AM, Pitt WG. Factors Affecting the Permeability of Pseudomonas aeruginosa Cell Walls toward Lipophilic Compounds: Effects of Ultrasound and Cell Age. Archives of Biochemistry and Biophysics. 1997;344(1):114-24.

[102] Carmen JC, Nelson JL, Beckstead BL, Runyan CM, Robison RA, Schaalje GB, et al. Ultrasonic-enhanced Gentamicin Transport Through Colony Biofilms of Pseudomonas aeruginosa and Escherichia coli. Journal of Infection and Chemotherapy. 2004;10(4): 193-9.

[103] Runyan CM, Carmen JC, Beckstead BL, Nelson JL, Robison RA, Pitt WG. Low-frequency Ultrasound Increases Outer Membrane Permeability of Pseudomonas aeruginosa. Journal of General and Applied Microbiology. 2006;52(5):295-301.

[104] Naghdi S, Ansari NN, Farhadi M. A Clinical Trial on the Treatment of Chronic Rhinosinusitis with Continuous Ultrasound. Journal of Physical Therapy Science. 2008;20(4):233-8.

[105] Ansari NN, Naghdi S, Farhadi M. Physiotherapy for Chronic Rhinosinusitis: The Use of Continuous Ultrasound. International Journal of Therapy & Rehabilitation. 2007 Jul;14(7):306-10.

[106] Høsøien E, Lund A, Vasseljen O. Similar Effect of Therapeutic Ultrasound and Antibiotics for Acute Bacterial Rhinosinusitis: a Randomised Trial. Journal of Physiotherapy. 2010;56(1):27.

[107] Ansari NN, Fathali M, Naghdi S, Hasson S. Effect of Pulsed Ultrasound on Chronic Rhinosinusitis: a Case Report. Physiotherapy Theory and Practice. 2010;26(8):558-63.

[108] Young D, Morton R, Bartley J. Therapeutic Ultrasound as Treatment for Chronic Rhinosinusitis: Preliminary Observations. The Journal of Laryngology and Otology. 2010;124(05):495-9.

[109] Sabelnikov AG, Cymbalyuk ES, Gongadze G, Borovyagin VL. Escherichia coli Membranes during Electrotransformation: an Electron Microscopy Study. Biochimica et Biophysica Acta (BBA) - Biomembranes. 1991;1066(1):21-8.

[110] Glaser RW, Leikin SL, Chernomordik LV, Pastushenko VF, Sokirko AI. Reversible Electrical Breakdown of Lipid Bilayers: Formation and Evolution of Pores. Biochimica et Biophysica Acta (BBA) - Biomembranes. 1988;940(2):275-87.

[111] Rajnicek AM, McCaig CD, Gow NAR. Electric Fields Induce Curved Growth of Enterobacter Cloacae, Escherichia coli, and Bacillus subtilis cells: Implications for Mechanisms of Galvanotropism and Bacterial growth. Journal of Bacteriology. 1994 Feb; 176(3):702-13.

[112] Shi WY, Lentz MJ, Adler J. Behavioral Responses of Escherichia coli to Changes in Temperature Caused by Electric Shock. Journal of Bacteriology. 1993 Sep;175(18): 5785-90.

[113] Applegate DH, Bryers JD. Effects of Carbon and Oxygen Limitations and Calcium Concentrations on Biofilm Removal Processes. Biotechnology and Bioengineering. 1991;37(1):17-25.

[114] del Pozo JL, Rouse MS, Mandrekar JN, Sampedro MF, Steckelberg JM, Patel R. Effect of Electrical Current on the Activities of Antimicrobial Agents against Pseudomonas aeruginosa, Staphylococcus aureus, and Staphylococcus epidermidis Biofilms. Antimicrobial Agents and Chemotherapy 2009 Jan;53(1):35-40.

[115] Wattanakaroon W, Stewart PS. Electrical Enhancement of Streptococcus gordonii Biofilm Killing by Gentamicin. Archives of Oral Biology. 2000 Feb;45(2):167-71.

[116] Caubet R, Pedarros-Caubet F, Chu M, Freye E, Rodrigues MD, Moreau JM, et al. A Radio Frequency Electric Current Enhances Antibiotic Efficacy Against Bacterial Biofilms. Antimicrobial Agents and Chemotherapy 2004 Dec;48(12):4662-4.

[117] Wellman N, Fortun SM, McLeod BR. Bacterial Biofilms and the Bioelectric Effect. Antimicrobial Agents and Chemotherapy 1996 Sep;40(9):2012-4.

[118] Blenkinsopp SA, Khoury AE, Costerton JW. Electrical Enhancement of Biocide Efficacy Against Pseudomonas aeruginosa Biofilms. Applied and Environmental Microbiology 1992 Nov;58(11):3770-3.

[119] Costerton JW, Ellis B, Lam K, Johnson F, Khoury AE. Mechanism of Electrical Enhancement of Efficacy of Antibiotics in Killing Biofilm Bacteria. Antimicrobial Agents and Chemotherapy 1994 Dec;38(12):2803-9.

[120] Pickering SAW, Bayston R, Scammell BE. Electromagnetic Augmentation of Antibiotic Efficacy in Infection of Orthopaedic Implants. J Bone Joint Surg-Br Vol. 2003 May; 85B(4):588-93.

[121] Del Pozo JL, Rouse MS, Patel R. Bioelectric Effect and Bacterial Biofilms. A Systematic Review. International Journal of Artificial Organs. 2008 Sep;31(9):786-95.

[122] Jass J, Costerton JW, Lappin-Scott HM. The Effect of Electrical Currents and Tobramycin on Pseudomonas aeruginosa Biofilms. Journal of Industrial Microbiology. 1995;15(3):234-42.

[123] Stewart PS, Wattanakaroon W, Goodrum L, Fortun SM, McLeod BR. Electrolytic Generation of Oxygen Partially Explains Electrical Enhancement of tobramycin Efficacy Against Pseudomonas aeruginosa Biofilm. Antimicrobial Agents and Chemotherapy 1999 Feb;43(2):292-6.

[124] Khoury AE, Lam K, Ellis B, Costerton JW. Prevention and Control of Bacterial Infections Associated with Medical Devices. American Society For Artificial Internal Organs Journal. 1992;38(3):M174-M8.

[125] McLeod BR, Fortun S, Costerton JW, Stewart PS. Enhanced bacterial biofilm control using electromagnetic fields in combination with antibiotics. Biofilms1999. p. 656-70.

[126] Jass J, Lappin-Scott HM. The Efficacy of Antibiotics Enhanced by Electrical Currents against Pseudomonas aeruginosa Biofilms. J Antimicrob Chemother. 1996 December 1, 1996;38(6):987-1000.

Chapter 5

Clinical Diagnosis and Severity Assessment in Immunocompetent Adult Patients with Community-Acquired Pneumonia

Fernando Peñafiel Saldías, Orlando Díaz Patiño and
Pablo Aguilera Fuenzalida

Additional information is available at the end of the chapter

http://dx.doi.org/10.5772/53475

1. Introduction

Community-acquired pneumonia (CAP) is a common and potentially serious illness [1]. It is defined as an acute infection of the pulmonary parenchyma, occurring outside the hospital, with clinical symptoms accompanied by the presence of pulmonary infiltrates on chest radiograph. With a prevalence estimated at nearly five million cases annually in United States, emergency physicians and general practitioners diagnose and treat CAP on a regular basis [2]; nearly one third of CAP patients arrived by emergency medical services, and half eventually were admitted [3].

Community-acquired pneumonia is the major infection-related cause of death in developed countries [4] and ranks as the third leading cause of all deaths in the world after ischaemic heart disease and cerebrovascular disease [5]. Mortality from CAP ranges from less than 1% in patients without risk factors treated as outpatients to 5-15% in hospital admitted patients to greater than 20-30% in intensive care unit patients [6]. Pneumonia increases in frequency with advancing age, and with associated comorbid medical illnesses (specially cardiovascular, metabolic, neoplastic, respiratory and neurological disease) there is a significant increase in morbidity and mortality [7].

Acute respiratory infections are a prevalent problem, affecting children, adults and the elderly, the main pathogens involved are respiratory viruses (*rhinovirus, influenza, parainfluenza, adenovirus, respiratory syncytial virus, metapneumovirus*) and secondly bacteria (*Streptococcus pneumoniae, Haemophilus influenzae, Mycoplasma pneumoniae, Chlamydophila pneumoniae, Le-*

gionella pneumophila, gram negative bacilli, and others), they are an important cause of school and labor absenteeism, especially during the cold seasons [1,8].

The clinical manifestations associated with respiratory infections, such as malaise, fever, chills, myalgia, sore throat, runny nose, cough, sputum production, chest pain and dyspnea, can occur in different clinical contexts that differ in etiology, pathogenesis, clinical course, treatment and prognosis [8,9]. Thus, the clinical picture may correspond to a mild self-limited upper respiratory tract infection to a severe lung parenchyma infection that requires specific treatment, as in cases of pneumonia and tuberculosis [10].

The reference standard to diagnose CAP is a new infiltrate on chest radiograph in the presence of recently acquired respiratory signs and symptoms [11]. These include cough, increased sputum production, dyspnea, fever and abnormal auscultatory findings [12]. Unfortunately, clinical findings do not reliably predict radiologically confirmed pneumonia [13]. Especially elderly people often present with atypical symptoms and without fever [14]. However physicians, especially in primary care, may not perform chest radiography and rely on the patient's history and physical examination [15].

The initial management of patients suspected of having community-acquired pneumonia is challenging because of the broad range of clinical presentations, comprehensive differential diagnosis, potential life-threatening nature of the illness, the need for antibiotic treatment and associated high costs of care [16,17]. The initial testing strategies should accurately establish a diagnosis and prognosis in order to determine the optimal treatment strategy, such as decisions about the site of care (ambulatory or in-hospital), extension of microbiology and laboratory assessments and antimicrobial recommendations.

The diagnosis is important to implement specific management measures, such as empirical antibiotic treatment and prevention of complications, and the prognosis is important in determining the site of care (ambulatory, general ward or intensive care facilities) and define treatment strategies to be implemented in each particular case [16,17]. This paper reviews the sensitivity, specificity and accuracy of the history, physical examination, and laboratory findings, individually and in combination, in diagnosing community-acquired pneumonia and predicting short-term risk for complications and death from the infection.

2. Diagnosis of pneumonia

Primary-care physicians usually rely on patient history, and signs and symptoms to diagnose or exclude pneumonia [10]. However, most signs and symptoms traditionally associated with pneumonia (e.g. malaise, fever, cough, sputum production and dyspnea) are not predictive of pneumonia in general practice [18]. Chest radiography (CXR) is the most frequently performed diagnostic investigation requested by general practitioners in the ambulatory setting (primary care and emergency department) [19]. The history and physical examination cannot provide a high level of certainty in the diagnosis of community-acquired pneumonia, but the absence of vital sign abnormalities and abnormal chest examination findings substantially reduces the probability of the infection [20].

The differential diagnosis of CAP includes several noninfectious causes, including pulmonary embolism, malignancy and congestive heart failure, among others [21]. The presence of a non-infectious differential diagnosis is usually suspected only after failure of antibiotic therapy, with the ensuing risks related to untreated, potentially life threatening non-bacterial disease [22]. Conversely, a delay of antibiotic treatment of more than 4-8 hours after hospital admission is associated with increased mortality [23]. Hence, both a rapid diagnosis of CAP and an accurate differentiation from viral respiratory illnesses and non-infectious causes has important therapeutic and prognostic implications [24].

2.1. Medical history

In the initial diagnosis of the patient who complains of acute respiratory symptoms or fever is necessary to establish the correct diagnosis based on clinical manifestations (history and physical examination) and laboratory tests (e.g., blood cell count, chest radiograph, C-reactive protein, procalcitonin, etc.) that are available in ambulatory practice. This requires knowledge of the epidemiology of respiratory infections in the geographic area, together with the sensitivity and specificity of the clinical history and physical signs abnormalities in diagnosing pneumonia [18].

The primary care physicians are often being confronted with patients presenting with non-specific constitutional symptoms (e.g., malaise, fever, chills, myalgia, headache, anorexia) or respiratory symptoms (e.g., cough, sputum production, chest pain, dyspnea), and must to establish a presumptive diagnosis based on their knowledge of the local epidemiology of acute respiratory infections and the main findings on clinical history and physical examination. Unfortunately clinical manifestations at presentation distinguish poorly between community-acquired pneumonia and other causes of respiratory illnesses (view differential diagnosis on Table 1). The likelihood ratio (LR) for these findings ranges between 1 and 3, which is not useful to confirm the diagnosis of pneumonia (Table 2) [25-29]. In general, the presence or absence of preexisting diseases, respiratory or constitutional symptoms does not have a substantial effect on the probability of pneumonia.

Five studies based in emergency departments have assessed the characteristics of individual items in the clinical history in the diagnosis of community-acquired pneumonia in adult patients [25-29]. In each of these studies, the reference standard for the diagnosis of pneumonia was a new infiltrate on a chest radiograph with or without clinical monitoring during one month. Table 2 summarizes the likelihood ratios associated to main clinical findings obtained from the history, including general manifestations, preexisting diseases and respiratory symptoms. Differences on results reflect, in part, variation in the selection criteria for each study. For example, chest radiographs were obtained for all patients presenting with acute cough in one study [25], while the other studies obtained chest radiographs only when the emergency physician previously determined a need for them, often to confirm or exclude a suspected diagnosis of pneumonia [26-29]. The latter approach provides a more highly selected population of patients with acute respiratory complaints that may change the measured test characteristics of individual clinical findings. Thus, the prevalence of pneumonia in study populations ranged from as low as 2.6% [25] to as high as 38.3% [26].

There are no individual items from the clinical history whose presence or absence would reduce or increase the odds of disease sufficiently to exclude or confirm the diagnosis of pneumonia without obtain a chest radiograph [18,20]. Though the presence of fever, comorbidities, history of dementia or immunosuppression may be helpful, they are not confirmatory, particularly given the typically low prevalence of pneumonia in the primary health services (2-5%) [1-3]. For example, when the estimated prevalence of pneumonia in primary care services is around 2-3%, the presence of subjective fever (LR^+=1.3-2.1) had a positive predictive value (PPV) ranging between 2.6% and 6.2% [25,28,29], reflecting the low prevalence of pneumonia in the ambulatory care setting. Meanwhile the presence of odynophagia or rhinorrhea (LR^+=0.5-0.7) in the same context had a positive predictive value ranging between 1.0% and 2.1% [25,29].

Common causes
Upper respiratory tract infections
Acute bronchitis and bronchiolitis
Influenza - Flu
Exacerbations of asthma and COPD
Pulmonary tuberculosis
Congestive heart failure
Pulmonary embolism
Primary neoplastic disease and metastatic lung disease
Pulmonary atelectasis
Rare causes
Hypersensitivity pneumonitis
Drug-induced lung diseases
Radiation-induced lung disease
Carcinomatous lymphangiosis
Collagen vascular disease: Systemic lupus erythematosus, rheumatoid arthritis, Wegener granulomatosis, Churg-Strauss syndrome.
Sarcoidosis
Eosinophilic pneumonia
Cryptogenic organizing pneumonia (COP)

Table 1. Differential diagnosis of adult patients with community-acquired pneumonia in the primary health care system.

http://dx.doi.org/10.5772/53475

Variables	Diehr et al	Gennis et al	Singal et al	Heckerling et al	Saldías et al
Cough	---	NS	1.8	NS	NS
Sputum production	1.3	NS	—	NS	1.2
Dyspnea	—	1.4	NS	NS	NS
Fever	2.1	NS	—	1.7	1.3
Chills	1.6	1.3	—	1.7	1.4
Myalgias	1.3	NS	—	—	NS
Odynophagia	0.7	NS	—	—	0.5
Rhinorrhea	0.7	NS	—	—	0.5
HR > 100/min	NS	1.6	NS	2.3	1.4
RR > 20/min	—	1.2	—	—	1.3
T > 37.8 °C	4.4	1.4	2.4	2.4	2.2
Normal vital signs	—	0.2	—	—	0.3
Dullness to percussion	NS	2.2	—	4.3	3.8
Ronchi	NS	1.5	—	1.4	NS
Bronchophony	—	—	—	3.5	9.5
Crackles	2.7	1.6	1.7	2.6	2.0
Normal lung exam	—	0.5	—	—	0.4

LR^+: positive likelihood ratio for pneumonia (sensitivity/1-specificity). HR: heart rate, RR: respiratory rate, T: temperature. Normal vital signs: heart rate < 100 beats/min, respiratory rate < 20 breaths/min and temperature < 37.8 °C. NS: result not significant.

Table 2. Predictive value of clinical manifestations (symptoms and signs) associated with the diagnosis of community-acquired pneumonia in adults (LR^+)[25-29].

2.2. Physical examination

The effect of vital sign abnormalities (e.g., tachycardia, tachypnea, fever) or pulmonary exam findings (e.g., decreased breath sound, bronchophony, dullness on percussion, rhonchus, crackles) on the probability of pneumonia depends on the cut-off value to define an abnormal result. For example, a respiratory rate greater than 20 breaths/min had a LR^+ of 1.2 to 1.3 [26,29], whereas a respiratory rate greater than 25 breaths/min had a LR^+ of 1.5 to 3.4 [25,28] (Table 2). When the estimated prevalence of pneumonia in primary care services is around 2-3%, the presence of crackles on pulmonary examination (LR^+=1.6-2.7) had a positive predictive value ranging between 3.2% and 8.1% [25-29]. In contrast, two studies have shown that having a normal heart rate (below 100 beats/min) without fever (temperature < 37.8 °C) and tachypnea (respiratory rate < 20 breaths/min) reduces significantly the probability of community-acquired pneumonia ($LR^- = 0.18$), thereby reducing the pretest odds of pneumonia by more than fivefold [26,29].

In the Chilean study [29], the major clinical predictors of pneumonia were fever (≥38 °C), tachypnea (≥20 breaths/min), mental confusion, orthopnea, cyanosis, dullness on percussion, bronchophony, crackles and oxygen saturation less than 90% breathing room air (LR $^+$: 2.0 to 9.5). In contrast, sore throat, runny nose, normal vital signs and lung auscultation without clinical abnormalities were less frequent in patients with final diagnosis of pneumonia (LR^+: 0.3-0.5). Unlike other studies, Saldías et al. examined some combinations of symptoms and signs showing that significantly increases the pretest probability. The combination of clinical variables increase the probability of pneumonia, such as the presence of fever and tachypnea associated with orthopnea, dullness on percussion, crackles or oxygen saturation below 90% (LR^+: 4.9 to 14.7). At the same time, the probability of pneumonia is very low in patients presenting with respiratory symptoms and normal vital signs and lung auscultation (LR^+: 0.1).

In summary, individual symptoms and signs at presentation distinguish poorly between community-acquired pneumonia and other causes of respiratory illnesses [13,18,20]. Thus, in 10-20% of ambulatory patients with a suspected lower respiratory tract infection CXR is requested [19]. CXR can diagnose pneumonia in cases with the presence of pulmonary infiltrates and differentiate pneumonia from other conditions that may present with similar symptoms (e.g., acute bronchitis or influenza) [2,3]. In addition, the results may suggest specific aetiologies (e.g., lung abscess, TB infection), identify coexisting conditions (e.g., bronchial obstruction, pleural effusion, neoplasms) and evaluate the severity of illness (e.g., multilobar or bilateral infiltrates, rapid progression of infiltrates, pleural effusion) [6,8]. Although chest radiography is frequently used for diagnosing pneumonia, little is known about the influence of CXR on the probability estimation of pneumonia by general practitioners and on change in patient management [18,20]. Chest radiography is considered the gold standard for pneumonia diagnosis; however, we do not know its sensitivity and specificity, and we have limited data on the clinical implications of false-positive and false-negative results [18]. In the absence of empirical evidence, the decision to order a chest radiograph needs to rely on expert opinion in seeking strategies to optimize the balance between harms and benefits [16,17].

2.3. Clinical judgment and decision guidelines

Although physicians often planning the diagnostic and laboratory exams considering the prevalence of the disease and its estimate of the probability in the population being evaluated, the diagnostic threshold of professionals varies considerably even when faced with similar clinical situations [30,31]. As the predictive value of individual signs and symptoms to the diagnosis of pneumonia is relatively low, to resolve this problem, it has been designed some predictive rules or decision guidelines incorporating the presence or absence of specific clinical findings intended to guide clinicians in the management of patients with similar clinical features [18,20]. In the literature we find several protocols or decision rules that are designed specifically to help primary care physicians in the assessment of adult patients with lower respiratory tract infections (Table 3) [25-29,32-34]. Thus, in the clinical practice guidelines is often recommended to primary care physicians request of chest radiography in patients presenting respiratory symptoms based on some of these decision rules, in order to optimize patient`s care [16,17,35].

Clinical prediction rules for pneumonia diagnosis in adults	
Diehr et al.	**Score**
Rhinorrhea	-2 points
Sore throat	-1 point
Night sweats	1 point
Mialgyas	1 point
Sputum production	1 point
RR > 25 breaths/min	2 points
T° ≥ 37.8 °C or 100 °F	2 points
Heckerling et al. Each variable scores a point.	
Heart rate > 100 beats/min	
Temperature > 37.8 °C or 100 °F	
Decreased breath sounds	
Crackles	
Absence of asthma	
Gennis et al. If one or more variables are present requesting chest radiograph.	
Heart rate > 100 beats/min	
Respiratory rate > 20 breaths/min	
Temperature > 37.8 °C	
Singal et al. Estimating the probability of pneumonia.	
Probability = $1/(1 + e^{-Y})$	
Where Y: -3.095 + 1.214 x Cough + 1.007 x Fever + 0.823 x Crackles	
Each variable = 1 if present	
Melbye et al. A logistic regression model is proposed for the diagnosis of pneumonia.	
Y= + 4.7 for fever (reported by patient) with duration of illness of one week or more; – 4.5 for coryza; – 2.1 for sore throat; + 5.0 for dyspnea; + 8.2 for lateral chest pain; + 0.9 for crackles.	
González Ortiz et al. A logistic regression model is proposed for the diagnosis of pneumonia.	
Y= –1.87; + 1.3 for pathologic auscultation; + 1.64 for neutrophilia; + 1.70 for pleural pain; + 1.21 for dyspnea.	
Hopstaken et al. A logistic regression model is proposed for the diagnosis of pneumonia.	
Y= –4.15; + 0.91 for dry cough; + 1.01 for diarrhea; + 0.64 for temperature ≥ 38 °C; + 2.78 for C-reactive protein ≥ 20 mg/L.	

Table 3. Clinical predictive rules for pneumonia diagnosed by chest radiography in the ambulatory care setting[25-28,32-34].

Prediction rules based on clinical information have been developed to support the diagnosis of pneumonia and help limit the use of expensive diagnostic tests [36,37]. However, these prediction rules need to be validated in the primary care setting. Several clinical prediction rules have been developed to predict pneumonia in adults but they were not superior to clinical judgment to predict pneumonia in the ambulatory setting [20,36,37]. In summary, combination of history and physical examination findings at presentation only moderately increase the probability of pneumonia. Thus, the clinical guidelines endorse the need for chest radiography to confirm all diagnoses of community-acquired pneumonia [16,17,35].

In two predictive rules, described by Diehr et al. [25] and Heckerling et al. [28], the pretest probability of pneumonia is amended according to the presence or absence of certain specific symptoms. While other rule, described by Singal et al. [27], was designed using a logistic regression analysis and provides a probability of pneumonia ranging from 4% (absence of symptoms and signs) to 49% (presence of cough, fever and crackles). On the other hand, Gennis et al. [26] suggested applying chest radiograph in patients with suspected of CAP and alteration in any vital signs (heart rate above 100 beats/min, respiratory rate above 20 breaths/min or temperature higher than 37.8 °C). Melbye et al [32], González Ortiz et al. [33] and Hospstaken et al. [34] proposed a logistic regression model for diagnosis of pneumonia based on clinical and laboratory variables.

Two prospective studies have examined the predictive value of clinical judgment and four clinical predictive rules in the diagnosis of community-acquired pneumonia in adults [37,38]. Emerman et al. [37] compared physician judgment in the use of chest radiographs for diagnosing pneumonia with decision rules developed by Diehr, Singal, Heckerling, and Gennis in the emergency department and medical outpatient clinic of a major urban teaching hospital. The prevalence of pneumonia in this study was 7%, they found that clinical judgment allowed to reduce the application of unnecessary chest radiographs better than the four predictive rules (LR^-= 0.25, 95%CI: 0.09 to 0.61) while clinical judgment allowed to increase the likelihood of pneumonia to around 13% (LR^+ = 2.0, 95%CI: 1.5 to 2.4), which would have led to demand many unnecessary radiographic examinations. Among the four examined predictive rules, the application of x-ray only to patients with abnormal vital signs recommended by Gennis et al. [26] had higher diagnostic yield with a LR^+ of 2.6 (95%CI: 1.6 to 3.7), which would have reduced by 40% the application of unnecessary radiographic examinations but would not have detected 38% of pneumonias confirmed by radiology (LR^- = 0.50, 95%CI: 0.27 to 0.78 compared with LR^- = 0.18 of the original study of Gennis et al.) [34]. The sensitivity of physician judgment (86%) exceeded that of all four decision rules (62-76%), but the higher specificity and accuracy of two of the decision rules [26,28] suggested that they may have a role in patient evaluation.

Saldías et al. [29,38] have shown that clinical diagnosis of pneumonia made by physicians in the emergency department had better sensitivity (range: 75-83%) than specificity (range: 47-83%) and better negative predictive value (NPV) (range: 85-91%) than PPV (range: 36-70%) (Table 4). In fact, a less experienced emergency physician had lower PPV and specificity compared to internal medicine and respiratory disease physicians (Table 5). The chance to change the initial diagnosis of pneumonia or positive likelihood ratio of three emergency physicians ranged between 1.5 and 4.8. Similar findings were described by Wipf et al. [39], who determined the accuracy of various physical examination maneuvers in diagnosing pneumonia and compared the interobserver reliability of the maneuvers among three examiners. The authors concluded that the clinical findings investigated in chest examination does not confirm or exclude with certainty the diagnosis of pneumonia, and the degree of interobserver agreement was highly variable for different physical examination findings.

Variables	Clinical diagnosis	Diehr et al	Singal et al	Heckerling et al	Gennis et al
	%, (95% CI)	%, (95% CI)	%, (95% CI)	%, (95% CI)	%, (95% CI)
Sensitivity	0.79 (0.72-0.84)	0.77 (0.70-0.83)	0.76 (0.69-0.82)	0.84 (0.78-0.90)	0.92 (0.87-0.96)
Specificity	0.66 (0.63-0.69)	0.64 (0.61-0.68)	0.54 (0.51-0.58)	0.41*(0.38-0.44)	0.31*(0.28-0.33)
PPV	0.55 (0.50-0.59)	0.54 (0.49-0.58)	0.46 (0.42-0.50)	0.43 (0.39-0,45)	0.42 (0.39-0.44)
NPV	0.85 (0.81-0.89)	0.84 (0.79-0.88)	0.81 (0.76-0.86)	0.84 (0.77-0.89)	0.88 (0.80-0.94)
Accuracy	0.70 (0.65-0.75)	0.69 (0.67-0.74)	0.62 (0.57-0.67)	0.56*(0.50-0.62)	0.53*(0.47-0.59)
LR^+	2.3 (1.9-2.7)	2.2 (1.8-2.6)	1.7 (1.4-1.9)	1.4* (1.2-1.6)	1.4* (1.2-1.4)

Note: 95% CI: confidence interval of 95%, PPV: positive predictive value; NPV: negative predictive value. * $p < 0.05$ compared with clinical judgment.

Table 4. Predictive value of clinical judgment and four predictive rules in the diagnosis of community-acquired pneumonia in adults[38].

Clinical diagnosis	Sensitivity	Specificity	PPV	NPV	LR^+
Physician A	**83%**	**83%**	**70%**	**91%**	**4.8**
Physician B	**75%**	**73%**	**56%**	**86%**	**2.8**
Physician C	**77%**	**47%**	**36%**	**85%**	**1.5**
Average	**79%**	**66%**	**55%**	**85%**	**2.3**

Note: Physicians A and B were specialists in internal medicine and respiratory disease over five years of professional practice. Physician C was an emergency medicine specialist with less than three years of clinical practice.

Table 5. Sensitivity, specificity, positive predictive value (PPV), negative predictive value (NPV) and positive likelihood ratio (LR^+) for clinical diagnosis of community-acquired pneumonia[29].

Lieberman et al. [40] evaluated the reliability of physicians' judgement relating to the presence of pneumonia in adult patients with acute respiratory symptoms by clinical assessment alone compared with chest X-ray. Physicians' judgements of pneumonia had a sensitivity of 74% (95% CI 49-90%), a specificity of 84% (95% CI 78-88%), a NPV of 97% (95% CI 94-99%)

and a PPV of only 27% (95% CI 16-42%). They concluded that the ability of physicians to negate radiologically confirmed pneumonia by clinical assessment in febrile adult respiratory tract infection patients was good, but that their ability to successfully predict this condition was poor.

In other study developed in two emergency departments from Madrid, Spain; Gonzalez et al. [33] showed that the clinical judgment had low sensitivity for the diagnosis of pneumonia (45%) with a moderate PPV (80%). The sensitivity and specificity of clinical diagnosis of pneumonia established by emergency medicine physicians were similar or slightly higher compared with the four clinical predictive rules described in the literature [37,38]. The area under the curve (AUC) of clinical judgment and the clinical decision rule described by Diehr et al. for diagnosis of pneumonia were similar (AUC = 0.79 and 0.75, respectively), and both were higher than those described by Heckerling (AUC = 0.70), Singal (AUC = 0.70) and Gennis et al. (AUC = 0.67) [38].

In summary, the clinical findings (history and physical examination) have only moderate sensitivity and specificity for diagnosis of pneumonia in immunocompetent adult patients presenting with fever or respiratory symptoms in the ambulatory care setting (Table 6). None of the decision rules described in the literature have been superior to clinical judgment in the diagnosis of pneumonia, yet no studies have examined its real contribution in the evaluation and management of patients presenting with respiratory symptoms or fever in the primary care services.

Clinical diagnosis	Sensitivity	Specificity	PPV	NPV	LR^{+}_{-}
González et al.	45%	93%	80%	74%	6.6
Wipf et al.	47-69%	58-75%	48-64%	57-72%	1.1-2.0
Emerman et al.	86%	58%	14%	98%	2.0
Lieberman et al.	49-90%	78-88%	16-42%	94-99%	___
Saldías et al.	75-83%	47-83%	36-70%	85-91%	1.5-4.8

Note: PPV: positive predictive value, NPV: negative predictive value, LR: likelihood ratio.

Table 6. Predictive value of clinical judgment in diagnosing community-acquired pneumonia in adults[29,37,39-41].

2.4. Biomarkers and lower respiratory tract infection diagnosis

Numerous non-infectious processes can produce respiratory symptoms and new pulmonary infiltrates with systemic inflammatory signs and symptoms that can be easily confused with bacterial pneumonia (Table 1). Typically, Gram stains of respiratory secretions are often unavailable or are difficult to evaluate, and microbiological culture reports take at least 24 to 48 hours. A negative sputum or blood culture in a patient suspected of having community-acquired pneumonia does not rule out the possibility of a severe lower respiratory tract infection [41]. Given these areas of uncertainty in clinical decision-making, a concerted effort has been undertaken to develop reliable and practical biomarkers for the diagnosis, risk prediction and management of CAP. To be helpful in routine clinical practice, a biomarker should provide additional actionable information – not already available by standard methods – that accomplishes at least one or more of the following: a) Assists in establishing a rapid and reliable diagnosis; b) Provides an indication of prognosis; c) Selects those patients most likely to benefit from a specific intervention; d) Reflects the efficacy or lack of efficacy of specific interventions.

The usefulness of biomarkers for diagnosing lower respiratory tract infections (LRTI), and identifying particular disease entities amongst LRTIs (e.g., acute bronchitis, influenza, COPD exacerbation, pneumonia) is still a matter of controversy.

2.4.1. C- reactive protein

Some observational studies indicate that C-reactive protein (CRP) may have some role in identifying patients with community-acquired pneumonia. Almirall et al. found significantly higher CRP values in adult patients with confirmed CAP compared to healthy controls and suspected CAP [42]. Flanders et al. evaluated CRP as a possible tool in the differential diagnosis of 168 adults with acute cough less than three weeks [43]. CRP levels correlated with the presence of pneumonia but not with its severity. A serum CRP level over 40 mg/L had a sensitivity of 70% and specificity of 90% to identify pneumonia. Holm et al. confirmed the low sensitivity (73%) and specificity (65%) of serum CRP in the differential diagnosis of LRTIs [44]. The authors concluded that only very high CRP levels (>100 mg/L) can be used as indicator for the presence of CAP. Accordingly, Stolz et al. showed that the specificity of CRP at the cut-off value of 100 mg/L to predict radiological confirmed pneumonia reaches 91.2% [45].

Falk et al. [46] assessed the diagnostic value of CRP in primary care and emergency departments in terms of ruling in or ruling out CAP. Eight studies incorporating 2,194 patients were included. The median prevalence of CAP was 14.6% (range 5%-89%). At a CRP cut-point of less than 20 mg/L, the pooled positive LR^+ was 2.1 (95%CI 1.8-2.4] and the pooled negative LR^- was 0.33 (95% CI 0.25-0.43). In conclusion, CRP may be of value in ruling out a diagnosis of CAP in situations where pneumonia probability exceeds 10%, typically in emergency departments. However, in primary care services, additional diagnostic testing with CRP is unlikely to alter the probability of CAP sufficiently to change subsequent management decisions such as antibiotic prescribing or referral to hospital.

2.4.2. Procalcitonin

Procalcitonin (PCT) is a 116 amino acid protein, precursor of calcitonin, which is physiologically produced by the C-cells of the thyroid after intracellular processing of the prohormone. The half-life of PCT is around 20-24 h and the plasma concentration in healthy individuals is typically below 0.1 μg/L. In some studies procalcitonin does not appear to be a significant marker for CAP [47,48]. However, a more recent evaluation of the role of highly sensitive CRP and PCT measurements showed a better discriminatory value of these biomarkers compared to clinical signs [49]. The diagnostic accuracy of clinical signs and symptoms and a range of laboratory markers were assessed in 545 patients with suspected lower respiratory tract infection admitted to the emergency department. The area under the curve of a clinical model including fever, cough, sputum production, abnormal chest auscultation and dyspnea was 0.79 (95%CI, 0.75-0.83). Combining the values for procalcitonin and highly sensitive C-reactive protein together increased the AUC to 0.92 (95%CI, 0.89-0.94), which was significantly better than the AUC for PCT, CRP and clinical signs and symptoms alone. The contribution to diagnostic reliability made by PCT was substantially greater than that made by CRP, which in turn performed better than the total leukocyte count. Clinical criteria such as sputum production and physical examination with chest auscultation were poor predictors for the diagnosis of CAP. To predict bacteremia, PCT also had a higher AUC (0.85, 95%CI 0.80-0.91) as compared to CRP (0.71, 95%CI 0.62-0.80; $p = 0.01$), leukocyte count (0.68, 95%CI 0.59-0.77; $p = 0.002$) and elevated body temperature (0.46, 95%CI 0.37-0.56; $p < 0.001$). The added value of the PCT biomarker as a clinical decision-making tool has been evidenced in several studies involving PCT measurement [50-57].

Circulating levels of the precursor hormone PCT, derived primarily from nonthyroidal tissues, can rise several thousand times above normal in various inflammatory conditions, but most notably in bacterial infection [54]. In differentiating bacterial infection from non-infective causes of inflammation in hospitalized patients, a meta-analysis concluded that PCT was both more sensitive (85% vs. 78%) and more specific (83% vs. 60%) compared with CRP. PCT was also more sensitive (92% vs. 86%) in differentiating between a bacterial etiology and a viral etiology [55].

PCT and ventilator-associated pneumonia: The utility of PCT levels to improve the early diagnosis of ventilator-associated pneumonia (VAP) has been evaluated in different studies. Due to the use of dissimilar thresholds the results were not consistent [56-58]. Ramirez et al. report a cohort study with sequential measurement of PCT and CRP in well characterized patients with VAP [59]. The results of this study showed that PCT and CRP plasma levels were statistically higher in patients with confirmed VAP, PCT being the more accurate marker. The combination of the simplified clinical pulmonary infection score (CPIS) and serum PCT was able to exclude all false-positive diagnosis of VAP thus resulting in 100% specificity.

2.4.3. Soluble triggering receptor expressed by myeloid cell

The soluble triggering receptor expressed by myeloid cells-1 (sTREM) has been proposed as another potentially useful diagnostic tool for CAP and VAP [58, 60-62]. The sTREM is upregulated by microbial products, it accurately identifies bacterial or fungal pneumonia in bronchoalveolar lavage fluid (BAL) from mechanically ventilated patients, and is superior in this regard to clinical findings or other laboratory values. Such intervention is not appropriate, however, in the routine care of patients with community-acquired pneumonia. In this setting, measurement of soluble triggering receptor expressed on myeloid cells-1 in plasma or serum has proved unhelpful as a guide to either etiology or outcome [61].

The first study on 148 patients suffering from suspected CAP or VAP and receiving mechanical ventilation, sTREM was assessed in the BAL fluid and its levels were a better predictor for bacterial infection than CPIS, TNF-alfa and IL-1 levels [58]. The authors also analyzed the behavior of PCT and did not find any role for this biomarker in identifying pneumonia. Another group evaluated the presence of sTREM in exhaled ventilator condensate (EVC) and in BAL fluid from 23 patients clinically suspected of having VAP [60]. In contrast with the first report, sTREM-1 was detected in the BAL fluid of all 14 VAP subjects but also in 8 of 9 subjects without pneumonia, and sTREM levels did not differ in the VAP subjects compared to the non-pneumonia subjects. However, sTREM-1 was detected in the EVC from 11 of 14 subjects with VAP, but from only 1 of 9 subjects without VAP, and was significantly higher in the pneumonia patients. Another study tends to rule out the value of sTREM detection in BAL as a useful tool in VAP diagnosis [62]. In this study, 105 consecutive patients receiving mechanical ventilation and undergoing BAL were enrolled. Of those, 19 patients (18.1%) met definite microbiologic criteria for bacterial or fungal VAP. All the statistical analysis performed showed that measurement of sTREM-1 was inferior to clinical parameters for the diagnosis of VAP.

In patients with community-acquired pneumonia, traditional criteria of infection based on clinical signs and symptoms, clinical scoring systems, and general inflammatory indicators (for example, leukocytosis, fever, sputum and blood cultures) are often of limited clinical value and remain an unreliable guide to diagnosis lower respiratory tract infections. Procalcitonin is superior to other commonly used markers in its specificity for bacterial infection, allowing alternative diagnoses to be excluded, mainly as a guide to the necessity for antibiotic therapy [63-65]. It can therefore be viewed as a diagnostic and prognostic test. It more closely matches the criteria for usefulness than other candidate biomarkers such as C-reactive protein, which is rather a nonspecific marker of acute phase inflammation, and proinflammatory cytokines such as plasma IL-6 levels that are highly variable, cumbersome to measure, and lack specificity for systemic infection.

2.5. Pneumonia in elderly

The clinical presentation of pneumonia in the elderly may be subtle, lacking the typical acute symptoms observed in younger adults. Riquelme et al. [66] reported the initial clinical presentation of 101 elderly patients with CAP (mean age, 78 years; 66.3% men) who were admitted to a 1000-bed teaching hospital in Barcelona, Spain. The most frequently observed symptoms were dyspnea (72.3%), cough (66.3%), fever (63.4%), asthenia (57.4%), purulent sputum (51.5%), anorexia (49.5%), altered mental status (44.6%), and pleuritic chest pain (33.7%). The classic triad of symptoms of pneumonia – cough, dyspnea, and fever – was observed in only 30.7% of these elderly patients. Nineteen patients (18.8%) did not have cough, purulent sputum, or pleuritic chest pain. In a prospective study [67] designed to assess the clinical characteristics of 503 elderly patients (mean age, 76.3 years; 63.4% men) admitted for CAP to 16 hospitals across Spain, the most frequently observed symptoms were cough

(80.9%), fever (75.5%), dyspnea (69.8%), sputum production (65.8%), chills (53.1%), pleuritic chest pain (43.3%), asthenia (38.6%), and altered mental status (25.8%). The typical constellation of symptoms of pneumonia (cough, purulent sputum, and pleural pain) was noted in only 152 patients (30.2%). Metlay et al. [68] studied the influence of age on symptoms at presentation in 1,812 patients with CAP. Cough, dyspnea, and pleuritic chest pain were significantly less common among elderly patients than among younger patients (81.7% vs. 87.8%, 68.8% vs. 73.9%, and 31.6% vs. 53.3%, respectively). After controlling for patient demographics, comorbidities, and severity of illness, elderly patients exhibited significantly fewer respiratory symptoms than did younger patients (respiratory symptom score, 7.21 vs. 9.79, respectively; $p < 0.01$). In other study, altered mental status and the absence of fever were observed more frequently in patients over 80 years of age than in those under 80 years of age (21.0% vs. 10.7%; $p < 0.001$ and 32.1% vs. 21.9%; $p < 0.001$, respectively). These findings are consistent with Saldías et al. study [69], which reported a higher incidence of dyspnea and confusion (71% vs. 53%; $p < 0.001$ and 28% vs. 8%; $p< 0.001$, respectively) but a lower incidence of fever, chills and pleuritic chest pain in the older patients (63% vs. 76%; $p = 0.007$, 21% vs. 41%; $p < 0.001$ and 12% vs. 32%; $p< 0.001$, respectively). Compared to adults below 65 years of age hospitalized for CAP during the same period, the following clinical findings were more prevalent among the elderly population: the presence of comorbidity, dyspnea, decreased level of consciousness, suspected aspiration, hypoxemia and high serum urea nitrogen on admission to hospital. In the elderly, admission to intermediate and intensive care units was more frequent (47.7% vs. 29.2%, $p< 0.001$), and the length of hospital stay was longer (10.6 vs. 8.6 days, $p= 0.03$). Multilobar radiographic involvement, pleural effusion, the hospital complication rate and the need for mechanical ventilation were similar in both groups, but mortality, both in-hospital and at 30-days follow-up, was higher in the elderly population (9.8% vs. 3.2%; $p= 0.03$ and 13.1% vs. 4.8%; $p= 0.02$, respectively). Furthermore, it has been suggested that the local inflammatory response to infection of the lungs is decreased in the elderly, resulting in less cough and sputum production [70]. The systemic inflammatory response (e.g., fever, leukocytosis, high serum C-reactive protein) is also reduced secondary to decreased production of cytokines. Nevertheless, the decrease in interleukin-6 (IL-6), the most prevalent mediator of fever, did not reach statistical significance in a study that measured IL-6 levels in 59 elderly patients and 21 younger patients with CAP (211.6 vs. 284.5 pg/mL, respectively) [71]. In contrast, tachypnea remains prevalent and appears to be a sensitive indicator of lower respiratory tract infection in the elderly [69,72]. Altered mental status, confusion, a sudden decline in functional physical capacity, and comorbidity decompensation may be the only symptoms of an infection (including pneumonia) in the elderly [66]. Clinicians should be cognizant of those symptoms to avoid delay in establishing the diagnosis and initiating antibiotic therapy.

2.6. Recommendation

The clinical diagnosis of pneumonia without radiological confirmation lacks specificity because the clinical feature (history and physical examination) does not allow differentiating the patient with pneumonia from other acute respiratory diseases (e.g., upper respiratory tract infections, bronchitis, bronchiolitis, influenza). The diagnosis of pneumonia based solely on clinical criteria is also hampered by the large variability in the ability to detect focal signs on chest examination between different examiners. Pneumonia remains foremost a clinical diagnosis. However, symptoms of lower respiratory infection, including fever, cough, purulent sputum, dyspnea, and pleuritic chest pain as well as the clinical findings of fever, tachypnea, tachycardia, hypoxemia, and auscultatory signs of consolidation, are not unique to pneumonia.

Although most patients with CAP can be managed successfully in the community by their general practitioner without additional investigations, distinguishing CAP from other causes of respiratory symptoms and signs can be difficult, particularly where the presence of comorbidities such as congestive heart failure, chronic lung disease, or COPD complicate the clinical picture. The elderly can present a particularly difficult diagnostic challenge because they more frequently present with non-specific or atypical symptoms and signs. Chest radiographs are therefore routinely required to confirm the clinical suspicion of pneumonia: The clinical history and physical examination suggest the presence of a lower respiratory tract infection, but the diagnosis is established when demonstrating the presence of new onset pulmonary infiltrates on chest radiography.

3. Prognosis of pneumonia

3.1. Severity assessment in adult patients with community acquired pneumonia

Once community-acquired pneumonia is diagnosed, a combination of history, physical examination, and laboratory exams can help estimate the short-term risk for torpid evolution or death and, along with the patient's psychosocial characteristics, determine the appropriate site of treatment [6,16,17,32]. These decisions, including the need for parenteral therapy and supportive care, ultimately relate to the decision on whether to hospitalize the patient.

The wide spectrum of severity in patients presenting in the ambulatory care setting explains the wide variation in case fatality rates for pneumonia reported in the national and international literature in different clinical contexts [1,4,6,8]. Thus adult patients with pneumonia without risk factors treated in the ambulatory setting has a low mortality risk (1-2%), rising to 5-15% in patients with comorbidities or specific risk factors that are admitted to hospital ward and increases to 20-50% in those admitted to the intensive care unit. The severity assessment allow us to decide the site of care (outpatient or in-hospital: general ward, intermediate care unit or ICU), the extension of laboratory and microbiological examination, coverage of empiric antibiotic treatment, route and length of treatment and level of medical and nursing care that requires the particular case. Recognition of patients at low risk of complications that can be managed as outpatients would significantly reduce the costs of health care, minimizing risks, without compromising the evolution and prognosis of CAP patients [73]. Hospital admission rates of adult patients with community-acquired pneumonia reported in the literature vary considerably, suggesting that physicians do not use uniform criteria to assess the risk of morbidity and mortality of patients. It has been reported that primary care physicians often overestimate the risk of complications and death in patients with CAP, hospitalizing consequently a significant number of patients at low risk [74]. The risk stratification of patients should help to reduce this variability and improve the decision of admission and cost effective management of the disease.

3.2. Clinical, radiographic and laboratory prognostic factors in community-acquired pneumonia

Numerous studies have examined hospital or ICU admission risk factors associated with complicated clinical course or poor prognosis in CAP patients, particularly related to hospital or short-term mortality [6,16,17,69]. Univariate studies have described more than 40 clinical and laboratory parameters associated with mortality [6,36,69,75-77]. However, an independent association with short-term risk of death or hospital complication rate was found only for some clinical variables using multivariate analysis.

To facilitate handling of short-term prognostic factors in pneumonia, it is convenient to group them in different categories: a) Sociodemographic factors: age, gender, origin, ethnicity, social factors; b) Clinical history: preexisting disease, immunosuppression, altered mental status, fever, cough, sputum production, dyspnea, chills, chest pain; c) Physical examination: tachycardia, hypotension, tachypnea, hypothermia, hyperthermia, confusion, or pulmonary exam abnormalities; d) Chest radiograph: multilobar or bilateral pulmonary infiltrates, cavitation or pleural effusion; e) Laboratory tests: hypoxemia, hypercapnia, acidosis, high blood urea nitrogen, anemia, leukopenia, leukocytosis, hypoalbuminemia, hyperglycemia, and raised biomarkers of inflammation; f) Microbiological exams: bacteremic pneumonia, lung infection by pneumococcus, anaerobic, atypical microorganisms, gram-negative bacilli or *S. aureus* [6].

Age: Several studies have demonstrated an association between extreme ages (below one year and over 65 years) and the risk of death in the hospital [4-6,14,23,78,79,82,83]. The community-acquired pneumonia in the elderly usually manifests with atypical or nonspecific symptoms (e.g., mental confusion, anorexia, arrhythmias, congestive heart failure), difficulting the diagnostic process and delaying specific treatment adversely compromising the prognosis of patients [14,66,69,70]. The absence of fever, prostration, multiple comorbidities, nutritional disorders and institutionalization are poor prognostic factors in the elderly [14,66,72]. However, based on evidence from clinical studies, there are not reasons that support the use of different clinical variables to assess the severity in elderly people.

Comorbidity: The presence of coronary heart disease, congestive heart failure, cerebrovascular disease with motor dysfunction or dementia, diabetes mellitus, chronic respiratory disease (COPD, bronchiectasis), cancer, immunosuppression, chronic renal failure, alcoholism, malnutrition and chronic hepatic disease are associated to increased hospital mortality in adult patients with pneumonia [6,69,75-77,83,85]. However, the contribution of different comorbidities to severity of community-acquired pneumonia in adults has been difficult to establish, due to lack of uniformity in the definition of chronic diseases in different studies and stratification problems with the severity of various comorbidities. This could partly explain the low predictive power of specific comorbidities as risk factors of death in multivariate analysis, despite that large number of studies have shown its importance in the univariate analysis.

Respiratory rate: Regardless of age of the patient, the presence of tachypnea is one of the most reliable indicators of severity of pneumonia in univariate and multivariate analysis [6,69,75-77,79,81-83,86,87]. There is a linear relationship between respiratory rate and mortality in pneumonia patients, but in the clinical practice, it is recommended that the respiratory rate above of 20 breaths/min should be considered a reliable sign of severity in patients with pneumonia.

Mental status: Altered mental status has been identified as an independent risk factor of death in several studies, including elderly population [6,14,66,69,72,79,82]. However, the definition of altered mental status has varied in different studies, thus complicating their integration as a prognostic factor. Despite this, the quantitative or qualitative impairment of consciousness are an excellent predictor of prognosis in patients with community-acquired pneumonia.

Blood pressure: Systolic hypotension (SBP <90 mmHg) or low diastolic blood pressure (DBP $\leq$ 60 mmHg) and the presence of septic shock on admission to hospital are independent factors of poor prognosis in multivariate analysis of several studies [6,69,75-82,84]. In the ICU, the presence of septic shock or prolonged systolic hypotension for more than 12 hours which does not improve with adequate volume replacement and/or vasopressor drugs prescription is another sign of poor prognosis.

Oxygenation: Hypoxemia and oxygen administration with a $FiO_2 \geq 0.5$ to maintain adequate tissue oxygenation or the application of PEEP are indicators of poor prognosis [6,78,79,83]. The severe acute respiratory failure and the need for mechanical ventilation in ICU admission or during hospital stay are also predictors of mortality. The presence of hypoxemia or hypercapnia should be corrected immediately and is a determining factor in deciding hospitalization of a particular case.

Chest radiography: Bilateral or multilobar pulmonary opacities, rapid progression of pulmonary infiltrates over 72 hours, the presence of cavitation or pleural effusion are poor prognostic factors associated to hospital complications and short-term mortality [6,74-77,82-84]. The performance of serial chest radiographs to assess the clinical evolution of hospitalized patients with pneumonia is not recommended outside the ICU, unless there is clinical evidence suggestive of treatment failure or a complication.

Leukocytes count: The presence of leukopenia (less than 4,000 leukocytes per mm^3) or leukocytosis (greater than 20,000 leukocytes per mm^3) on admission to hospital was associated with high mortality in univariate analysis. However, multivariate analysis results have been controversial and suggest that leukopenia may be a better predictor of mortality [6,79].

Renal function: The high blood urea nitrogen on admission to hospital has been recognized as a poor prognostic factor in patients with community acquired pneumonia in the univariate and multivariate analysis, probably reflecting the deterioration of tissue perfusion [6,69,75-77, 79,81,82]. It is important to emphasize, the main prognostic laboratory tests measured at admission in hospitalized adult patients with community-acquired pneumonia are the arterial blood gases and measurement of uremia.

Microbiology: Bacteremic pneumonia with positive blood cultures has two to three times greater risk of death [6,75-77,83]. Pneumonia caused by gram negative bacilli, *Staphylococcus aureus* and *Pseudomonas aeruginosa* tend to have more complications during the evolution and increased lethality [6,83]. Pulmonary infection by *Legionella spp* is a common cause of severe pneumonia and admission to the intensive care unit, specially reported in Europe. However, the clinical-radiographic features has failed to differentiate between the different etiologic agents of pneumonia; in this way, the late microbiological information has not been useful for assessing the severity of the individual patient on admission to hospital or in the context of attention in primary health care services (outpatient clinics or emergency departments). Nevertheless, microbiological tests are useful for evaluating the severity and guide antimicrobial therapy in patients hospitalized with community-acquired pneumonia.

3.3. Clinical predictive rules to assess the severity of the patient with pneumonia

The evaluation of the severity of the patient with pneumonia depends on the experience of the clinician, who has been reported often underestimate the seriousness of the disease [78]. No prognostic factor is sufficiently sensitive and specific for predicting the evolution of the individual patient. Thus, in the medical literature have been described several prognostic indices that would help the clinician to identify patients with community acquired pneumonia that have low or high risk of complications and/or death during the evolution (Table 7) [76,79-82]. None of the developed predictive models has allowed stratifying patients into well-defined risk categories. The development and dissemination of clinical guidelines that examine the severity of the patient with pneumonia by objective criteria, have reduced the hospitalization of low risk patients, significantly reducing the cost of medical resources without affecting the evolution and prognosis of patients [16,17,35,88,89]. Severity predictive models based on clinical and laboratory exams are best viewed as adjunctive tools for the clinical evaluation of patients. In general, predictive models should be used with care and should never override clinical judgment. The periodic assessment of severity during the course of hospital stay is mandatory to allow adjustment of empirical antibiotic treatment to avoid adverse events associated to it.

Significant variation in admission rates among hospitals and among individual physicians has been well documented. Physicians often overestimate severity and hospitalize a significant number of patients at low risk for death [90,91]. Because of these issues, interest in developing simple and objective clinical criterias available at primary health care has stimulated to develop such predictive rules by several research groups [76,79-82]. The relative merits and limitations of various proposed criteria have been carefully evaluated [92]. The two most interesting predictive rules are the Pneumonia Severity Index (PSI) described by Fine et al. [81] for screening of patients at low risk for outpatient treatment, and the British Thoracic Society criteria (CURB-65) for screening of high risk patients with severe CAP [79,80].

http://dx.doi.org/10.5772/53475

Patient characteristics	Score (points)
Demographic factors	
Age (in years)	
Male	Age
Female	Age - 10
Nursing home resident	10
Coexisting conditions	
Neoplastic disease	30
Liver disease	20
Congestive heart failure	10
Cerebrovascular disease	10
Renal disease	10
Initial physical examination findings	
Altered mental status	20
Respiratory rate ≥30 breaths/min	20
Systolic blood pressure < 90 mmHg	20
Temperature < 35 °C or ≥40 °C	15
Heart rate ≥125 beats/min	10
Initial laboratory findings	
pH < 7.35	30
BUN > 30 mg/dL	20
Sodium < 130 mEq/L	20
Glucose ≥250 mg/dL	10
Hematocrit < 30%	l10
PaO_2 < 60 mmHg or O_2 sat < 90%	10
Pleural effusion	10

Risk class	Score	Mortality	Site of care recommendation
I	50	0.1 – 0.4%	Outpatient
II	51 – 70	0.6 – 0.7%	Outpatient
III	71 – 90	0.9 – 2.8%	Short stay inpatient
IV	91 – 130	8.2 – 12.5	Inpatient
V	> 130	27.1 – 31.1%	Inpatient
British Thoracic Society criteria (CURB-65)			
Confusion			
BUN > 7 mmol/L or 20 mg/dL			
Systolic BP < 90 mmHg or Diastolic BP ≤60 mmHg			
Respiratory rate ≥30 breaths/min			
Age ≥65 years			

Risk categories	Score	Mortality	Site of care recommendation
I	0 – 1	1.5%	Outpatient
II	2	9.2%	Inpatient
III	3	22%	Inpatient (ICU admission)

Severe Community Acquired Pneumonia score (SCAP)		
Variables	*Score*	
Age ≥80 years	5	
Systolic blood pressure < 90 mmHg	11	
Respiratory rate > 30 breaths/min	9	
Confusion	5	
Blood urea nitrogen > 30 mg/dL	5	
Multilobar or bilateral pulmonary infiltrates	5	
PaO_2 < 54 mmHg or PaO_2/FiO_2 < 250	6	
pH < 7.30	13	
Risk categories	**Score**	**Severe CAP ***
Low	0 – 9	0.19 - 3.4%
Intermediate	10 – 19	9.2 - 11.2%
High	20	36.6 - 75.8%

* *Severe CAP was defined by hospital* mortality, mechanical ventilation use and/or septic shock.

Table 7. Prognostic rules in adults patients with community-acquired pneumonia[79-81].

3.3.1. Pneumonia severity index

The PSI is based on derivation and validation cohorts of 14,199 and 38,039 hospitalized patients with CAP, respectively, plus an additional 2,287 combined inpatients and outpatients [81]. The Pneumonia Severity Index allows us stratify patients into five risk categories. Patients with pneumonia risk class I have low risk of death and adverse events, with a mortality rate ranging between 0.1% and 0.4%. In an observational study, low-risk patients susceptible to ambulatory care had a 30-days hospitalization rate around 5.5% [93]. The model described by Fine et al. was developed as a two-stage predictive tool to identify low risk patients for ambulatory management. In a first step, we consider some epidemiological variables (age, gender, nursing home residence), the presence of certain specific comorbidities (congestive heart failure, malignancy, chronic liver disease, cerebrovascular disease and chronic kidney disease) and some physical examination abnormalities (mental status, heart rate, blood pressure, respiratory rate and temperature). In a second step, we consider some laboratory and radiographic findings (for example, anemia, hypoxemia, azotemia, hyperglycemia and pleural effusion). On the basis of associated mortality rates, it has been suggested that risk class I and II patients should be treated as outpatients, risk class III patients should be treated in an observation unit or with a short hospitalization, and risk class IV and V patients should be treated as inpatients (Table 7). In general, patients younger than 60 years without comorbidities and abnormalities in mental status and vital signs are classified into low risk categories, which could be treated as outpatients unless there are social factors that hinder their control or adherence to treatment (e.g., alcoholism, drug addiction, psychiatric disorders or, rural origin).

http://dx.doi.org/10.5772/53475

3.3.2. British thoracic society rule

To identify high-risk patients has been useful the discriminant rule developed by the British Thoracic Society, confirming that advanced age, altered mental status or confusion, respiratory rate above 30 breaths/min, diastolic blood pressure below 60 mmHg and blood urea nitrogen greater than 20 mg/dL are associated with increased mortality [79,80]. The BTS original criteria of 1987 have subsequently been modified [78-80]. In the initial study, risk of death was increased 21-fold if a patient, at the time of admission, had at least 2 of the following 3 conditions: tachypnea, diastolic hypotension, and an elevated blood urea nitrogen level. These criteria appear to function well except among patients with chronic renal failure and among elderly patients [94,95]. The most recent modification of the BTS criteria includes five easily measurable factors [80]. Multivariate analysis of 1,068 patients identified the following factors as indicators of increased mortality: confusion (based on a specific mental test or disorientation to person, place, or time), BUN level above 17 mmol/L (20 mg/dL), respiratory rate over 30 breaths/min, low blood pressure (systolic, below 90 mm Hg; or diastolic, below 60 mmHg), and age over 65 years; this gave rise to the acronym CURB-65. In the derivation and validation cohorts, the 30-day mortality among patients with 0, 1, or 2 factors was 0.7%, 2.1%, and 9.2%, respectively. Mortality was higher when 3, 4, or 5 factors were present and was reported as 14.5%, 40%, and 57%, respectively. The authors suggested that patients with a CURB-65 score of 0-1 be treated as outpatients, that those with a score of 2 be admitted to the wards, and that patients with a score of ≥ 3 often required ICU care. A simplified version (CRB-65), which does not require testing for BUN level, may be appropriate for decision making in the primary care practitioner's office [96].

3.3.3. Severe CAP rule

Severe CAP (SCAP) is a life-threatening condition that requires intensive care. Estimates of the frequency of severe CAP range from 5 to 35%, with mortality ranging from 20 to 50% [6]. These relatively wide ranges indicate disparities between definitions of SCAP. There is no universally accepted definition of SCAP. During the last decade, the term has been used for cases that ultimately result in death, and/or patients requiring admission to an intensive care unit. Such practical definitions seem to be insufficient because the risk of death from CAP is not the same as the need for inpatient care. On the other hand, the decision to admit a patient to the ICU depends on the clinical judgment of individual clinicians and the local practices of their hospitals, differences that could account for much of the variability regarding ICU admission. Studies focused on the evaluation of patients admitted to the ICU mix some variables evident at the time of admission with other potentially evolutionary criteria, which are not applicable to early hospital admission. Other criteria, such as mechanical ventilation and septic shock, are less subject to interpretive variability and better reflect illness severity [97]. España et al. [82] developed a clinical prediction rule for severe community-acquired pneumonia (SCAP) in 1,057 adult patients visiting the emergency department from one hospital, which was then validated in two different populations: 719 patients from the same center and 1,121 patients from four other hospitals. In the multivariate analyses, eight independent predictive factors were correlated with severe community-acquired pneumonia: arterial pH below 7.30, systolic blood pressure under 90 mmHg, respiratory rate above 30 breaths/min, altered mental status, blood urea nitrogen over 30 mg/dL, oxygen arterial pressure under 54 mmHg or ratio of arterial oxygen tension to fraction of inspired oxygen under 250 mmHg, age greater than or equal to 80 years, and multilobar or bilateral lung affectation. The SCAP score was designed to identify high risk patients at admission, by predicting the hospital mortality, need for mechanical ventilation, and risk for septic shock.

The Severe Community Acquired Pneumonia score described by España et al. was validated to predict 30-day mortality in an internal validation cohort of consecutive adult patients admitted to one hospital [98]. Consecutive inpatients from other three hospitals were used to externally validate the score and compare the SCAP with the PSI and CURB-65. The discriminatory power of these rules to predict 30-day mortality was tested by the area under curve (AUC), and their predictive accuracy with the sensitivity, specificity and predictive values. The 30-day mortality rate increased directly with increasing SCAP score (class 0: 0.5%, to class 4: 66.5% risk) in the internal validation cohort, and from 1.3% to 29.2% in external cohort (p <0.001) with an AUC of 0.83 and 0.75, respectively (p= 0.024). The SCAP score identified 62.4% (95%CI 58.8-66.0) low-risk patients, 52.5% (95%CI 48.8-56.2) the PSI and 46.2% (95%CI 42.5-49.9) the CURB-65 in the external cohort. Patients classified as low risk by the three rules had similar 30-day mortality (SCAP: 2.5%, PSI: 1.6% and CURB-65: 2.7%). The SCAP score was valid to predict 30-day mortality among low-risk patients and to identify patients at low-risk was similar or greater than the other studied rules.

3.3.4. Generic sepsis scores

Generic scoring systems such as the systemic inflammatory response syndrome (SIRS) criteria and standardized early warning score (SEWS) have been extensively assessed in critically ill patients and are relatively simple to calculate [99,100]. However, it has been reported that SIRS and SEWS perform less favourably than CURB-65 and PSI scores for severity assessment in CAP and prediction of progression to sepsis in severe CAP [101,102]. Considering the limited number of studies to date does not support use of generic sepsis scores over pneumonia-specific scores in CAP.

The clinical pulmonary infection score (CPIS) - original or modified - has been proposed for the diagnosis and management of ventilator-associated pneumonia [103, 104]. The clinical pulmonary infection score has low diagnostic accuracy; however, incorporating gram stains results into the score may help clinical decision making in patients with clinically suspected pneumonia [105].

The use of APACHE II predictive model in the evaluation of patients with severe pneumonia in the ICU has demonstrated its usefulness as a predictor of mortality [106,107]. However, it has not been proved applicable in units of lower complexity of the hospital. The application of this prognostic tool out of the ICU is difficult, time consuming and impractical.

3.3.5. Clinically relevant adverse outcome prediction

Severity scores provide pivotal direction for the management of community-acquired pneumonia, helping guide decisions such as the appropriate venue for care, diagnostic strategies, and antibiotic therapies. The most popular severity scores, the pneumonia severity index and CURB-65 are accurate for predicting pneumonia-related mortality [108-114]. But clinical care should be based on a broader set of medical outcomes than just mortality, such as ICU admission, need for mechanical ventilation, progression to severe sepsis, or treatment failure [115,116]. Unfortunately, there is no consensus surrounding serious complications that warrant hospitalization for patients with pneumonia.

It has been reported that the SCAP score is slightly better than the PSI and CURB-65 in predicting adverse outcomes other than mortality in two independent cohorts [117]. In the external validation cohort, the rate of adverse outcomes increased steadily from low- to high-risk classes for the SCAP score as well as for the PSI and CURB-65 ($p < 0.001$). In the internal validation cohort, there were no significant differences in outcomes such as ICU admission and mechanical ventilation for the PSI and CURB-65. All three scores predicted treatment failure with low to moderate discrimination in the external validation cohort. It must be noted that the initial severity of CAP is only one factor predicting treatment failure. Other factors, such as the causal microorganism and treatment-related factors, are not part of the three prediction tools. The SCAP score classified a significantly higher proportion of patients as low risk in both cohorts than the PSI and CURB-65, with lower rates of all adverse outcomes. Another goal of the tool is its negative predictive value. If the score is low, ICU admission and others adverse outcomes are very unlikely. In addition, patients identified as high risk by the SCAP score had somewhat higher rates of ICU admissions, need for mechanical ventilation, and severe sepsis compared with the PSI and CURB-65. Thus, applying the SCAP score would identify CAP patients who should receive closer monitoring and more aggressive treatment. Given the somewhat poorer predictive power of the PSI and CURB-65 in the internal validation cohort, the sensitivity, specificity, and AUC of the three scores were compared in the external validation cohort. Although the SCAP score had significantly better sensitivities and specificities than the PSI and CURB-65, the differences were small and of uncertain clinical relevance.

Saldías et al. [77] assessed the accuracy and discriminatory power of three validated rules (PSI, CURB-65 and SCAP) for predicting clinically relevant adverse outcomes (ICU admission, need for mechanical ventilation and hospital complications rate) in patients hospitalized with community-acquired pneumococcal pneumonia. The rate of all adverse outcomes and hospital length of stay increased directly with increasing PSI, CURB-65 and SCAP scores. The three severity scores allowed us to predict the risk of in-hospital complications and 30-day mortality. The PSI score was more sensitive and the SCAP was more specific to predict hospital complications and the risk of death. However, the SCAP was more sensitive and specific in predicting the use of mechanical ventilation. Thus, the severity scores validated in the literature allow us to predict the risk of complications and death in adult patients hospitalized with pneumococcal pneumonia. Nevertheless, the clinical indexes differ in their sensitivity, specificity and discriminatory power to predict different adverse events.

3.4. Biomarkers of inflammation for the severity assessment of CAP

The clinical guidelines for the management of adult patients with CAP suggest the use of severity-based approach for the purpose of guiding therapeutic options, such as the need for hospital or ICU admission, suitability for ambulatory care, and choice and route of antimicrobial agents. The use of prognostic scores, like CURB-65 and PSI, is recommended to support clinical judgment [16,17,35]. Despite their widespread use in clinical routine, traditional markers, such as severity of disease assessment by the patient`s fever, white blood cell count and also CRP level are not reliable for the assessment of disease severity and mortality risk in CAP. The pneumonia severity index (PSI) is a widely accepted and validated severity scoring system that assesses the risk of mortality for pneumonia patients in a two step algorithm, combining clinical signs, demographic data and laboratory values [81]. However, its complexity is high, jeopardizing its dissemination and implementation, especially in everyday clinical practice. Therefore, the CURB-65 score has been proposed as a simpler alternative [79,80].

A number of studies have explored the prognostic value of biomarkers in patients with CAP. Muller et al. [49] reported a significant relationship between procalcitonin levels and PSI categories, with PCT being markedly elevated in the highest PSI class. However, it must be taken into account that many PSI class V patients had low PCT values. Huang et al. [118], report a multicenter, prospective, observational cohort study in a large population of 1,651 patients admitted to 28 community or teaching emergency departments for CAP to determine whether procalcitonin can provide prognostic information beyond the Pneumonia Severity Index and CURB-65. In this study procalcitonin levels did not add relevant prognostic information for most pneumonia patients. Used alone, procalcitonin had modest test characteristics: specificity (35%), sensitivity (92%), positive likelihood ratio (1.41), and negative likelihood ratio (0.22). However, among higher-risk groups as assessed by the Pneumonia Severity Index score, low procalcitonin level reliably predicted lower mortality.

The predictive value of procalcitonin was compared to CRP, leukocyte count and CRB-65 score in a large study of the CAPNETZ competence network [119] involving 1,671 patients with proven CAP, clinical and laboratory variables were determined at admission and patients were followed-up for 28 days for outcome. The PCT levels at admission were a better predictor of CAP severity and outcome than leukocyte count and CRP levels, with a similar prognostic accuracy as the CRB-65 score. The area under the curve for PCT and CRB-65 was comparable (0.80, 95%CI 0.75-0.84 versus 0.79, 95%CI 0.74-0.84), but each significantly higher compared with CRP (0.62, 95%CI 0.54-0.68) and leukocyte count (0.61, 95%CI 0.54-0.68). Another finding from this study, a PCT threshold of ≤ 0.228 ng/mL identified low-risk patients within all CRB-65 risk groups.

Another study from the CAPNETZ network explored the role of pro-atrial natriuretic peptide (MR-proANP), pro-vasopressin (CT-proAVP), PCT and CRP for severity assessment and outcome prediction in 589 adult patients with CAP [120]. MR-proANP, CT-proAVP and PCT levels, but not CRP, increased with increasing severity of CAP, classified according to the CRB-65 score. The area under the curve values for CT-proAVP (0.86, 95%CI 0.83-0.89) and MR-proANP (0.76, 95%CI 0.72-0.80) were similar to the AUC of CRB-65 (0.73, 95%CI 0.70-0.77). In multivariate Cox proportional hazards regression analyses high levels of MR-proANP and CT-proAVP were the strongest predictors of mortality. Thus, the authors concluded that MR-proANP and CT-proAVP are predictors of CAP severity and 28-day mortality comparable to the clinical CRB-65 score.

4. Conclusion

In assessing the probability of death in adult patients with community-acquired pneumonia, the clinical history and physical examination abnormalities significantly influenced the prognosis [4,6,49,69,75-87]. In medical history, advanced age (over 65-70 years), specific comorbidities, symptoms of dyspnea and confusion were associated with increased risk of death. Among comorbid conditions, the strongest predictors of death were neurologic disease, cancer, immunosuppression, alcoholism, malnutrition, renal disease, liver disease and congestive heart failure. In physical examination, altered mental status, hypotension, tachypnea and hypothermia were associated with increased odds of death. Laboratory abnormalities significantly associated to bad prognosis are azotemia (blood urea nitrogen level above 20 mg/dL), hypoxemia, leukopenia (≤ 4,000 cells/mm^3) and leukocytosis (≥ 20,000 cells/mm^3). Pleural effusion, rapid progression of pulmonary infiltrates and multilobar or bilateral infiltrates on chest radiograph were also associated to increased risk of complications and death.

Individual clinical and laboratory abnormalities are associated with only moderate increases in the odds of death [6,49,75-87]. Thus, combinations of factors are necessary to accurately assess short-term risk for death and guide site-of-care decisions. These prognosis rules include demographic factors (age, gender and nursing home residence), comorbid conditions (for example, neoplastic disease, diabetes, pulmonary disease, and heart disease), symptoms and signs (for example, altered mental status, lack of pleuritic chest pain or fever, tachypnea, and hypotension), and laboratory and radiographic findings (for example, hypoxemia, azotemia, leukopenia, acidosis, hypoalbuminemia and multilobar infiltrates). The Pneumonia Patient Outcomes Research Team (PORT) Severity Index and CURB-65 are well validated prognostic rules recommended in the clinical guidelines [16,17,35] to assess severity of pneumonia patients in the ambulatory care setting. In evaluating clinical findings as a guide to initial site of treatment, most studies on prognosis have focused on mortality as the sole outcome, which is problematic because a high risk for death may not be the only reason for hospitalization. Increased risk for other serious adverse events (e.g., ICU admission, mechanical ventilation support, progression to septic shock), reliability in adhering to therapy, returning for follow-up, and availability of supportive care at home are also important determinants for hospitalization. Therefore, clinical judgment should always prevail over the severity index calculation in clinical decision for site of care and treatment planning.

4.1. Pneumonia severity assessment in the ambulatory setting

Clinicians are advised to implement a simple and practical strategy for assessing the severity and risk of complications in patients with community-acquired pneumonia assisted in the ambulatory care setting (outpatient clinics and emergency departments). It is suggested to classify patients into three risk categories:

a. Low-risk patients (short-term mortality less than 1-2%) susceptible to ambulatory treatment or brief hospitalization.

b. High-risk patients (short-term mortality around 20-30%) that must be managed in the hospital and probably in specialized units (Intermediate Care Unit or ICU) with severe pneumonia criteria.

c. Intermediate-risk patients with advanced age, comorbidities or independent risk factors of death, but they cannot be classified into a specific category.

Clinical judgment is essential to decide the setting of care and treatment of patients with community-acquired pneumonia, especially those located in the intermediate risk category. In general, patients younger than 65 years without preexisting diseases, abnormal vital signs or altered mental status at admission, could be managed as outpatients considering its low risk of death and complications. Elderly patients (aged above 65 years) with specific comorbidities and two or more risk factors from the British Thoracic Society rule (CURB-65), it is recommended to handle them in the hospital with severe pneumonia criteria.

In primary health care services, we recommend to assess the severity of adult patients with community acquired pneumonia considering only clinical variables available in primary care services:

- Age over 65 years.
- Comorbidity: coronary heart disease, congestive heart failure, chronic pulmonary disease (COPD, bronchiectasis), diabetes mellitus, cerebrovascular disease with motor dysfunction or dementia, chronic renal failure, chronic liver disease, alcoholism, malignancies, malnutrition.
- Altered mental status: drowsiness, stupor, coma or mental confusion.
- Tachycardia or heart rate ≥ 120 beats/min.
- Low blood pressure or hypotension (BP < 90/60 mmHg).
- Tachypnea or respiratory rate ≥ 20 breaths/min.
- Chest X-ray: bilateral or multilobar pulmonary infiltrates, cavitation or pleural effusion.
- Pulse oximetry: SpO_2 saturation less than 90% on room air.
- Presence of decompensated comorbidity (e.g., COPD exacerbation, congestive heart failure, myocardial infarction, hyperglycemia, arrhythmias).

In general terms, in young adults without risk factors it is recommended outpatient management, in presence of one risk factor it is recommended ambulatory or short-term hospital care depending on previous experience and clinical judgment, in presence of two or more risk factors it is recommended to refer the patient to the hospital (Figure 1).

http://dx.doi.org/10.5772/53475

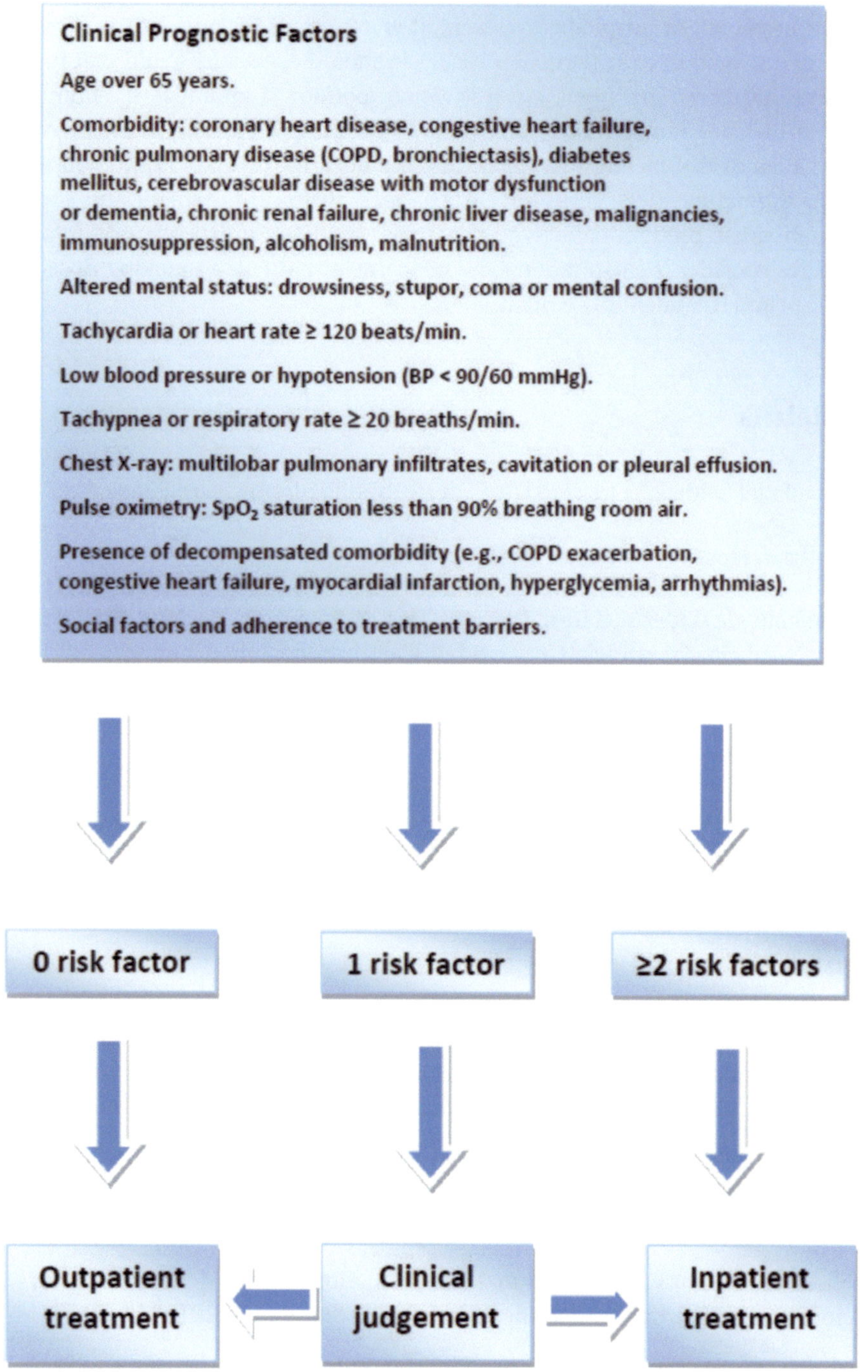

Figure 1. Severity assessment in adult patients with community-acquired pneumonia attended in primary health care services (outpatient clinics and emergency departments).

Nevertheless, after evaluating the severity of the case, when the clinician needs to decide the site of care (outpatient or hospital admission), it is important to consider the clinical and social variables involved in each particular case. We should especially avoid that high-risk patients receive outpatient treatment, but it is also important to minimize the number of low-risk patients that are unnecessarily admitted to hospital. Different studies have allowed developing a list of risk factors that determine the need for hospital admission and aid the clinicians in estimating the severity of CAP patients. Clinical judgment and experience of the physician must predominate over predictive models, which are not infallible, and should always consider the aspirations and concerns of patients in making decisions about the site of care and treatment prescribed.

Author details

Fernando Peñafiel Saldías[1*], Orlando Díaz Patiño[2] and Pablo Aguilera Fuenzalida[3]

*Address all correspondence to: fsaldias@med.puc.cl

1 Departamento de Enfermedades Respiratorias y Programa de Medicina de Urgencia, Facultad de Medicina, Pontificia Universidad Católica de Chile, Chile

2 Departamento de Enfermedades Respiratorias y Medicina Intensiva, Facultad de Medicina, Pontificia Universidad Católica de Chile, Chile

3 Programa de Medicina de Urgencia, Facultad de Medicina, Pontificia Universidad Católica de Chile, Chile

References

[1] Gotfried MH. Epidemiology of clinically diagnosed community-acquired pneumonia in the primary care setting: results from the 1999-2000 respiratory surveillance program. Am J Med 2001;111(Suppl 9A):25S-29S.

[2] Schappert SM, Burt CW. Ambulatory care visits to physician offices, hospital outpatient departments, and emergency departments: United States, 2001-02. Vital Health Stat 2006;159:1-66.

[3] Niska R, Bhuiya F, Xu J. National Hospital Ambulatory Medical Care Survey: 2007 emergency department summary. Natl Health Stat Report 2010;26:1-32.

[4] Mortensen EM, Coley CM, Singer DE, Marrie TJ, Obrosky DS, Kapoor WN, Fine MJ. Causes of death for patients with community-acquired pneumonia: results from the Pneumonia Patient Outcomes Research Team cohort study. Arch Intern Med 2002; 162:1059-64.

[5] The top ten causes of death – World Health Organization. Updated June 2011. http://www.who.int/mediacentre/factsheets/fs310/en/index.html

[6] Fine MJ, Smith MA, Carson CA, Mutha SS, Sankey SS, Weissfeld LA, Kapoor WN. Prognosis and outcomes of patients with community-acquired pneumonia: a meta-analysis. JAMA 1996;275:134-41.

[7] Marrie TJ. Community-acquired pneumonia in the elderly. Clin Infect Dis 2000;31:1066-78.

[8] File TM. The epidemiology of respiratory tract infections. Semin Respir Infect 2000;15: 184-94.

[9] Gonzalez R, Steiner JF, Sande MA. Antibiotic prescribing for adults with colds, upper respiratory tract infections, and bronchitis by ambulatory care physicians. JAMA 1997; 278:901-4.

[10] Metlay JP, Stafford RS, Singer DE. National trends in the use of antibiotics by primary care physicians for adult patients with cough. Arch Intern Med 1998;158:1813-18.

[11] Dalhoff K. Worldwide guidelines for respiratory tract infections: community-acquired pneumonia. Int J Antimicrob Agents 2001;18(Suppl 1):S39-44.

[12] Hoare Z, Lim WS. Pneumonia: update on diagnosis and management. BMJ 2006; 332: 1077-9.

[13] Aagaard E, Maselli J, Gonzales R. Physician practice patterns: chest X-ray ordering for the evaluation of acute cough illness in adults. Med Decis Making 2006;26:599-605.

[14] Janssens JP, Krause KH. Pneumonia in the very old. Lancet Infect Dis 2004;4:112-24.

[15] Goossens H, Little P. Community acquired pneumonia in primary care. BMJ 2006; 332:1045-6.

[16] Mandell LA, Wunderink RG, Anzueto A, Bartlett JG, Campbell GD, Dean NC, et al; Infectious Diseases Society of America; American Thoracic Society. Infectious Diseases Society of America/American Thoracic Society consensus guidelines on the management of community-acquired pneumonia in adults. Clin Infect Dis 2007;44 (Suppl 2):S27-72.

[17] Lim WS, Baudouin SV, George RC, Hill AT, Jamieson C, Le Jeune I, et al. Pneumonia Guidelines Committee of the British Thoracic Society Standards of Care Committee. British Thoracic Society guidelines for the management of community acquired pneumonia in adults: update 2009. Thorax 2009;64(Suppl 3):1-55.

[18] Metlay JP, Kapoor WN, Fine MJ. Does this patient have community-acquired pneumonia? Diagnosing pneumonia by history and physical examination. JAMA 1997; 278:1440-5.

[19] Woodhead M, Gialdroni Grassi G, Huchon GJ, Léophonte P, Manresa F, Schaberg T. Use of investigations in lower respiratory tract infection in the community: a European survey. Eur Respir J 1996;9:1596-600.

[20] Saldías F, Méndez JI, Ramírez D, Díaz O. Predictive value of history and physical examination for the diagnosis of community-acquired pneumonia in adults: a literature review. Rev Med Chile 2007;135:517-28.

[21] O'Donnell WJ, Kradin RL, Evins AE, Wittram C. Case records of the Massachusetts General Hospital. Weekly clinicopathological exercises. Case 39-2004. A 52-year-old woman with recurrent episodes of atypical pneumonia. N Engl J Med 2004;351:2741-9.

[22] Genne D, Kaiser L, Kinge TN, Lew D. Community-acquired pneumonia: causes of treatment failure in patients enrolled in clinical trials. Clin Microbiol Infect 2003;9:949-54.

[23] Meehan TP, Fine MJ, Krumholz HM, Scinto JD, Galusha DH, Mockalis JT, et al. Quality of care, process, and outcomes in elderly patients with pneumonia. JAMA 1997;278: 2080-4.

[24] Evans AT, Husain S, Durairaj L, Sadowski LS, Charles-Damte M, Wang Y. Azithromycin for acute bronchitis: a randomised, double-blind, controlled trial. Lancet 2002;359:1648-54.

[25] Diehr P, Wood RW, Bushyhead J, Krueger L, Wolcott B, Tompkins RK. Prediction of pneumonia in outpatients with acute cough – a statistical approach. J Chron Dis 1984;37: 215-25.

[26] Gennis P, Gallagher J, Falvo C, Baker S, Than W. Clinical criteria for the detection of pneumonia in adults: guidelines for ordering chest roentgenograms in the emergency department. J Emerg Med 1989;7:263-8.

[27] Singal BM, Hedges JR, Radack KL. Decision rules and clinical prediction of pneumonia: evaluation of low-yield criteria. Ann Emerg Med 1989;18:13-20.

[28] Heckerling PS, Tape TG, Wigton RS, Hissong KK, Leikin JB, Ornato JP, et al. Clinical prediction rule for pulmonary infiltrates. Ann Intern Med 1990;113:664-70.

[29] Saldías F, Cabrera D, De Solminihac I, Hernández P, Gederlini A, Díaz A. Predictive value of history and physical examination for the diagnosis of community-acquired pneumonia in adults. Rev Med Chile 2007;135:143-52.

[30] Pauker SG, Kassirer JP. The threshold approach to clinical decision making. N Engl J Med 1980;302:1109-17.

[31] Bushyhead JB, Christensen-Szalanski JJ. Feedback and the illusion of validity in a medical clinic. Med Decis Making 1981;1:115-23.

[32] Melbye H, Straume B, Aasebo U, Dale K. Diagnosis of pneumonia in adults in general practice. Relative importance of typical symptoms and abnormal chest signs evalu-

ated against a radiographic reference standard. Scand J Prim Health Care 1992;10:226-33.

[33] González Ortiz MA, Carnicero Bujarrabal M, Verela Entrecanales M. Prediction of the presence of pneumonia in adults with fever. Med Clin (Barc) 1995;105:521-4.

[34] Hopstaken RM, Muris JW, Knottnerus JA, Kester AD, Rinkens PE, Dinant GJ. Contributions of symptoms, signs, erythrocyte sedimentation rate, and C-reactive protein to a diagnosis of pneumonia in acute lower respiratory tract infection. Br J Gen Pract 2003;53:358-64.

[35] Chilean Respiratory Disease Society and Chilean Infectious Disease Society. Chilean consensus for management of community-acquired pneumonia in adults. Rev Chil Enf Respir 2005;21:69-140.

[36] Metlay JP, Fine MJ. Testing strategies in the initial management of patients with community-acquired pneumonia. Ann Intern Med 2003;138:109-18.

[37] Emerman CL, Dawson N, Speroff T, Siciliano C, Effron D, Rashad F, et al. Comparison of physician judgment and decision aids for ordering chest radiographs for pneumonia in outpatients. Ann Emerg Med 1991;20:1215-9.

[38] Saldías F, Cabrera D, de Solminihac I, Gederlini A, Agar V, Díaz A. Evaluación del juicio clínico y las guías de decisión en la pesquisa de pacientes adultos con neumonía adquirida en la comunidad en la unidad de emergencia. Rev Chil Enf Respir 2007;23:87-93.

[39] Wipf JE, Lipsky BA, Hirschmann JV, Boyko EJ, Takasugi J, Peugeot RL, et al. Diagnosing pneumonia by physical examination: relevant or relic? Arch Intern Med 1999;159:1082-7.

[40] Lieberman D, Shvartzman P, Korsonsky I, Lieberman D. Diagnosis of ambulatory community-acquired pneumonia. Comparison of clinical assessment versus chest X-ray. Scand J Prim Health Care 2003;21:57-60.

[41] Nair GB, Niederman MS. Community-acquired pneumonia: an unfinished battle. Med Clin N Am 2011;95:1143-61.

[42] Almirall J, Bolibar I, Toran P, Pera G, Boquet X, Balanzó X, et al. Contribution of C-reactive protein to the diagnosis and assessment of severity of community-acquired pneumonia. Chest 2004;125:1335-42.

[43] Flanders SA, Stein J, Shochat G, Sellers K, Holland M, Maselli J, et al. Performance of a bedside C-reactive protein test in the diagnosis of community-acquired pneumonia in adults with acute cough. Am J Med 2004;116:529-35.

[44] Holm A, Nexoe J, Bistrup LA, Pedersen SS, Obel N, Nielsen LP, et al. Aetiology and prediction of pneumonia in lower respiratory tract infection in primary care. Br J Gen Pract 2007;57:547-54.

[45] Stolz D, Christ-Crain M, Gencay MM, Bingisser R, Huber PR, Müller B, et al. Diagnostic value of signs, symptoms and laboratory values in lower respiratory tract infection. Swiss Med Wkly 2006;136:434-40.

[46] Falk G, Fahey T. C-reactive protein and community-acquired pneumonia in ambulatory care: systematic review of diagnostic accuracy studies. Fam Pract 2009;26:10-21.

[47] Boussekey N, Leroy O, Georges H, Georges H, Devos P, d'Escrivan T, Guery B. Diagnostic and prognostic values of admission procalcitonin levels in community-acquired pneumonia in an intensive care unit. Infection 2005;33:257-63.

[48] Polzin A, Pletz M, Erbes R, Raffenberg M, Mauch H, Wagner S, et al. Procalcitonin as a diagnostic tool in lower respiratory tract infections and tuberculosis. Eur Respir J 2003; 21:939-43.

[49] Muller B, Harbarth S, Stolz D, Bingisser R, Mueller C, Leuppi J, et al. Diagnostic and prognostic accuracy of clinical and laboratory parameters in community-acquired pneumonia. BMC Infect Dis 2007;7:10.

[50] Muller B, Becker KL, Schachinger H, Rickenbacher PR, Huber PR, Zimmerli W, Ritz R. Calcitonin precursors are reliable markers of sepsis in a medical intensive care unit. Crit Care Med 2000;28:977-83.

[51] Weglohner W, Struck J, Fischer-Schulz C, Morgenthaler NG, Otto A, Bohuon C, Bergmann A. Isolation and characterization of serum procalcitonin from patients with sepsis. Peptides 2001;22:2099-103.

[52] Assicot M, Gendrel D, Carsin H, Raymond J, Guilbaud J, Bohuon C. High serum procalcitonin concentrations in patients with sepsis and infection. Lancet 1993;341:515-8.

[53] Uzzan B, Cohen R, Nicolas P, Cucherat M, Perret GY. Procalcitonin as a diagnostic test for sepsis in critically ill adults and after surgery or trauma: a systematic review and meta-analysis. Crit Care Med 2006;34:1996-2003.

[54] Joyce CD, Fiscus RR, Wang X, Dries DJ, Morris RC, Prinz RA. Calcitonin gene-related peptide levels are elevated in patients with sepsis. Surgery 1990;108:1097-101.

[55] Simon L, Gauvin F, Amre DK, Saint-Louis P, Lacroix J. Serum procalcitonin and C-reactive protein levels as markers of bacterial infection: a systematic review and meta-analysis. Clin Infect Dis 2004;39:206-17.

[56] Oppert M, Reinicke A, Muller C, Barckow D, Frei U, Eckardt KU. Elevations in procalcitonin but not C-reactive protein are associated with pneumonia after cardiopulmonary resuscitation. Resuscitation 2002;53:167-70.

[57] Duflo F, Debon R, Monneret G, Bienvenu J, Chassard D, Allaouchiche B. Alveolar and serum procalcitonin: diagnostic and prognostic value in ventilator-associated pneumonia. Anesthesiology 2002;96:74-9.

[58] Gibot S, Cravoisy A, Levy B, Bene MC, Faure G, Bollaert PE. Soluble triggering receptor expressed on myeloid cells and the diagnosis of pneumonia. N Engl J Med 2004; 350:451-8.

[59] Ramirez P, Garcia MA, Ferrer M, Aznar J, Valencia M, Sahuquillo JM, et al. Sequential measurements of procalcitonin levels in diagnosing ventilator-associated pneumonia. Eur Respir J 2008;31:356-62.

[60] Horonenko G, Hoyt JC, Robbins RA, Singarajah CU, Umar A, Pattengill J, Hayden JM. Soluble triggering receptor expressed on myeloid cell-1 is increased in patients with ventilator-associated pneumonia: a preliminary report. Chest 2007;132:58-63.

[61] Muller B, Gencay MM, Gibot S, Stolz D, Hunziker L, Tamm M, Christ-Crain M. Circulating levels of soluble triggering receptor expressed on myeloid cells (sTREM)-1 in community-acquired pneumonia. Crit Care Med 2007;35:990-1.

[62] Anand NJ, Zuick S, Klesney-Tait J, Kollef MH. Diagnostic implications of soluble triggering receptor expressed on myeloid cells-1 in BAL fluid of patients with pulmonary infiltrates in the ICU. Chest 2009;135:641-7.

[63] Christ-Crain M, Jaccard-Stolz D, Bingisser R, Gencay MM, Huber PR, Tamm M, Muller B. Effect of procalcitonin-guided treatment on antibiotic use and outcome in lower respiratory tract infections: cluster-randomised, single-blinded intervention trial. Lancet 2004;363:600-7.

[64] Christ-Crain M, Stolz D, Bingisser R, Muller C, Miedinger D, Huber PR, et al. Procalcitonin guidance of antibiotic therapy in community-acquired pneumonia: a randomized trial. Am J Respir Crit Care Med 2006;174:84-93.

[65] Briel M, Schuetz P, Mueller B, Young J, Schild U, Nusbaumer C, et al. Procalcitonin-guided antibiotic use vs a standard approach for acute respiratory tract infections in primary care. Arch Intern Med 2008;168:2000-7.

[66] Riquelme R, Torres A, el-Ebiary M, Mensa J, Estruch R, Ruiz M, et al. Community-acquired pneumonia in the elderly. Clinical and nutritional aspects. Am J Respir Crit Care Med 1997;156:1908-14.

[67] Zalacain R, Torres A, Celis R, Blanquer J, Aspa J, Esteban L, et al; for the Pneumonia in the Elderly Working Group, Area de Tuberculosis e Infecciones Respiratorias. Community-acquired pneumonia in the elderly: Spanish multicentre study. Eur Respir J 2003;21:294-302.

[68] Metlay JP, Schulz R, Li YH, Singer DE, Marrie TJ, Coley CM, et al. Influence of age on symptoms at presentation in patients with community-acquired pneumonia. Arch Intern Med 1997;157:1453-9.

[69] Saldías F, O`Brien A, Gederlini A, Farías G, Díaz A. Community-acquired pneumonia requiring hospitalization in immunocompetent elderly patients: clinical features, prognostic factors and treatment. Arch Bronconeumol 2003;39:333-40.

[70] Ahkee S, Srinath L, Ramirez J. Community-acquired pneumonia in the elderly: association of mortality with lack of fever and leukocytosis. South Med J 1997;90:296-8.

[71] Kelly E, MacRedmond RE, Cullen G, Greene CM, McElvaney NG, O'Neill SJ. Community-acquired pneumonia in older patients: does age influence systemic cytokine levels in community-acquired pneumonia? Respirology 2009;14:210-6.

[72] Kaplan V, Angus DC. Community-acquired pneumonia in the elderly. Crit Care Clin 2003;19:729-48.

[73] Guest JF, Morris A. Community-acquired pneumonia: the annual cost to the National Health Service in the United Kingdom. Eur Respir J 1997;10:1530-4

[74] Fine MJ, Hough LJ, Medsger AR, Li YH, Ricci EM, Singer DE, et al. The hospital admission decision for patients with community-acquired pneumonia. Results from the pneumonia Patient Outcomes Research Team cohort study. Arch Intern Med 1997;157: 36-44.

[75] Saldías F, Mardónez JM, Marchesse M, Viviani P, Farías G, Díaz A. Community-acquired pneumonia in hospitalized adult patients. Clinical presentation and prognostic factors. Rev Med Chile 2002;130:1373-82.

[76] Saldías F, Farías G, Villarroel L, Valdivia G, Mardónez JM, Díaz A. Development of an instrument to assess the severity of community acquired pneumonia among hospitalized patients. Rev Med Chile 2004;132:1037-46.

[77] Saldías F, Díaz O. Severity scores for predicting clinically relevant outcomes for immunocompetent adult patients hospitalized with community-acquired pneumococcal pneumonia. Rev Chilena Infectol 2011;28:303-9.

[78] Neill AM, Martin IR, Weir R, Anderson R, Chereshsky A, Epton MJ, et al. Community acquired pneumonia: aetiology and usefulness of severity criteria on admission. Thorax 1996;51:1010-6.

[79] Harrison BD, Farr BM, Pugh S, Selkon JB. British Thoracic Society Research Committee. Community-acquired pneumonia in adults in British hospitals in 1982-1983: a survey of aetiology, mortality, prognostic factors and outcome. Q J Med 1987;62:195-220.

[80] Lim WS, Van Der Eerden MM, Laing R, Boersma WG, Karalus N, Town GI, et al. Defining community acquired pneumonia severity on presentation to hospital: an international derivation and validation study. Thorax 2003;58:377-82.

[81] Fine MJ, Auble TE, Yealy DM, Hanusa BH, Weissfeld LA, Singer DE, et al. A prediction rule to identify low-risk patients with community-acquired pneumonia. N Engl J Med 1997;336:243-50.

[82] España PP, Capelastegui A, Gorordo I, Esteban C, Oribe M, Ortega M, et al. Development and validation of a clinical prediction rule for severe community-acquired pneumonia. Am J Respir Crit Care Med 2006;174:1249-56.

[83] Marrie TJ, Durant H, Yates L. Community-acquired pneumonia requiring hospitalization: 5-year prospective study. Rev Infect Dis 1989;11:586-99.

[84] Riquelme R, Torres A, El-Ebiary M, de la Bellacasa JP, Estruch R, Mensa J, et al. Community-acquired pneumonia in the elderly: a multivariate analysis of risk and prognostic factors. Am J Respir Crit Care Med 1996;154:1450-5.

[85] Fine MJ, Hanusa BH, Lave JR, Singer DE, Stone RA, Weissfeld LA, et al. Comparison of a disease-specific and a generic severity of illness measure for patients with community-acquired pneumonia. J Gen Intern Med 1995;10:359-68.

[86] Ortqvist A, Hedlund J, Grillner L, Jalonen E, Kallings I, Leinonen M, Kalin M. Aetiology, outcome and prognostic factors in community-acquired pneumonia requiring hospitalization. Eur Respir J 1990;3:1105-13.

[87] Van Eeden SF, Coetzee AR, Joubert JR. Community-acquired pneumonia: factors influencing intensive care admission. S AfrMed J 1988;73:77-81.

[88] Atlas SJ, Benzer TI, Borowsky LH, Chang Y, Burnham DC, Metlay JP, et al. Safely increasing the proportion of patients with community-acquired pneumonia treated as outpatients: an interventional trial. Arch Intern Med 1998;158:1350-6.

[89] Martínez R, Reyes S, Lorenzo MJ, Menéndez R. Impact of guidelines on outcome: the evidence. Semin Respir Crit Care Med 2009;30:172-8.

[90] McMahon LF Jr, Wolfe RA, Tedeschi PJ. Variation in hospital admissions among small areas. A comparison of Maine and Michigan. Med Care 1989;27:623-31.

[91] Marrie TJ, Lau CY, Wheeler SL, Wong CJ, Vandervoort MK, Feagan BG. A controlled trial of a critical pathway for treatment of community-acquired pneumonia. CAPITAL Study Investigators. Community-Acquired Pneumonia Intervention Trial Assessing Levofloxacin. JAMA 2000;283:749-55.

[92] Auble TE, Yealy DM, Fine MJ. Assessing prognosis and selecting an initial site of care for adults with community-acquired pneumonia. Infect Dis Clin North Am 1998;12:741-59.

[93] Minogue MF, Coley CM, Fine MJ, Marrie TJ, Kapoor WN, Singer DE. Patients hospitalized after initial outpatient treatment for community acquired pneumonia. Ann Emerg Med 1998;31:376-80.

[94] Dean NC. Use of prognostic scoring and outcome assessment tools in the admission decision for community-acquired pneumonia. Clin Chest Med 1999;20:521-9.

[95] Woodhead M. Assessment of illness severity in community acquired pneumonia: a useful new prediction tool? Thorax 2003;58:371-2.

[96] Capelastegui A, España PP, Quintana JM, Areitio I, Gorordo I, Egurrola M, Bilbao A. Validation of a predictive rule for the management of community-acquired pneumonia. Eur Respir J 2006;27:151-7.

[97] Ewig S, Ruiz M, Mensa J, Marcos MA, Martinez JA, Arancibia F, et al. Severe community-acquired pneumonia. Assessment of severity criteria. Am J Respir Crit Care Med 1998;158:1102-8.

[98] España PP, Capelastegui A, Quintana JM, Bilbao A, Diez R, Pascual S, et al. Validation and comparison of SCAP as a predictive score for identifying low-risk patients in community-acquired pneumonia. J Infect 2010;60:106-13.

[99] Rangel-Frausto MS, Pittet D, Costigan M, Hwang T, Davis CS, Wenzel RP. The natural history of the systemic inflammatory response syndrome (SIRS). A prospective study. JAMA 1995;273:117-23.

[100] Subbe CP, Kruger M, Rutherford P, Gemmel L. Validation of a modified Early Warning Score in medical admissions. QJM 2001;94:521-6.

[101] Barlow G, Nathwani D, Davey P. The CURB65 pneumonia severity score outperforms generic sepsis and early warning scores in predicting mortality in community-acquired pneumonia. Thorax 2007;62:253-9.

[102] Dremsizov T, Clermont G, Kellum JA, Kalassian KG, Fine MJ, Angus DC. Severe sepsis in community-acquired pneumonia: when does it happen, and do systemic inflammatory response syndrome criteria help predict course? Chest 2006;129:968-78.

[103] Pugin J, Auckenthaler R, Mili N, Janssens JP, Lew PD, Suter PM. Diagnosis of ventilator-associated pneumonia by bacteriologic analysis of bronchoscopic and non-bronchoscopic "blind" bronchoalveolar lavage fluid. Am Rev Respir Dis 1991;143:1121-9.

[104] Singh N, Rogers P, Atwood CW, Wagener MM, Yu VL. Short-course empiric antibiotic therapy for patients with pulmonary infiltrates in the intensive care unit. A proposed solution for indiscriminate antibiotic prescription. Am J Respir Crit Care Med 2000;162:505-11.

[105] Fartoukh M, Maitre B, Honoré S, Cerf C, Zahar JR, Brun-Buisson C. Diagnosing pneumonia during mechanical ventilation: the clinical pulmonary infection score revisited. Am J Respir Crit Care Med 2003;168:173-9.

[106] Alvarez-Sánchez B, Alvarez-Lerma F, Jordà R, Serra J, López-Cambra MJ, Sandar MD. Prognostic factors and etiology in patients with severe community-acquired pneumonia admitted at the ICU. Spanish multicenter study. Study Group on Severe Community-Acquired Pneumonia in Spain. Med Clin (Barc) 1998;111:650-4.

[107] Richards G, Levy H, Laterre PF, Feldman C, Woodward B, Bates BM, Qualy RL. CURB-65, PSI, and APACHE II to assess mortality risk in patients with severe sepsis and community acquired pneumonia in PROWESS. J Intensive Care Med 2011;26:34-40.

[108] España PP, Capelastegui A, Quintana JM, Soto A, Gorordo I, García-Urbaneja M, et al. A prediction rule to identify allocation of inpatient care in community-acquired pneumonia. Eur Respir J 2003;21:695-701.

http://dx.doi.org/10.5772/53475

[109] Marras TK, Gutierrez C, Chan CK. Applying a prediction rule to identify low-risk patients with community-acquired pneumonia. Chest 2000;118:1339-43.

[110] Aujesky D, Auble TE, Yealy DM, Stone RA, Obrosky DS, Meehan TP, et al. Prospective comparison of three validated prediction rules for prognosis in community-acquired pneumonia. Am J Med 2005;118: 384-92.

[111] Man SY, Lee N, Ip M, Antonio GE, Chau SS, Mak P, et al. Prospective comparison of three predictive rules for assessing severity of community-acquired pneumonia in Hong Kong. Thorax 2007;62:348-53.

[112] Buising KL, Thursky KA, Black JF, MacGregor L, Street AC, Kennedy MP, et al. A prospective comparison of severity scores for identifying patients with severe community acquired pneumonia: reconsidering what is meant by severe pneumonia. Thorax 2006;61:419-24.

[113] Ananda-Rajah MR, Charles PG, Melvani S, Burrell LL, Johnson PD, Grayson ML. Comparing the pneumonia severity index with CURB-65 in patients admitted with community acquired pneumonia. Scand J Infect Dis 2008;40:293-300.

[114] Ewig S, de Roux A, Bauer T, Garcia E, Mensa J, Niederman M, Torres A. Validation of predictive rules and indices of severity for community acquired pneumonia. Thorax 2004; 59:421-7.

[115] Marrie TJ, Huang JQ. Low-risk patients admitted with community-acquired pneumonia. Am J Med 2005;118:1357-63.

[116] Siegel RE. Clinical opinion prevails over the pneumonia severity index. Am J Med 2005;118:1312-3.

[117] España PP, Capelastegui A, Quintana J, Diez R, Gorordo I, Bilbao A, et al. Prospective comparison of severity scores for predicting clinically relevant outcomes for patients hospitalized with community-acquired pneumonia. Chest 2009;135:1572-9.

[118] Huang DT, Weissfeld LA, Kellum JA, Yealy DM, Kong L, Martino M, Angus DC; GenIMS Investigators. Risk prediction with procalcitonin and clinical rules in community-acquired pneumonia. Ann Emerg Med 2008;52:48-58.

[119] Kruger S, Ewig S, Marre S, Papassotiriou J, Richter K, von Baum H, et al. Procalcitonin predicts patients at low risk of death from community-acquired pneumonia across all CRB-65 classes. Eur Respir J 2008;31:349-55.

[120] Kruger S, Papassotiriou J, Marre R, Richter K, Schumann C, von Baum H, Morgenthaler NG, Suttorp N, Welte T; CAPNETZ Study Group. Pro-atrial natriuretic peptide and pro-vasopressin to predict severity and prognosis in community-acquired pneumonia: results from the German competence network CAPNETZ. Intensive Care Med 2007;33:2069-78.

Chapter 6

Pneumonia in Children

Irena Wojsyk-Banaszak and Anna Bręborowicz

Additional information is available at the end of the chapter

http://dx.doi.org/10.5772/54052

1. Introduction

Pneumonia causes substantial morbidity in children worldwide and is a leading cause of death in children in the developing world. The incidence of pneumonia is the highest in children under 5 years of age and in recent years the incidence of complicated and severe pneumonia seems to be increasing.

Etiological factors vary with age, source of infection (community vs. hospital acquired pneumonia) and underlying host defects (e.g immunodeficiency). Viruses are the most common etiological factors in preschool children, although in many cases more than one causative agents can be identified. There are several emerging pathogens in community acquired pneumonia in children: virulent strains of *Streptococcus pneumoniae* that are not present in currently available vaccines, Panton-Velentine leucocidin producing *Staphylococcus aureus*, human Bocaviruses and metapneumoviruses being the most important.

Diagnosis in most of milder cases of community acquired pneumonia is based on clinical judgement alone, since laboratory tests and radiologic examination do not provide clues concerning etiology. Children with severe pneumonia, hospital acquired pneumonia and immunocompromised children require invasive diagnostic approach.

Treatment of mild and moderate cases consists in supportive care and antibiotic treatment. First-line recommended therapy in previously healthy children regardless of age is amoxicillin, as it provides sufficient coverage against the most common invasive bacterial pathogen, namely *Streptococcus pneumoniae*. For hospital acquired pneumonia initial empiric treatment should be based on local antimicrobial susceptibility patterns, and modified adequately as soon as the results of microbiological tests are available.

Despite the fact, that if properly diagnosed and treated pneumonia resolves with no residual changes, in some cases due to pathogen virulence and/or host susceptibility its course might be complicated with pleural effusion and empyema, pneumoatocele, lung abscess or necrotizing pneumonia. A recognized complication of severe pneumonia is hyponatremia and SIADH (Syndrome of Inappropriate Antidiuretic Hormone Secretion).

Burden of pneumonia can be diminished using preventive measures ranging from the simplest infection control methods like hand washing, limiting exposure to infectious cases, limiting exposure to tobacco smoke, vaccinations to passive immunization in selected cases.

2. Definition

Pneumonia is defined as an inflammation of lung tissue due to an infectious agent. Commonly used clinical World Health Organization operational definition is based solely on clinical symptoms (cough or difficulties in breathing and tachypnoea) [1]. In the developing world the term Lower Respiratory Tract Infection (LRTI) is widely used instead of pneumonia, because of poor access to x-ray and difficulties in radiological confirmation of diagnosis.

Depending on the place of acquisition pneumonia can be divided into:

a. Community Acqiured Pneumonia (CAP)

b. Hospital Acquired Pneumonia (HAP).

Recently a third type - Health Care Associated Pneumonia (HCAP) has been distinguished in adult patients.

The significance of this classification is based on its clinical utility since in most cases pathogens responsible for CAP and HAP are different, warranting varying approach and empiric treatment.

3. Community acquired pneumonia

CAP can be defined as pneumonia in previously healthy children caused by an infectious agent contracted outside the hospital. The common clinical practice is to confirm the diagnosis by radiological findings of consolidations.

4. Epidemiology

Globally the incidence of pneumonia in children < 5 years in developing countries is 0.28 episodes per child - year (150 mln/year), compared to 0.05 episodes per child - year in developed countries [2]. Pneumonia is responsible for 18% of death (2 mln/year) in young children worldwide, mostly occurring in impoverished countries with limited access to healthcare system. In more affluent societies pneumonia is rarely fatal, it leads however to substantial morbidity. Incidence of radiologically confirmed pneumonia in previously healthy children in Europe is 144-147/100,000 children/year and decreases with age, being the highest in children <5 years (328-338/100,000/year and 421/100,000/year in those aged 0-2 years) [3,4]. The rates of hospitalization due to pneumonia in this age group were 122/100,00/year in children ≤ 16 and 287/100,000/year in those ≤ 5 [4]. British studies show the rate of CAP presenting to General Practitioners in children < 5 to be 191/100, 000 person - years [5], probably due to the fact that more severely sick children would present directly to the hospital. In a German study incidence of hospitalized pneumonia was 300/100,000/year in children 0-16 and 658/100,000/year in those aged 0-5. In 23% of those cases underlying conditions were present, and it is possible that many children with bronchiolitis were classified as having pneumonia [6].

Since introduction of conjugate pneumococcal vaccine (PCV7) to national immunization programs in the USA and Europe the incidence of pneumococcal pneumonia has decreased (by 65% in the USA) and rates of CAP hospitalizations have decreased for children <1 but seem to be increasing for children > 5 [7-9]. At the same time the incidence of severe pneumonia requiring hospital management as well as complicated pneumonia seems to be increasing. Between 1997 and 2006, the rate of local complications of CAP increased by 77.8% (5.4 and 9.6 cases per 100 000 population, respectively). Empyema accounted for >97% of all local complications [8,9].

5. Etiology

Organisms causing pneumonia are varied and include bacteria, viruses, fungi and protozoans. Most cases of pneumonia are preceded by acute viral bronchitis. Viruses facilitate infections with pathogenic microorganisms colonizing nasopharynx. These pathogens include *Streptococcus pneumoniae, Haemophilus influenzae* and *Moraxella catarrhalis*. Previous colonisation with *Streptococcus mitis* and anaerobic cocci *Peptostreptococcus anaerobius* may have protective effect against pathogenic strains.

Etiological factor of pneumonia can be identified in no more than 65-86% patients combining multiple diagnostic tools including culture, serology and PCR [7,11]. In everyday clinical practice these methods are rarely used and treatment remains empiric based on national and international guidelines.

Viruses are responsible for 30-67% cases of CAP, and are the most common in children <2. The most frequently identified are respiratory syncytial virus (RSV) isolated in 13-29% and rhinovirus (3-45%) either in combination with bacteria or alone. Other viruses responsible for pneumonia comprise adenovirus (1-13%), influenza (4-22%) and parainfluenza virus (3-10%), rhinovirus (3-45%), human metapneumovirus (5-12%), human bocaviruses (5-15%). The less common are enterovirus, varicella-, herpes- and cytomegalovirus [7,11-13]. In older children bacterial infections are more frequent: *Streptococcus pneumoniae* being the leader (30-44% of CAP) followed by *Mycoplasma pneumoniae* (22-36%) and *Chlamydophila pneumoniae* (5-27%) [7,11,13-16]. *Streptococcus pneumoniae* remains the leading cause of severe pneumonia requiring hospitalization even in countries with reduced rates of invasive pneumococcal disease [17]. Since introduction of PCV7 the most common pneumococcal isolates are 1 (predominantly responsible for empyema), 19A, 3, 6A and 7F (all included in 13-valent vaccine) [18]. Contrary to previous reports *Mycoplasma pneumoniae* seems to be equally frequent in school and preschool children [11,13]. Less common bacterial causes of CAP in children include *Haemophilus influenzae* type B (5-9%), *Staphylococcus aureus, Moraxella catarrhalis* (1.5-4%), *Bordatella pertussis, Streptococcus pyogenes* (1-7%), *Chlamydia trachomatis* and a new pathogen identified in the 1990ies – *Simkania negevensis* [7,12]. Unlike in adults *Legionella pneumophila* is a rare cause of CAP in children [19].

In malaria–endemic regions of tropical Africa a challenging etiological factor of pneumonia is multidrug–resistant non typhoidal Salmonella, and in regions where tuberculosis is endemic it is increasingly being recognized as a cause of acute pneumonia [20].

8-40% of cases represent a mixed viral - bacterial or bacterial - bacterial infection [3,4,7,12,16,19]. Primary viral infection predisposes to bacterial pneumonia: influenza epidemics in developed countries coincide with epidemics of *Streptococcus pneumoniae* and *Staphylococcus aureus* pneumonias and measles or RSV infections contribute to increased pneumonia mortality in developing countries [2].

6. Risk factors for cap

There are several known risk factors for CAP to consider in addition to immunization status, epidemiological data and exposure to other children, especially preschoolers. Underlying comorbidities like diabetes mellitus, asplenia or splenic dysfunction, chronic cardiac disease, nephrotic syndrome, severe liver disease are risk factors for invasive pneumococcal disease including pneumonia. Other risk factors for CAP include: asthma, history of wheezing episodes, otitis media treated by tympanocentesis in the first 2 years of life (risk factor for children <5), tobacco smoke exposure, malnutrition, immunological deficits (primary or secondary), mucocilliary dysfunction (cystic fibrosis, cilliary dyskinesia), congenital malformation of airways, impaired swallowing, microaspiration, gastroesophageal reflux, neuromuscular disorders, treatment with gastric acid inhibitors (risk factor in adults, in children its role was confirmed in one study). Environmental factors like indoor air pollution caused by cooking and heating with biomass fuels (like wood or dung), living in crowded conditions and parental smoking also increase a child's susceptibility to pneumonia [1,7]. Tobacco smoke exposure has been found to increase risk of hospitalization for pneumonia in children < 5 [21]. Conditions predisposing to severe pneumonia include age <5 and prematurity (24-28 GA) [11]. Viral infections, especially influenza and prior antibiotic exposure additionally predispose to pneumococcal and staphylococcal pneumonia. Antibiotics alter bacterial microflora in the airways destroying commensal bacteria like alfa-hemolytic Streptococci while viruses release neuraminidase and other enzymes promoting adherence and expression of pneumococcal receptors on host cells like platelet activating factor receptor or CD14 [17,22].

http://dx.doi.org/10.5772/54052

7. Clinical manifestations

Typical clinical symptoms of pneumonia consist of:

- cough (30% of children presenting to outpatient clinic with cough, after excluding those with wheeze, have radiographic signs of pneumonia, and cough was reported in 76% of children with CAP) [13,23]. It should be noted that sputum production in preschool children is rare, because they tend to swallow it.
- fever (present in 88-96% of children with radiologically confirmed pneumonia) [13]
- toxic appearance
- signs of respiratory distress: tachypnoe (table 1), history of breathlessness or difficulty in breathing – chest retractions, nasal flaring, grunting, use of accessory muscles of respiration. Tachypnoe is a very sensitive marker of pneumonia. 50-80% of children with WHO defined tachypnoe had radiological signs of pneumonia, and the absence of tachypnoe is the best single finding for ruling out the disease [13,23]. In children <5 tachypnoe had sensitivity of 74% and specificity of 67% for radiologically confirmed pneumonia, but its clinical value was lower in the first 3 days of illness. In infants < 12 months respiratory rate of 70 breaths/min had a sensitivity of 63% and specificity of 89% for hypoxemia [7].

Age	Respiratory rate/minute
0-2 months	"/>60
2-12 months	"/>50
1-4 years	"/>40
≥ 5 years	"/>30

Table 1. Tachypnoe defined according to WHO criteria [1]

- chest pain,
- abdominal pain (referred pain from the diaphragmatic pleura might be the first sign of pneumonia in little children) and/or vomiting
- headache

Based on clinical symptoms pneumonia can be divided into severe pneumonia that warrants hospitalization and mild, moderate or non-severe. Signs of severe pneumonia differ with age and according to BTS comprise of: temperature 38,5 ^{0}C, respiratory rate > 70 breaths/minute in infants and > 50 breaths/minute in older children, moderate to severe recessions in infants and severe difficulty in breathing in older children, nasal flaring, cyanosis, intermittent apnoea, grunting, not feeding in infants and signs of dehydration in older children, tachycardia, capillary refill time ≥2s [7]. Agitation may be the sign of hypoxemia. Table 2 presents a simplified approach recommended by WHO to be implemented in developing world to help field healthcare workers assess the need for hospital referral.

Physical examination:

- crackles (present in 33-90% of children with pneumonia), diminished breath sounds over affected site, bronchial breath sounds specific for lobar consolidation, absent breath sounds and dullness to percussion suggestive of effusion. A pleural rub may be heard if pneumonia is accompanied by pleuritis. Crackles and bronchial breath sounds have sensitivity of 75% and specificity of 57% in pneumonia diagnosis [7].
- presence of wheeze, especially in the absence of fever, makes the diagnosis of typical bacterial pneumonia unlikely [24]. It is however a common sign in viral and *Mycoplasma pneumonia* (up to 30%) infection [7].
- combining several clinical symptoms into diagnostic algorithm improves sensitivity and specificity of diagnosis. WHO criteria for defining pneumonia (cough or difficulties in breathing and tachypnoea) investigated in a Brasilian study of 390 children have sensitivity of 94% for children <2, and 62% for children ≥2 and specificities of 20% and 16% respectively. Adding fever improved specificity to 44% and 50% [25]. In an Australian study of febrile children < 5 presenting to tertiary emergency department, clinical indicators of pneumonia confirmed radiologically and microbiologically comprised an unwell appearance, fever ≥ 39 0 C, breathing difficulties, chronic disease, prolonged capillary refill time, tachypnoe, crackles on auscultation and lack of antipneumococcal vaccination [26].

It is important to note that no clinical or radiological sign either alone or in combination, is sensitive and specific enough to differentiate between viral, atypical or typical bacterial etiology of pneumonia.

Pneumonia/non severe pneumonia	Cough Problems with breathing Tachypnoe * No signs of severe pneumonia present
Severe pneumonia	Signs of pneumonia & ≥1 - lower chest wall indrawing - nasal flaming - expiratory grunting - no signs of very severe pneumonia
Very severe pneumonia	Signs of severe pneumonia & ≥1 - inability to feed - cyanosis - severe respiratory distress - impaired consciousness or convulsions

*Look table 1

Table 2. Severity of pneumonia – WHO classification [2,27]

http://dx.doi.org/10.5772/54052

8. Additional tests

1. Pulsoximetry should be performed in all children with pneumonia since its results facilitate assessment of severity and therefore the need for hospital referral. Pulsoximetry should be definitely performed in all children admitted to hospital [7].
2. Laboratory studies
3. Determination of etiology – microbiological investigations

Determining the specific pathogen in children with CAP is difficult. Little children do not expectorate sputum, nasopharyngeal swabs are not reliable since bacteria present in the upper airways are not necessarily the same as those causing pneumonia. Invasive diagnostic tools, though efficacious are hardly acceptable in otherwise healthy children most of whom improve with empiric treatment. British Thoracic Society (BTS) standards, Pediatric Infectious Diseases Society guidelines as well as American Academy of Pediatrics Policy statements do not recommend microbiological investigation of the child with pneumonia treated as an outpatient. For patients admitted to the hospital, especially those admitted to ICU and those with complications of CAP, microbiological diagnosis should be attempted.

- blood cultures are positive in <10% of patients with pneumonia and < 2% of patients treated in the outpatient setting. They should nevertheless be performed since if positive, they provide information on CAP etiology and antibiotic resistance [7,19]. In children with complicated pneumonia prevalence of bacteremia vary from 7.8% to 26.5% in pneumonia with parapneumonic effusion [19].
- nasopharyngeal aspirates or nasal lavage samples may be helpful in identifying respiratory viruses including respiratory syncytial virus, parainfluenza virus, influenza virus and adenovirus by immunofluorescence method. The results of these tests are particularly useful for cohorting infected children during outbreaks and for epidemic purposes [7].
- sputum is difficult to obtain in small children. A reliable sputum sample, as opposed to saliva, contains <10 epithelial cells per low-powered field [35]. Sputum induced by inhalation with 5% hypertonic saline has much higher bacterial yield and seems to be a valuable tool in microbiological diagnosis in children with CAP [36].
- children who require mechanical ventilation should have tracheal aspirates taken for Gram stain and culture at the time of endotracheal tube placement [19].
- aspirated pleural fluid should be sent for microscopy, culture and antigen detection. Cultures are positive in 9% - 18% of cases (sensitivity 23%, specificity 100%) [7, 37]. Pneumococcal antigen detection in pleural fluid has sensitivity of 90% and specificity of 95% [38]. Pleural fluid should be checked for *Mycobacteria*.
- pneumococcal antigens detection in urine is not specific, as it is often positive in young children with nasopharyngeal colonization
- Serological testing: fourfold rise in antibody titers in complement fixation test is a golden diagnostics standard, unfortunately not useful for treatment guidance. In many laborato-

ries enzyme linked immunosorbent assays (ELISA) has replaced complement fixation tests as less time consuming. Positive anti *Mycoplasma* IgM antibody titer 9-11 days from the onset of illness is also suggestive of recent infection. Cross reactions with adenovirus and *Legionella pneumophila* have been described [23]. Cold agglutinins measurement value is limited – in school children the positive predictive value for *Mycoplasma* of a rapid cold agglutinin test was 70% [7]. In *Chlamydophila pneumoniae* infection IgM rise is observed after 3 weeks and IgG rise after 6-8 weeks.

- *Legionella pneumophila* urinary antigen detection remains golden standard for the diagnosis of legionellosis. The test remains positive for weeks after acute infection. Urinary antigen is positive only in case of infection with serogroup 1. Antigens are excreted in urine at the beginning of the second week of illness. Quick diagnostic tests are commercially available with sensitivity of 80% and specificity of 99-100%. Infection with serogroup 1 can be excluded when the results of 3 consecutive urine samples are negative.

- real time Reverse Transcriptase Polymerase Chain Reaction (RT-PCR) can be used for investigating the etiology of pneumonia. The advantage of this method is the availability of results on the same day. It does not however provide information on bacterial sensitivity nor is readily available outside research settings. Pneumolysin based PCR has been increasingly used to detect *Streptococcus pneumoniae* in blood and pleural fluid with sensitivity of 100% and specificity of 95% [7]. Measuring bacterial load with RT-PCR may help predict the outcome of CAP as adult patients with bacterial load > 1000 copies/mL were at higher risk for sepsis, respiratory insufficiency and death [39].

4. Chest radiography

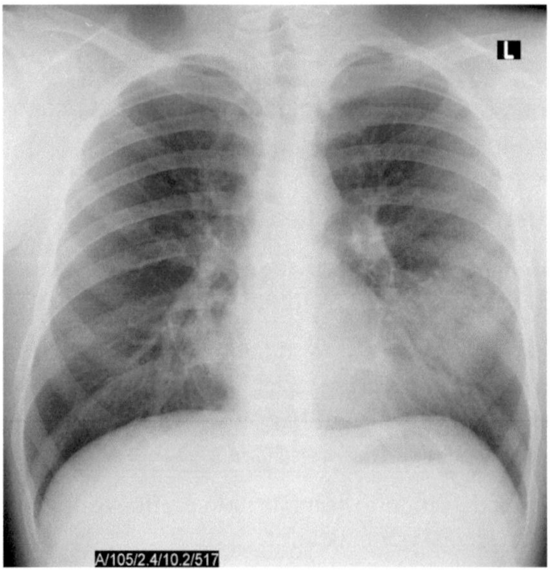

Figure 1. Alveolar consolidations in the left lower lobe and in the right lower lobe. *Mycoplasma pneumoniae* pneumonia

http://dx.doi.org/10.5772/54052

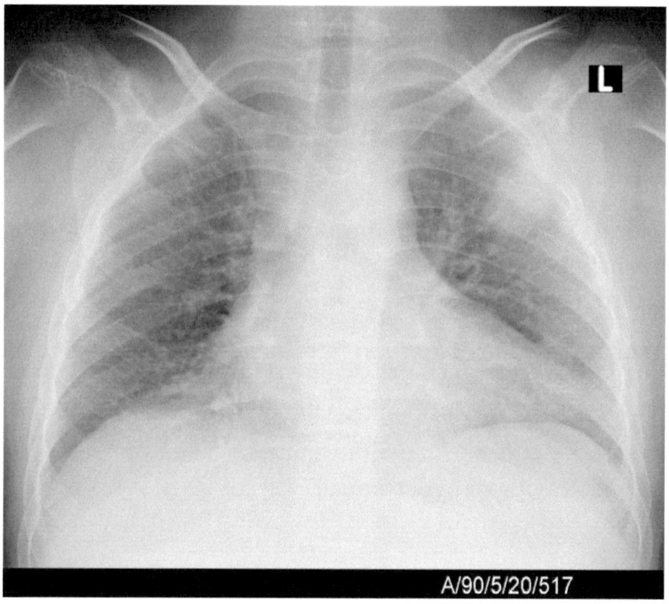

Figure 2. Round focus of consolidation in the left upper lobe. Pneumonia.

9. Management

Most children with CAP can be safely managed on outpatient basis. Indications for hospital referral comprise:

- clinical signs of severe pneumonia (listed above),
- signs of sepsis or septic shock
- young age – < 6 months of life
- hypoxemia – oxygen saturation < 92% (according to BTS) or <90% (according to AAP and PIDS), PaO_2 <60 mmHg and $PaCO_2$ >50 mmHg, central cyanosis
- underlying conditions eg. congenital heart defect, cystic fibrosis, bronchopulmonary dysplasia, immune deficiencies
- diffuse radiological changes: multilobar pneumonia, pleural effusion
- outpatient treatment failure
- CAP caused by pathogen with increased virulence eg. MRSA(PIDS)
- parents' inability to manage the illness at home

Children who are not improving despite treatment and present with impeding respiratory failure or shock should be admitted to Intensive Care Unit. Criteria for ICU admission comprise:

- need for invasive mechanical ventilation or non-invasive positive pressure ventilation,
- fluid refractory shock
- hypoxemia requiring FiO_2 greater than inspired concentration or flow feasible in general care area; pulsoximetry measurements ≤92% with inspired oxygen of ≥0.5 (according to BTS) or ≥0.6 (according to PIDS)
- altered mental status due to hypercarbia, hypoxemia or as a result of pneumonia
- recurrent apnea, grunting or slow irregular breathing
- rising respiratory rate and heart rate with clinical evidence of severe respiratory distress and exhaustion with or without hypercarbia [7,19]

10. General management

All children treated for pneumonia should be reassessed in 48 hours if there is no clinical improvement or deterioration and persistence of fever. It is important that parents of children treated at home have clear written instructions on fever management, preventing dehydration, recognizing signs of deterioration as well as further access to healthcare professionals [7].

Hospitalized hypoxemic children should be given oxygen to maintain oxygen saturation > 92%. Dehydrated children should be provided adequate amount of oral fluids and if unable to drink should receive intravenous fluids. Their electrolytes and creatinine serum levels should be measured on daily basis. Up to date there have been no studies proving beneficial effects of chest physiotherapy in children with pneumonia and therefore chest physiotherapy should not be performed.

A child should improve as evaluated by clinical symptoms and laboratory inflammatory markers in 48-72 hours after initiation of adequate treatment. Failure to improve warrants further investigation for possible complications, resistant microorganisms or alternative diagnosis.

11. Antibiotic treatment

There is no consensus between experts whether all children with CAP should receive antibiotics. According to BTS guidelines issued in 2011 all children diagnosed with pneumonia should be treated with antibiotics. This is in contrast to previous guidelines stating that if viral etiology is suspected antibiotics might be withheld provided that the child is reassessed in 24-48 hours. The reason for this change, despite the obvious concerns of increasing antibiotic resistance among bacteria as well as possible adverse reactions in children unnecessarily treated with antibiotics, is the fact that based on clinical, laboratory and radiological markers, either alone or in combination, a reliable distinction between viral and bacterial infection is impossible. Children <2 especially with a history of conjugate pneumococcal vaccination and with mild symptoms of lower respiratory tract infection are unlikely to have pneumonia. In these children antibiotics might be withheld provided reassessment of the child is made if the symptoms persist or deterioration occurs [7]. PIDS guidelines, on the contrary, state that preschool children with CAP do not routinely require antibiotic therapy since pneumonia in this age group is predominantly of viral origin [19].

Antibiotic of choice for CAP treated in community is amoxicillin 90 mg/kg/day applied in two doses for 5-10 days. Results from two randomized trials on short course (3 days) oral antibiotics performed on infants in developing countries are difficult to interpret since many of these children had bronchiolitis with wheeze or upper respiratory tract infection and did not need antibiotics at all [43,44]. Amoxicillin is effective against the majority pathogens responsible for CAP in children. It is well tolerated and affordable. Alternatives are co-amoxiclav, cefaclor and macrolides. For *Streptococcus pneumoniae* resistant to penicillin with MICs up to 4.0 μg/mL preferred treatment consists in ceftriaxone, and for MICs >4.0 μg/mL in vancomycin, linezolid or clindamycin though resistance to clindamycin seems to be increasing amounting to 15-40% in certain geographic regions [19]. It should be noted that interpretation of *in vitro* susceptibility tests to penicillin depends on the route of administration. Intravenously administered penicillin can achieve tissue concentrations effective against organisms with minimal inhibitory concentration (MICs) ≤2.0 μg/mL, possibly effective for strains with MICS of 4 μg/mL and not likely to be effective for strains with MICS ≥ 8 μg/mL. For orally administered penicillin corresponding values are <0.06 μg/mL, 0.12 – 1.0 μg/mL, and ≥2.0 μg/mL for resistant strains [19]. Clinical laboratory standards vary depending on the region. Those given above, were issued jointly by Infectious Diseases Society of America (IDSA) and American Thoracic Society (ATS). BTS recommends cut off values for intravenously administered penicillin of <0.1 mg/L; 0.1-1.0 mg/L and > 1.0-4.0 mg/L and European Respiratory Society (ERS) recommends MIC breakpoints <0.5 mg/L; 0.5 – 2.0 mg/L and >2.0 mg/L respectively [17,19]. PIDS recommends levofloxacin for children from 6 months of age as preferred choice for oral therapy [19]. Macrolide antibiotics may be added if *Mycoplasma pneumoniae* or *Chlamydophila pneumonia* are suspected when the child is not improving after 24 - 48 hours or in very severe cases. They are not recommended as first choice antibiotics because up to 40% of currently isolated in USA strains of *S. pneumoniae* are resistant to macrolides [19].

As is the case with indications for antibiotics in CAP there is no consensus as to how they should be administered. According to BTS guidelines if the child is feeding well and not vomiting, antibiotics should be given orally. Children with moderate pneumonia admitted because of respiratory distress can be treated with oral antibiotics and discharged when fever and respiratory distress subside [7,45]. Intravenous route of antibiotic administration is reserved for children with severe, complicated pneumonia or sepsis for whom intravenous amoxicillin, co-amoxiclav, cefuroxime, cefotaxime or ceftriaxone are recommended. According to PIDS guidelines however all children treated in hospital should receive antibiotics intravenously to provide reliable blood and tissue concentrations [19]. In hospitalized children suspected of *S. aureus* infection vancomycin or clindamycin should be added to beta-lactam therapy. For children with penicillin allergy recommended drugs are cephalosporins and in case of type-I allergic reactions macrolides, vancomycin or clindamycin are suggested. In children who do not tolerate vancomycin or clindamycin, linezolid may be administered [19]. Antibiotic should be changed according to results of culture and sensitivity if these tests are positive. As soon as the child's condition improves, a switch to oral antibiotics should be considered [7].

12. Complications

12.1. Empyema and parapneumonic effusion

Parapneumonic effusion is defined as pleural fluid collection in association with underlying pneumonia and empyema is defined as the accumulation of purulent fluid in the pleural cavity [46]. Incidence of parapneumonic effusion is increasing (by 70-100% between 1990s and the beginning of the present century), affecting 0.6% of all children with CAP, 2 - 10% of pneumonia hospitalizations and 1/3 of pneumococcal pneumonia hospitalizations [47-50]. Predominant etiological factors are *S. pneumonia* (serotype 1,3,14,19A) responsible for 10-66% of empyema cases, *S. aureus* including MRSA (4-30%) and *S. pyogenes.* The less common include *Haemophilus influenzae, Mycobacterium* spp, *Pseudomonas aeruginosa,* anaerobes, *Mycoplasma pneumonia* and fungi [28,46,47,51,52]. Fluid collection is usually unilateral. Empyema classically exhibits three stages:

- Exudative – pleural space contains free flowing fluid with a low white cell count, so called parapneumonic effusion that results from increased vascular permeability and migration of neutrophils, lymphocytes and eosinophils in the course of inflammatory process.

- Fibrinopurulent occurs 5-10 days from the onset of the disease and consists in the deposition of fibrin in the pleural space that leads to septation and formation of loculations. The number of white cells increases (empyema) in response to bacterial invasion across the damaged epithelium and if left untreated it progresses into

- Organizing - includes infiltration of fibroblasts and evolution of thick elastic membrane in the pleural cavity (the "peel"). These membranes may impair lung function and prevent lung re-expansion. Empyema at this stage may heal spontaneously or a chronic empyema may develop [46].

Some authors distinguish "pleuritis sicca stage" that precedes exudative stage, not necessarily leading to it [53].

Empyema should be suspected in every child with pneumonia with a history of prolonged fever, tachypnoe, pain on abdominal palpation, pleuritic chest pain, splinting of the affected side and persistence of high serum C-reactive protein levels [50]. On physical examination asymmetry of breath sounds, unilateral decreased chest wall expansion, dullness to percussion might be appreciated [27]. In some children with pneumonia empyema may develop during intravenous antibiotic treatment [50]. One of the identified risk factors for bacterial empyema is precedent varicella [49].

Chest radiographs show homogenous opacity over the entire lung (large effusion) (Figure 3). In smaller effusions an ascending rim of fluid along the lateral chest wall (meniscus sign) occurs. Costophrenical angle obliteration is the first sign of pleural effusion. Based on radiograph it is not possible to distinguish effusion from empyema [47]. A method of choice for radiologic evaluation of patients with parapneumonic effusion and empyema is ultrasonography. It helps estimate the amount of fluid, its echogenicity, detects loculations and fibrin strands and is used to guide invasive procedures [28]. Chest CT should not be routinely performed, it may be useful however for diagnosis of underlying pathology eg. tumor in the mediastinum or lung abscess [46,53].

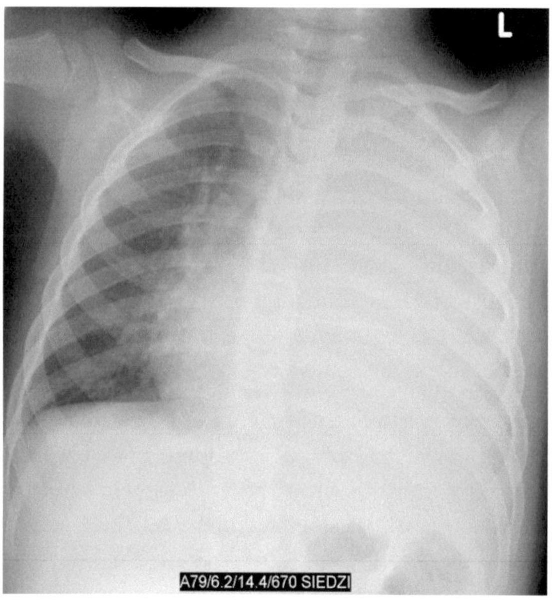

Figure 3. Opacification of left hemithorax with mediastinal shift to the opposite side. Alveolar consolidations in the central field of the right lobe. Lobar pneumonia with pleural effusion caused by *Streptococcus pneumoniae*

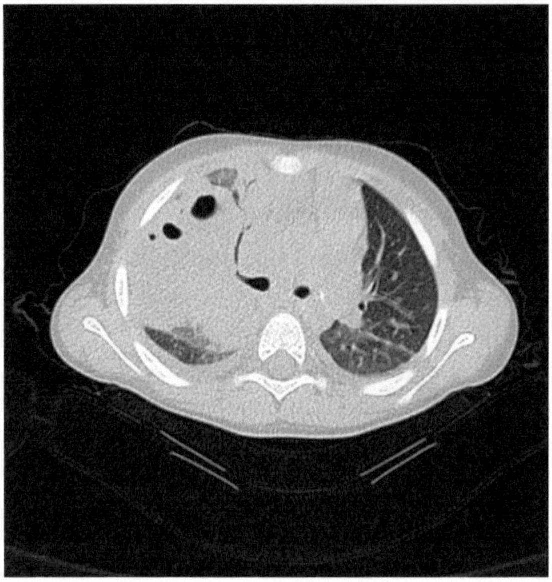

Figure 4. Multiple abscesses in the right upper lobe. Diffuse alveolar consolidations with thickening of intraalveolar spaces in the middle and lower right lobes. Fluid in the right pleural space. *Staphylococcus aureus* pneumonia with lung abscesses and pleural effusion.

Pleural fluid, if obtained during thoracocentesis or video-assisted thoracoscopic surgery (VATS), should be sent for culture, Gram stain, cytology and molecular techniques if available. Bacteriological investigations should always be undertaken even though they are positive in ¼ of cases since they may provide useful information guiding antibiotic therapy. Stain for acid-fast bacilli, culture and PCR should also be performed [46]. In most cases of bacterial empyema polymorphonuclear leukocytes are the predominant cells. In case of malignancy the fluid may be blood stained with lymphocytic predominance, although malignant cells may not be present. In tuberculosis there is also predominance of lymphocytes in pleural fluid although in 10% of cases effusion might be neutrophilic [46]. Light criteria, useful for treatment guidance in adult patients, have not been properly validated in children and their routine use is not recommended [46,53].

All children with empyema or pleural effusion should be treated as inpatients [46]. There is no consensus however as to what is optimal treatment of empyema: antibiotics alone for small to moderate effusions, chest tube insertion with or without fibrinolytics or VATS for moderate to severe cases. Differences in management result to some extent from personal experience and availability of different treatment modalities, including experienced interventional radiologists and pediatric thoracic surgeons. Generally, two most important factors determining the need for chest tube insertion are the size of effusion and the child's degree of respiratory compromise [19]. There is agreement that due to an invasive nature of the procedure and the need for general anesthesia in younger children, a drain should be inserted instead of repeated needle thoracocenteses [46]. According to PIDS, pleural effusions can be divided depending on their size into:

http://dx.doi.org/10.5772/54052

- Small: < 10 mm on lateral decubitus radiograph or opacifies < ¼ hemithorax
- Moderate: >10 mm rim of fluid and opacifies < ½ hemithorax
- Large: opacifies > ½ hemithorax

Conservative treatment with antibiotics is recommended for small effusions. Antibiotic selection is based on blood or pleural fluid culture results, and if these are not available, on treatment guidelines. Many patients improve with conservative treatment alone. In an American study over 50% of all patients with moderate to severe effusions recovered with antibiotic treatment alone [54]. Management of moderate effusions depends on child's degree of respiratory compromise: if clinical condition is good, treatment with antibiotics is appropriate and if the child presents signs of respiratory distress, treatment is the same as for large effusions: fluid should be removed either by tube thoracocentesis (for not loculated fluid) or chest tube with fibrinolytics or VATS (both for loculated fluid) [19]. Once the chest tube is inserted, no more than 10 ml/kg of fluid in little children and 1.5 liters of fluid in older children and adolescents should be removed in order to avoid re-expansion pulmonary edema. When this volume is reached, the drain should be clamped for an hour [46]. There is no clear evidence on advantage in clinical outcome of children treated with fibrinolytic agents versus VATS [55,56]. The recommended doses for fibrinolytic agents are [19,57,58]:

- Urokinase (not available in USA) 10,000 U every 12 hours for 3 days in children < 1 year and 40,000 U every 12 hours for 3 days in children > 1 year
- Streptokinase 12,000 - 25,000 IU/kg/dose daily for 3-5 days
- Tissue plasminogen activator 0.1 mg/kg; maximum of 3 mg three times a day for 3 to 4 days or 4 mg every 24 hours

With streptokinase and urokinase there is risk of hypersensitivity reactions.

Children who fail to improve despite antibiotics, drainage and fibrinolytics, should undergo VATS in order to debride fibrinous adhesions and remove dense loculated fluid. It seems prudent to ask for surgical opinion if the patient is not improving after 7 days of treatment. Another indication for surgery is bronchopleural fistula with pyopneumothorax [46]. As an alternative to VATS, especially in organized empyema in a child with non-resolving signs of systemic infection with fever, formal thoracotomy with decortications should be considered [19]. According to BTS guidelines indications for surgery referral are clinical signs and symptoms and not aberrant radiologic picture in an asymptomatic child [46]. Risk factors for the failure of tube thoracostomy include duration of symptoms > 7 days before the procedure, complex multiloculated empyema, pneumatocele, pulmonary necrosis and an underlying medical condition [59,60]. A chest tube can be removed if fluid output is < 1 ml/kg/day calculated over the last 12 hours or 50-60 ml/day and there is no air leak [19].

A more aggressive approach is to perform VATS in the first 48 hours of treatment. That gives a chance for bacteriological diagnosis and shorter hospital stay, though not all studies confirm the latter observation [54].

The optimal duration of antibiotic treatment for parapneumonic effusion and empyema depends on clinical response. Recommended route of administration is intravenous until the chest tube is removed, and then can be switched to oral route for 1 to 4 weeks or longer if the child has not fully recovered. However, there are no randomized clinical trials to support this approach [19,46]. Long-term outcome in children is favorable. Radiological evidence of pleural disease completely resolves within 3 months in up to 80% of children and by 18 months in all children. Lung function tests results as well as exercise tolerance in most patients are normal 12 months after discharge [46,52,53]. Conditions predisposing to severe pneumonia with pleural effusion and empyema include immunodeficiencies and cystic fibrosis and they should be excluded during follow-up period [46].

12.2. Lung abscess

Lung abscess is a thick-walled cavity containing necrotic tissue 2 cm or greater in diameter caused by an infection [28]. It may be either primary – occurring in healthy children without lung abnormalities or secondary – occurring in children with underlying condition predisposing to lung disease. The most important mechanism of lung abscess formation is aspiration, especially in children with neuromuscular disorders. Other risk factors include immunodeficiencies, underlying lung disease like congenital malformations, cystic fibrosis, swallowing problems, eg. achalasia, poor dental hygiene. Abscesses may also ensue by hematogenous spread from septicemia or right-sided bacterial endocarditis, extension from foci in abdominal cavity or retropharyngeal space or from airway obstruction by foreign body [61,62].

The main causative organisms are usually streptococci, anaerobic bacteria, *S. aureus* and *Klebsiella pneumonia*, however there are rare reports of other causative organisms including *Mycoplasma pneumoniae* [63]. Mixed infections are common. The most frequent sites for lung abscess formation in recumbent position are: the right upper lobe, the left lower lobe and the apical segments of both lower lobes. When the patient aspirates in supine position the posterior segments of the upper lobes are usually involved.

Clinical symptoms include cough, purulent sputum production, fever, dyspnea, chest pain, tachypnoe, weight loss, hemoptysis, malaise/lethargy. Physical signs do not differ from uncomplicated pneumonia, decreased breath sounds and dull note on percussion may be appreciated. Symptoms may persist for several weeks [61].

Diagnosis is usually made by chest radiograph showing an inflammatory infiltrate of the pulmonary parenchyma with a cavity containing an air-fluid level. Initially it may appear as a solid lesion surrounded by an alveolar infiltrate. Bulging fissure representing increased volume of the affected lobe may be present. CT is usually performed to exclude other complications like empyema, pneumatocoele, underlying congenital abnormality like sequestration, bronchogenic cyst or adenomatoid malformation. Features distinguishing abscess from other entities include well-marginated walls, density greater than water, contrast enhancement in adjacent tissues (Figure 4, Figure 5) [61].

http://dx.doi.org/10.5772/54052

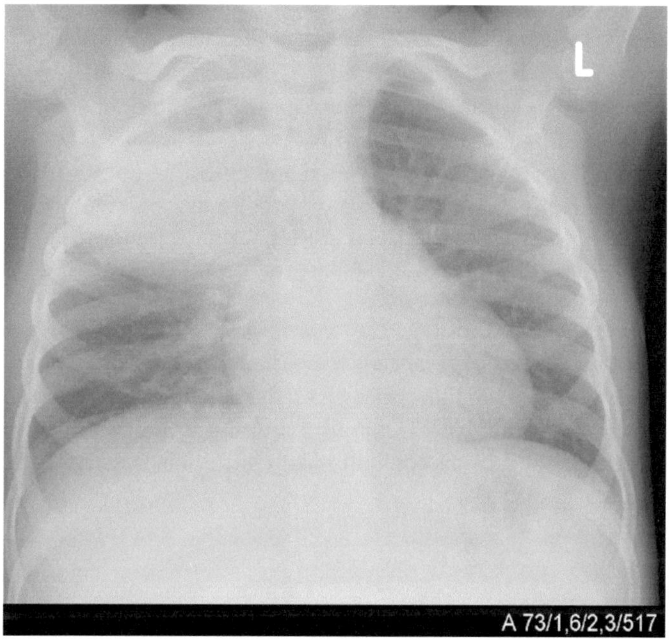

Figure 5. Infiltrate with air-fluid level in the upper field of the right lobe. Lung abscess.

The mainstay of treatment is conservative antibiotic therapy with spectrum covering *S. pneumoniae, S. aureus* and Gram-negative bacilli and anaerobes in case of secondary abscess. For immunocompromised patients antibiotics should cover fungal pathogens. Antibiotic of choice is penicillin with clindamycin or metronidazole. Other experts recommend third-generation cephalosporin and flucloxacillin, ticarcillin, ampicillin/clavulanic acid and piperacillin/tazobactam. One should consider the possibility of MRSA infection, especially if the abscess complicates pneumonia or results from hematogenous spread from other organs [61,62]. A 2-3 week course of intravenous therapy followed by oral treatment for 4 to 8 weeks is usually recommended [28]. In experienced interventional radiology centers CT-guided aspiration of the lung abscess and placement of pigtail catheter is performed for diagnostic and therapeutic reasons. Surgical intervention is indicated for abscesses failing to improve despite medical treatment.

The overall outcome is favorable, mortality being much lower than in adults: <5% and mostly occurring in children with secondary lung abscesses or underlying medical problems. The complications include empyema or pyopneumothorax if abscess ruptures into pleural cavity, bronchopleural fistula if connection between the abscess cavity and pleural space persists and localized bronchiectasis.

12.3. Necrotising pneumonia

Necrotizing pneumonia (NP), defined as multiple cavitary lesions in consolidated areas, is a rare, though increasingly detected complication in children. It is characterized by liquefaction and cavitation of pulmonary tissue [63]. The most frequently associated pathogen is *Streptococcus pneumoniae,* especially serotypes 3 and 14. Other pathogens involved include group A *Streptococci, Staphylococcus aureus* and *Mycoplasma pneumoniae* [64-68]. The majority of patients have no prior medical history. Necrotizing pneumonia should be suspected in patients with complicated pneumonia who do not improve despite optimal medical treatment. Diagnosis can be established by computed tomography. Radiographic criteria for necrotizing pneumonia include the loss of normal pulmonary parenchymal architecture and the presence of areas of liquefaction replaced within 1-2 days by multiple small cavities [64]. Necrotizing pneumonia often coexists with pleural effusion.

Treatment consists in prolonged course of intravenous antibiotics active against CAP pathogens including resistant strains of *S. pneumoniae.* Interventional procedures are contraindicated in children with NP, as they may increase the risk of complications such as bronchopleural fistula formation [35]. Generally, despite prolonged hospital course and associated morbidity, the long term outcome in most children is favorable. Mortality rates are 5.5-7% [28,65].

13. Prevention

In order to prevent pneumonia several measures can be taken, starting with general recommendations like improving nourishment, housing conditions, heating systems, reducing tobacco smoke exposure, promoting breast-feeding for the first 6 months of age, to more specific infection control measures like hand-washing, avoiding individuals with signs of respiratory tract infections, and vaccinations. For prevention of pneumonia immunization against the following microorganisms is recommended:

- influenza virus
- *Streptococcus pneumoniae* (conjugate and non-conjugate vaccine)
- *Haemophilus influenzae* (conjugate vaccine)
- measles virus
- varicella virus
- *Bordatella pertussiss*
- *Mycobacterium tuberculosis*

High risk infants: prematurely born (<35 week of GA), with hemodynamically significant congenital heart disease, bronchopulmonary dysplasia, congenital abnormalities of the airways and neuromuscular diseases should receive immune prophylaxis with RSV specific monoclonal antibody (palivizumab) in RSV season [68].

AAP recommends the routine use of 13-valent pneumococcal conjugate vaccine (PCV13) for healthy children 2 through 59 months of age and for children 60 through 71 months of age with an underlying medical condition that increases the risk of invasive pneumococcal disease (IPD) [69]. Underlying medical conditions that indicate the need for pneumococcal immunization comprise:

- chronic heart disease, in particular cyanotic congenital heart disease and cardiac failure
- chronic lung disease including asthma if treated with prolonged high-dose oral corticosteroids
- diabetes mellitus
- cerebrospinal fluid leaks
- cochlear implant
- functional or anatomical asplenia including children with sickle cell disease and other hemoglobinopathies
- immunocompromising conditions: HIV infection, chronic renal failure and nephrotic syndrome, diseases associated with treatment with immunosuppressive drugs or radiation therapy (including malignant neoplasms, leukemias, lymphomas, Hodgkin disease, solid organ transplantation) and congenital immunodeficiency (including B- (humoral) or T-lymphocyte deficiency; complement deficiencies, particularly C1, C2, C3 and C4 and phagocytic disorders excluding chronic granulomatous disease).

Healthy children <5 and children with underlying medical conditions <6, who are fully immunized with PCV7 should receive a single supplemental dose of PCV13. Children between 6 and 18 with medical conditions favoring IPD (listed above) should receive a single dose of PCV13 regardless of whether they have previously received PCV7 or PPSV23 (2 doses of PPSV23 recommended). PCV13 which in addition to the 7 serotypes included in PCV7 (4,6B,9V,14,18C,19F,23F) contains the 6 pneumococcal serotypes (1,3,5,6A,7F,19A) responsible for 63% of cases of invasive pneumococcal disease occurring in children <5 in the USA has been licensed by the US Food and Drug Administration in 2010 for use in children between 2 and 71 months of age. Because of the expended coverage provided it is meant to replace PCV7 [69].

14. Specific bacterial causes of pneumonia

14.1. *Streptococcus pneumoniae*

Streptococcus pneumoniae is the most common pathogen in CAP in children and the most common cause of pneumonia mortality in children worldwide. It is responsible for at least 1.2 million deaths in infants annually, mostly in sub-Saharan Africa and Asia [45]. There are 92 known pneumococcal serotypes that differ by polysaccharide capsule. It was found that serotypes are correlated with different pneumonia outcomes, study results are not however equivocal. In pediatric patients serotypes 7F, 23F and 3 were correlated with the highest risk of death in the course of invasive pneumococcal disease [70]. In another study serotypes

1,6,14,19 were the most prevalent among children with complicated pneumonia, with serotype 1 causing 24.4% of the complicated cases versus 3.6% of the uncomplicated cases [71].

S. pneumoniae commonly colonizes epithelium of nasopharynx in 20 - 40% of healthy children and > 60% of infants and children in day-care settings. After colonization a new strain eliminates other competing pneumococcal serotypes and persists for months in a carrier state. Bacteria with so called "persistent colonization phenotype", with low risk of tissue invasion are responsible for perpetual transmission within human populations and induce acquired B-cell mediated immunity to reinfection. To facilitate their stay within nasopharynx and evade host defenses they use different mechanisms like surface adhesions, IgA1 protease and inhibitors of antibacterial peptides. Defects in host defense mechanisms can destroy the balance and lead to infection in immunocompromised host. Another phenotype – so called "invasive pneumococcal disease phenotype" is able to spread efficiently from person to person by coughing and rapidly induce the disease. Its main virulence factor is polysaccharide capsule that prevents mechanical clearance by mucous secretions, restricts autolysis, reduces exposure to antibiotics and facilitates invasion and dissemination. Other virulence factors include: pore-forming cytotoxin – pneumolysin that among other pathological effects is able to inhibit cilliary movement of epithelial cells and impairs respiratory burst of phagocytic cells. Recent acquisition of an invasive serotype is more important in terms of further infection than long-term colonization and is in fact recognized as one of definite risk factors for pneumococcal pneumonia [45].

Some of the host immune mechanisms essential for defense against pneumococcal pneumonia are toll-like receptors (TLRs). Children with genetic deficiency of the common TLR-adaptor protein – myeloid differentiation primary-response protein 88 (MyD88) or interleukin-1 receptor – associated kinase 4 (IRAK4), a kinase acting directly downstream from MyD88, are especially susceptible to invasive pneumococcal disease. Another genetic factor predisposing to invasive pneumococcal disease is polymorphism of genes coding inhibitors of nuclear factor κB and defects in the complement C3 pathway crucial for opsonization and consequently clearance of pneumococci [45].

Pneumonia usually begins with viral upper respiratory tract infection. The pathogen most commonly associated with dual infections with *Streptococcus pneumonia* is influenza virus. Co-infection with influenza virus attenuates host immune response diminishing its ability to clear pneumococcus. Influenza virus possesses neuraminidase that by exposing certain receptors facilitates pneumococcus' adherence to respiratory epithelium [72]. Local innate immune defense systems like mucociliary clearance, cough reflex, antimicrobial peptides usually succeed in eliminating the pathogen. Should they fail, pneumonia ensues. Clinical symptoms are characteristic for bacterial pneumonia with high fever, chills, malaise, cough and dyspnoea. Cough becomes productive in older children, with purulent, blood tinged sputum. Pleural involvement is quite common. Untreated pneumococcal pneumonia may progress to respiratory failure, septic shock and consequently death.

The usual radiological presentation of pneumococcal pneumonia is lobar pneumonia, frequently accompanied by small pleural effusion. Changes may be confined to a single segment or involve several segments or lobes or present as bronchopneumonia [41].

Since universal introduction of pneumococcal conjugated 7-valent vaccine in 2000, there has been a decrease in incidence of pneumococcal pneumonia in children <5 [7]. There is, however, concern that the serotypes included in the vaccine can be replaced with previously rare, potentially more virulent serotypes like serotype 1 or 19A [73,74]. Fortunately, these serotypes have been included in the newer conjugated 13-valent vaccine.

There is a problem of increasing antibacterial resistance – up to 10% of cultured pneumococcal isolates in 2008 in Europe are not susceptible to penicillin, though the impact of *in vitro* resistance on clinical outcome of patients is not that clear. Fortunately, there was no increase in mortality or complication rate reported in children infected with resistant strains [71,73,74].

14.2. *Staphylococcus aureus*

The incidence of *Staphylococcus aureus* pneumonia has increased significantly during the past 20 years. An increasing number (up to 76% in Texas) of community-associated *S. aureus* is methicillin resistant (CA-MRSA) and in some regions it has become the main cause of complicated CAP in children [75-77]. CA-MRSA were described for the first time in the 1990s as a cause of infection in previously healthy young children and adolescents with no prior hospitalization or record with chronic healthcare facilities [77]. There is also significant increase in nasal colonization of healthy children with MRSA – in another study from the USA 36.4% of healthy children were colonized with *S. aureus* and 9.2% with MRSA. CA-MRSA has its own genotype different from hospital acquired strains [77]. It is worth noticing that 22% of MRSA strains had gene locus for PVL, and in a British study 11% of all *S. aureus* isolates from pneumonia patients carried the gene [78,79]. Even if the impact of nasal colonization on the risk of pneumonia is not clear, since 1/3 of patients with staphylococcal infection had no prior colonization documented [80], these data show a wide distribution of MRSA in the community.

Primary *S. aureus* pneumonia results from direct invasion of the lungs through the tracheobronchial tree, and secondary pneumonia results from hematogenous spread. *S. aureus* CAP typically occurs in very young infants: 30% of cases occur in children younger than 3 months of age and 70% in those <1 year of age, more often in boys [60].CA-MRSA CAP frequently occurs in previously healthy children and adolescents and in many cases is preceded by influenza or flu-like illness or skin and soft tissue infection. Severe respiratory symptoms and hypotension develop rapidly. The USA300 clone is associated with venous thrombosis and subsequent septic pulmonary emboli [77].

S. aureus possesses a variety of virulence factors including surface proteins (eg. protein A) that promote adherence and hence colonization of host tissues, invasions (leukocidin, kinases and hyaluronidase) that promote bacterial spread in tissues and membrane damaging toxins (eg. mentioned above leukocidin). There have been several reports in previously healthy children and adolescents of pneumonia caused by Panton – Valentine leukocidin producing *Staphylococcus aureus*. The pore–forming toxin encoded by *luk-S-PV* and *luk-F-PV* genes lyses neutrophils causing exaggerated though ineffective inflammatory response. Patients present with rapidly progressing necrotizing pneumonia manifested by fever, leucopenia and hemoptysis preceded by viral infection, most common influenza [75]. Leucopenia is characteristic for PVL and is thought to be secondary to leukocidin destroying white blood cells [77]. Radiographic appearance is multiple nodular infiltrates, usually unilateral that may transform into cavitary lesions and pneumatocele. Radiographic progression of infiltrates may be very rapid and should raise possibility of *S. aureus* pneumonia. Another characteristic radiographic sign – pneumatoceles – occurs in over half of cases and both its size and number may change hourly [61]. Staphylococcal pneumonia is often complicated with empyema, formation of lung abscesses, pneumothorax and acute respiratory distress syndrome (ARDS).

Given the severe and potentially fatal nature of the infection, prompt initiation of appropriate antibiotic therapy is crucial. For hospitalized patients with pneumonia caused by methicillin susceptible *S. aureus* PIDS recommends intravenous therapy with β-lactamase stable penicillin (oxacillin, cloxacillin, flucloxacillin or nafcillin) or the first generation cephalosporin (cefazolin). For more severe infections some experts recommend combination therapy with an aminoglycoside or rifampin although data from controlled clinical studies supporting these recommendations are lacking [19]. The first line treatment for hospitalized children suspected of CA-MRSA is vancomycin. There is a concern, however, of adequate concentration of the drug in lung epithelial lining fluid – in adults it has been shown to achieve 18% of serum levels [77]. Alternative choices are linezolid and clindamycin that have an additional advantage of blocking the production of PVL toxin and staphylococcal exotoxins so they are the drugs of choice in treatment of PVL-CA infections. Clindamycin should be used with care considering local susceptibility data and it should not be used in high inoculum infections such as empyema since in that case there is high risk that the bacteria will constitutively produce methylase [19]. Linezolid achieves higher concentrations in epithelial lining of the lung [80].

14.3. *Mycoplasma pneumoniae*

Mycoplsamas are the smallest self-replicating organisms able to live outside the host cells. They do not have cell wall, but a cell membrane containing sterols and do not stain well with Gram stain and antibiotics disrupting bacterial cell wall like β-lactams are inactive against these organisms. *Mycoplasma pneumonia*e pneumonia is usually a mild disease. Transmission occurs via person to person contact and incubation period is usually 1 to 2 weeks. Epidemics occur in approximately 4 - 7 year cycles. Recurrent infections are usual.

Infections with *Mycoplasma pneumonia* are common. Antibodies are present in 1/3 of all infants between 7 to 12 month of life and over 90% of adolescents. Very few infections occur in infants in the first 6 months of life probably due to presence of maternal antibodies. Recent studies show that contrary to previous reports *M. pneumoniae* CAP is also quite common in children <4 years. These microorganism are responsible for ¼ of infections in this age group [81].

Microorganisms are acquired via respiratory route. In the airways they attach to a receptor on respiratory epithelium via adhesions. Lung injury in *M. pneumoniae* pneumonia is associated with cell-mediated immunity of the host and it is also accompanied by ciliostasis [81].

http://dx.doi.org/10.5772/54052

Patients present with symptoms of upper respiratory tract infection, fever, malaise, headache. Symptoms ensue gradually. Cough, which is initially unproductive, appears 3 to 5 days from the onset of disease. Associated symptoms include hoarsness, chills, chest pain, vomiting, nausea, diarrhea and myalgia. Coryza is a rare finding, and pleural effusion occurs in 5-20% of patients. On auscultation crackles, wheezes and bronchial breathing may be present. *Mycoplasma pneumonie* may present with extrapulmonary involvement including: nonexudative pharyngitis, cervical lymphadenopathy, otitis media, conjunctivitis, arthritis and rash. Illness usually resolves within 3 - 4 weeks, but it might be more severe in children with sickle cell disease and in Down syndrome. *Mycoplasma* may cause exacerbations in asthmatic patients [28].

Radiological findings vary from reticular and interstitial pattern to lobar consolidations. Hilar adenopathy is present in 1/3 of patients. Characteristic is poor correlation between clinical symptoms and physical and radiological findings.

Treatment of choice consists in macrolide antibiotics.

In rare cases *Mycoplasma pneumoniae* pneumonia may be severe with massive lobar consolidation, pleural effusion, lung abscess or pneumatocele formation. Occasionally, fever and radiological changes progress, despite standard macrolide therapy. There is one report of successful treatment of refractory pneumonia with methylprednisolone in children [82]. Rare complications – obliterative bronchiolitis and diffuse interstitial fibrosis – have been described. In 1/3 of children 1 - 2 years after *Mycoplasma pneumoniae* infection abnormal findings including mosaic perfusion, bronchiectasis, bronchial wall thickening, decreased vascularity and air trapping are observed [81]. Extrapulmonary complications of *Mycoplasma* pneumonia provoke signs from a variety of organs and systems. These include:

- neural system: meningoencephalitis, transverse myelitis, cranial neuropathy, myeloradiculopathy, a poliomyelitis-like syndrome, psychosis, Guillain-Barré syndrome
- skin: erythematous maculopapular or vesicular exanthems, erythema multiforme, Stevens – Johnson syndrome
- heart: pericarditis, myocarditis, congestive heart failure, heart block
- gastrointestinal tract: nausea, vomiting, diarrhea, hepatic dysfunction, jaundice
- hematologic: hemolytic anemia, thrombocytopenia, disseminated intravascular coagulation
- musculoskeletal: myalgias, arthralgias
- genitourinary: glomerulonephritis, interstitial tubulonephritis

15. Hospital acquired pneumonia

Hospital acquired pneumonia (HAP) is defined as pneumonia that occurs 48 hours or more after admission in a patient who had no signs of disease at the time he or she was presenting to the hospital [83]. It may be further divided into early onset (48-96 hours after admission) usually caused by pathogens responsible for CAP and late onset (> 96 hours after admission) caused by multidrug resistant nosocomial pathogens [84].

Ventilator associated pneumonia (VAP), a type of HAP affecting mechanically ventilated patients is defined as pneumonia that occurs more than 48 hours after intubation [83].

A third type, only recently described, represents health-care associated pneumonia (HCAP) that develops in patients who fulfill one of the following conditions:

- hospitalization for 2 or more days within 90 days of the infection
- residence in a nursing home or long-term care facility
- antibiotic therapy or chemotherapy or wound care within 30 days of the infection
- attending haemodialisis center [83].

Definition of HCAP has not been validated in children, although, due to a growing number of pediatric patients with chronic medical conditions (eg. cerebral palsy, congenital malformation syndromes, chronic pulmonary, heart and renal disease) who frequently have contacts with healthcare personnel, HCAP poses a significant problem in this population.

HAP occurs in 16-29% of pediatric patients and accounts for 10-15% of all nosocomial infections in children and up to 67% of nosocomial infections in children admitted to pediatric intensive care units [85-87]. VAP occurs in about 3 to 32% of ventilated pediatric ICU patients [87,88]. In Europe it is the most common and in the USA second most common nosocomial infection in children treated in intensive care units [88-90]. Mortality in HAP is much higher than in CAP and ranges from 10 to 70% depending on the etiological factors and comorbidities [85,86,88]. HAP and VAP in particular increase length of hospital stay and hospital costs [86,88,91].

The most common etiological factors of pediatric HAP are respiratory viruses including respiratory syncytial virus, adenovirus, influenza and parainfluenza viruses. Bacteria responsible for late onset HAP comprise Gram-negative bacilli: *Pseudomonas aeruginosa, Escherichia coli, Klebsiella pneumonia, Acinetobacter* spp., *Serratia* spp.., Gram positive organisms esp. *Staphylococcus aureus* and coagulase - negative *Staphylococci. P. aeruginosa* is the most common bacterial pathogen in pediatric intensive care units associated with mortality rates up to 80% [90]. Most bacteria responsible for nosocomial infections are multidrug resistant, among them methicillin resistant *Staphylococci* (MRSA) and extended spectrum β-lactamase (ESBL) producing Gram negative bacilli. Immunocompromised children are at particular risk of infection caused by fungi, esp. *Aspergillus, Candida* and *Pneumocystis jiroveci.* In 38% of cases etiology of VAP in children is polymicrobial [88].

Risk factors for hospital acquired pneumonia comprise intubation and mechanical ventilation (increases the risk 6 to 21-fold increased risk), neuromuscular blockade, length of hospital stay, immunosuppression, recent treatment with antibiotics and H2 blockers as well as overcrowding and understaffing of hospital wards [85,86]. Genetic syndrome, female gender, reintubation, transport out of the intensive care unit, surgery before ICU admission, enteral feeds, use of narcotic medications were found to be independent risk factors of VAP in children [88,91].

Nosocomial pneumonia should be suspected in any child with new respiratory symptoms during hospital stay, hypoxemia, increased oxygen or ventilation requirements, increased amount or altered characteristic of respiratory secretions. Most definitions include clinical and radiological signs, some additional bacteriological and laboratory data [83,92]. According to National Healthcare Safety Network of Centers for Disease Control (CDC), HAP can be diagnosed in patients with new radiological changes (infiltrate, consolidation, cavitation, pneumatocele in infants in the 1st year of life) and at least three clinical criteria (clinically defined pneumonia) or two clinical and one laboratory criteria. For children with underlying pulmonary or heart disease radiologic changes must be confirmed in at least two serial x-rays. Clinical criteria, that must be fulfilled include:

- fever > 38⁰C with no other cause or
- leucopenia (<4,000/mm^3) or leucocytosis (≥12,000/mm^3) and at least one (or two for clinically defined pneumonia) of the following:
- new onset of purulent sputum,
- increase in respiratory secretions,
- change in the character of sputum or respiratory secretions,
- new onset or worsening of respiratory symptoms: cough, tachypnea, dyspnea,
- auscultary findings: rales, bronchial sounds,
- increased oxygen requirements, $PaO_2/FiO_2 \leq 240$.

In children up to12 years of age clinical criteria are slightly different and at least three (two in infants ≤1 year of age) must be fulfilled. These include:

- fever > 38^{0}C or hypothermia < 36.5^{0}C (or temperature instability for infants ≤1 year of age) with no other cause or
- leucopenia (<4,000/mm^3) or leukocytosis (≥15,000/mm^3) and ≥10% immature forms (infants ≤1 year of age)
- new onset of purulent sputum,
- increase in respiratory secretions,
- change in the character of sputum or respiratory secretions,
- new onset or worsening of respiratory symptoms: apnea, cough, tachypnea, dyspnea,
- nasal flaring with chest wall retractions or grunting, wheezing - infants ≤1 year of age
- auscultary findings: rales, bronchial sounds,
- bradycardia (<100 beats/minute) or tachycardia (>170 beats per minute) - infants ≤1 year of age

- increased ventilation requirements, hypoxemia (Sat <94%) – this condition is obligatory for infants ≤1 year of age.

Laboratory criteria include positive cultures of blood (not related to other infections), pleural fluid or specimens from lower respiratory tract (bronchoalveolar lavage - BAL or protected specimen brushing), intracellular bacteria seen in ≥5% of cells obtained from BAL on direct microscopic exam, histopathologic evidence of abscess formation, focal consolidations, intensive polymorphonuclear cell accumulation in the small airways, lung parenchyma invasion by hyphae or pseudohyphae. Diagnostic value of BAL in children with VAP is found to be 50-72% and specificity 80-88%, and of quantification of intracellular organisms in BAL samples 30-55% and 89-95% respectively [93-96]. Laboratory criteria for HAP caused by atypical bacteria (*Mycoplasma* spp., *Chlamydophila* spp., *Legionella* spp.) or viruses include: positive culture from respiratory secretions, positive detection of antigen or antibody in respiratory secretions, 4-fold IgG rise in paired sera, positive PCR, detection of *Legionella pneumophila* serogroup 1 antigens in urine [92].

Bacteriological diagnosis is often difficult, since hospitalized patients are commonly colonized with pathogenic flora. Therefore a quantitative criterion of bacterial yield (≥10^4 cfu/mL, or ≥10^4cfu/g tissue in case of lung parenchyma specimen) has been established to aid the etiological diagnosis of pneumonia [92]. Applicability of invasive diagnostic techniques (lung biopsy) remains controversial for the fear of complications in unstable or severely sick patients and lack of data confirming their influence on clinical course or mortality rates.

Patients with HAP are most often debilitated individuals with multiple underlying conditions. HAP is a severe disease with high mortality rates. Therefore diagnosis should be established as quickly as possible using a wide array of diagnostic tools and techniques and empiric treatment should be implemented promptly while cultures and other microbiological studies are pending. Antibiotics should have spectrum broad enough to cover gram negative and gram positive bacteria considering previous antibiotic exposure, local flora, antimicrobial susceptibility patterns and guidelines from the infectious diseases specialist. Risk factors for acquisition of antibiotic-resistant gram negative bacteria in pediatric intensive care unit (PICU) patients include younger age, severe general condition (appreciated based on PRISM {pediatric risk of mortality} score), intravenous antibiotics administration in the previous 12 months, PICU admission in the past, contacts with chronic care facilities [87,94]. Inappropriate antibiotic treatment is associated with increased mortality in patients with HAP [90]. Children with early onset HAP might be treated as those with CAP provided they do not have specific risk factors for HCAP, VAP or colonization with multi-drug resistant bacteria. PICU patients should receive coverage against *Pseudomonas aeruginosa* (aminoglycoside with an appropriate β-lactam: piperacillin, ceftazidime or cefepime) and in hospital wards where incidence of methicillin resistant staphylococci or ESBL producing gram negative bacilli exceeds 5% vancomycin and carbapenems or ureidopenicillin derivative plus β-lactamase inhibitor respectively should be included in empiric treatment regimes [92]. In children with immunodeficiencies antifungals should be administered. As soon as the causative organism and its sensitivity is known, therapy should be tailored using the agent of the narrowest spectrum available. Antibiotics should be administered intravenously and switched to oral route if possible once the patient improves.

Infection control measures that should be meticulously implemented in order to decrease the number of HAP include:

- appropriate hand hygiene, use of gloves
- personal protective equipment – face masks, especially in the periods of increased incidence of respiratory viruses
- cohorting patients infected or colonized with resistant microorganisms
- nursing practices: semirecumbent position for ventilated patients, mouth care
- use of non-invasive ventilation instead of mechanical ventilation in appropriate patients
- care of medical equipment: ventilator circuits, suction devices, pulmonary function testing equipment
- avoiding overcrowding and understaffing
- avoiding H_2 antagonists
- judicious use of antibiotics
- immunization practices (as described above for CAP).

Acknowledgements

The authors wish to thank Katarzyna Jończyk-Potoczna MD, PHD for her excellent assistance with radiological examinations.

Author details

Irena Wojsyk-Banaszak and Anna Bręborowicz

*Address all correspondence to: iwojsyk@ump.edu.pl

Department of Pulmonology, Pediatric Allergy and Clinical Immunology, Karol Marcinkowski University of Medical Sciences, Szpitalna, Poznań, Poland

References

[1] World Health Organization. Pneumonia. Fact sheet No. 331.2011. Available at www.who.int/mediacentre/factsheets/fs331/en. Accessed 03.08.2012

[2] Singh V, Aneja S. Pneumonia – management in the developing World. Pediatr Respir Rev 2011;12:52-59

[3] Senstad AC, Suren P, Brauteset L, Eriksson JR, Hoiby EA, Wathne KO. Community acquired pneumonia (CAP) in children in Oslo. Norway. Acta Paediatr 2009;98:332-336

[4] Clark JE, Hammal D, Hampton F, Spencer D, Parker L. Epidemiology of community acquired pneumonia in children seen in hospital. Epidemiol Infect 2007;135:262-9

[5] Myles PR, MC Keever TM, Pogson Z, Smith CJ, Hubbard RB. The incidence of pneumonia using data from a computerized general practice database. Epidemiol Infect 2009; 137:709-716

[6] Weigl JA, Puppe W, Belke O, Neususs J, Bagci F, Schmitt HJ. Population-based incidence of severe pneumonia in children in Kiel, Germany. Klin Pediatr 2005;217:211-9

[7] Harris M, Clark J, Coote N, Fletcher P, Harnden A, McKean M, Thomson A. on behalf of the British Thoracic Society Standards of Care Committee. British Thoracic Society guidelines for the management of community acquired pneumonia in children: update 2011. Thorax 2011; 66:ii1-ii23

[8] Grijalva CG. Recognising pneumonia burden through prevention. Vaccine 2009;27S:C6-C8

[9] Lee GE, Lorch SA, Sheffler-Collins S, Kronman MP, Shah SS. National hospitalization trends for pediatric pneumonia and associated complications. Pediatrics 2010;126:204-213

[10] Roxburgh CS, Youngson GG, Townend JA, Turner SW. Trends in pneumonia and empyema in Scottish children in the past 25 years. Arch Dis Child 2008;93:316-318

[11] Michelow IC, Olsen K, Lozano J, Rollins NK, Duffy LB, Ziegler T, Kauppila J, Leinonen M, McCracken GH Jr.. Epidemiology and clinical characteristic of community acquired pneumonia in hospitalized children. Pediatrics 2004;113:701-7

[12] Virkki R, Juven T, Rikalainen H, Svedestrom E, Mertsola J, Ruuskanen O. Differentiation of bacterial and viral pneumonia in children. Thorax 2002;57:438-41

[13] Don M, Canciani M, Korppi M. Community – acquired pneumonia in children: what's old? What's new? Acta paediatrica 2010;99:1602-1608

[14] Principi N, Esposito S, Blasi F, Allegra L; Mowgli study group. Role of Mycoplasma pneumoniae and Chlamydia pneumoniae in children with community - acquired lower respiratory tract infections. Clin Infect Dis 2001;32:1281-9

[15] Baer G, Engelcke G, Able-Horn M, Schaad UB, Heininger U. Role of Chlamydia pneumoniae and Mycoplasma pneumoniae as causative agents of community – acquired pneumonia in hospitalised children and adolescents. Eur J Clin Microbiol Infect Dis 2003;22:742-5

[16] Tsolia MN, Psarras S, Bossios A, Audi H, Paldanius M, Gourgioyis D, Kallergi K, Kafetzis DA, Constantopoulos A, Papadopoulos NG. Etiology of community acquired pneumonia in hospitalized school-age children: Evidence for high prevalence of viral infections. Clin Infect Dis 2004;39:681-686

[17] Van der Poll T, Opal SM. Pathogenesis, treatment and prevention of pneumococcal pneumonia. Lancet 2009;274:1543-56

[18] Isaacman DJ, McIntosh ED, Reinert RR. Burden of invasive pneumococcal disease and serotype distribution among Streptococcus pneumoniae isolates in young children in Europe: impact of the 7-valent pneumococcal conjugate vaccine and considerations for future conjugate vaccines. Int J Infect Dis 2010;14:e197-209

[19] Bradley JS, Byington CL, Shah SS, Alverson B, Carter ER, Harrison C, Kaplan SL, Mace SE, McCracken GH Jr, Moore MR, St Peter SD, Stockwell JA, Swanson JT, Pediatric Infectious Diseases Society and the Infectious Diseases Society of America. The management of community – acquired pneumonia in infants and children older than 3 months of age: Clinical Practice Guidelines by the Pediatric Infectious Diseases Society and the Infectious Diseases Society of America. Published by Oxford University Press on behalf of the Infectious Diseases Society of America. DOI: 10.1093/cid/cir531

[20] Graham SM. Child pneumonia: current status, future prospects. Int J Tuberc Lung Dis 2010;14:1357-61

[21] Suzuki M, Thiem VD, Yanai H, Matsubayashi T, Yoshida L-M, Tho LH, Minh TT, Anh DD, Kilgore PE, Ariyoshi K. Association of environment tobacco smoking exposure with an increased risk of hospital admissions for pneumonia in children under 5 years of age in Vietnam. Thorax 2009; 64:484-489

[22] Talbot TR, Hartet TV, Mitchel E, Halasa N, Arbogast PG, Poehling KA, Schaffner W, Craig AS, Griffin MR. Asthma as a risk factor for invasive pneumococcal disease. N Engl J Med. 2005;352:2082-2090

[23] Coote N, McKenzie S. Diagnosis and investigation of bacterial pneumonia. Pediatric Respir Rev. 2000;1:8-13

[24] Mathews B, Shah S, Cleveland RH, Lee EY, Bachur RG, Neuman MI. Clinical predictors of pneumonia among children with wheezing. Pediatrics 2009;124:e29-36

[25] Cardoso MRA, Nascimento – Carvalho CM, Ferrero F, Alves F, Cousens SN. Adding fever to WHO criteria for diagnosing pneumonia enhances the ability to identify pneumonia cases among wheezing children. Arch Dis Child doi:10.1136/adc. 2010.189894

[26] Craig JC, Williams GJ, Jones M, Codarini M, Macaskill P, Hayen A, Irwig L, Fitzgerald DA, Isaacs D, McCaskill M. The accuracy of clinical symptoms and signs for the diagnosis of serious bacterial infection in young febrile children: prospective cohort study of 15 781 febrile illnesses. BMJ 2010;340:c1594

[27] Thomson AH. Treatment of community-acquired pneumonia in children. Clin Pulm Med 2008;15:283-292

[28] Light M.J. Pneumonia. In: Light M.J. (ed.) Pediatric Pulmonology. Policy of the American Academy of Pediatrics. American Academy of Pediatrics; 2011. p 392-421

[29] Don M, Valent F, Korppi M, Canciani M. Differentiation of bacterial and viral community – acquired pneumonia in children. Pediatr Int 2009;51:91-96

[30] Korppi M, Remes S, Heiskanen – Kosma T. Serum procalcitonin concentrations in bacterial pneumonia in children: a negative result in primary healthcare settings. Pediatr Pulm 2003;35:56-61

[31] Khan DA, Rahman A, Khan FA. Is procalcitonin better than C-reactive protein for early diagnosis of bacterial pneumonia in children? J Clin Lab Anal 2010;24 (1):1-5

[32] Flood RG, Badik J, Aronoff SC. The utility of serum C- reactive protein in differentiating bacterial from non-bacterial pneumonia in children: a meta-analysis of 1230 children. Pediatr Infect Dis J 2008;27:95-9

[33] Schuetz P, Christ-Crain M, Thomann R, Falconnier C, Wolbers M, Widmer I, Neidert S, Fricker T, Blum C, Schild U, Regez K, Schenenberger R, Henzez C, Bregenzer T, Hoess C, Krause M, Bucher HC, Zimmerli W, Mueller B. for the proHOSP Study Group. Effect of procalcitonin-based guidelines vs standard guidelines on antibiotic use in lower respiratory tract infections. The ProHOSP randomized controlled trial. JAMA 2009;302:1059-1066

[34] Muller F, Christ-Crain M, Bregenzer T, Krause M, Zimmerli W, Mueller B, Schuetz P, for the proHOSP Study Group. Procalcitonin levels predict bacteremia in patients with community – acquired pneumonia. CHEST 2010;138:121-129

[35] Sandora TJ, Harper MB. Pneumonia in hospitalized children. Pediatr Clin N Am 2005;52:1059-81

[36] Lahti E, Peltola V, Waris M, Virkki R, Rantakokko – Jalava K, Jalava J, Eerola E, Ruuskanen O. Induced sputum in the diagnosis of childhood community – acquired pneumonia. Thorax 2009;64:252-257

[37] Requejo HI, Guerra ML, Dos Santos M, Cocozza AM. Immunodiagnoses of community – acquired pneumonia in childhood. J Trop Pediatr 1997;43:208-12

[38] Le Monnier A, Carbonnelle E, Zahar JR, Le Bourgeois M, Abachin E, Quesne G, Varon E, Descamps P, De Blic J, Scheinmann P, Berche P, Ferroni A. Microbiological diagnosis of empyema in children: comparative evaluations by culture, polymerase chain reaction and pneumococcal antigen detection in pleural fluids. Clin Infect Dis 2006;42:1135-40

[39] Rello J, Lisboa T, Lujan M, Gallego M, Kee C, Kay I, Lopez D, Waterer GW; DNA-Neumococo Study Group. Severity of pneumococcal pneumonia associated with genomic bacterial load. Chest 2009;136:832-40

[40] Ferrero F, Nascimento – Carvalho CM, Cardoso MR, Camargos P, March M-Fp, Berezin E, Ruvinsky R, Sant'Anna C, Feris-Iglesias J, Maggi R, Benguigui Y, CARIBE group. Radiographic findings among children hospitalized with severe community – acquired pneumonia. Pediatr Pulm 2010;45:1009-13

[41] Vilar J, Domingo ML, Doto C, Cogollos J. Radiology of bacterial pneumonia. Eur J Radiol 2004;51:102-13

[42] Gibson NA, Hollman AS, Payton JY. Value of radiological follow up of childhood pneumonia. BMJ 1993;307:1117

[43] Argawal D, Awasthi S, Kabra SK, Kaul A, Singhi S, Walter SD; ISCAP Study Group. Three day versus five day treatment with amoxicillin for non-severe pneumonia in young children: a multicentre randomized controlled trial BMJ 2004;328:791 (erratum BMJ 2004;328:1066)

[44] Quazi S. Clinical efficacy of 3 days versus 5 days of oral amoxicillin for treatment of childhood pneumonia: a multicentre double-blind trial. Lancet 2002;360:835-41

[45] Atkinson M, Lakhanpaul M, Smyth A. Comparison of oral amoxicillin and intravenous benzyl penicillin for community acquired pneumonia in children (PIVOT trial): a multicentre pragmatic randomized controlled equivalence trial. Thorax 2007;62:1102-6

[46] Balfour –Lynn IM, Abrahamson E, Cohen G, Hartley J, King S, Parikh D, Spencer D, Thomson AH, Urquhart D, on behalf of the Pediatric Pleural Diseases Subcommittee of the BTS Standards of Care Committee. BTS guidelines for the management of pleural infection in children. Thorax 2005;60(Suppl I):i1-i21

[47] Puligandla PS, Laberge JM. Respiratory infections: Pneumonia, lung abscess and empyema. Sem Pediatr Surg 2008;17:42-52

[48] Li S-TT, Tancredi DJ. Empyema hospitalization increased in US children despite pneumococcal conjugate vaccine. Pediatrics 2010;125:26-33

[49] Byington CL, Spencer LY, Johnson TA, Pavia AT, Allen D, Mason EO, Kaplan S, Carroll KC, Daly JA, Christenson JC, Samore MH. An epidemiological investigation of a sustained high rate of pediatric parapneumonic empyema: risk factors and microbiological associations. Clin Infect Dis 2002;34:434-40

[50] Lahti E, Peltola V, Virkki R, Alanen M, Ruuskanen O. Development of parapneumonic empyema in children. Acta Paediatr 2007:96:1686-92

[51] Buckingham SC, King MD, Miller ML. Incidence and etiologies of complicated parapneumonic effusions in children 1996 to 2001. Pediatr Infect Dis J 2003;22:499-504

[52] Barnes NP, Hull J, Thomson AH. Medical management of parapneumonic pleural disease. Pediatr Pulmon 2005;39:127-134

[53] Jaffe A, Balfour –Lynn IM. Management of empyema in children. Pediatr Pulmon 2005;40:148-156

[54] Carter E, Waldhausen J, Zhang W, Hoffman L, Redding G. Management of children with empyema: plural drainage is not always necessary. Pediatr Pulmon 2010;45:475-480

[55] Sonnappa S, Cohen G, Owens CM, van Doorn C, Cairns J, Stanojevic S, Elliott MJ, Jaffe A. Comparison of urokinase and video – assisted thoracoscopic surgery for treatment of childhood empyema. Am J Respir Crit Care Med 2006;174:221-227

[56] St Peter SD, Tsao K, Harrison C, Jackson MA, Spilde TL, Keckler SJ, Sharp SW, Andrews WS, Holcomb GW, Ostile DJ. Thoracoscopic decortications vs tube thoracostomy with fibrinolysis for empyema in children: a prospective, randomized trial. J Pediatr Surg 2009;44:106-111

[57] Yao C-T, Wu J-M, liu C-C, Wu M-H, Chuang H-Y, Wang J-N. Treatment of complicated parapneumonic pleural effusion with intrapleural streptokinase in children. Chest 2004;125:566-71

[58] Feola GP, Shaw CA, Coburn L. Management of complicated parapneumonic effusions in children. Techniques Vasc Radiol 2003;6:197-204

[59] Jamal M, Reebye SC, Zamakhshary M, Skarsgard ED, Blair GK. Can we predict the failure of thoracostomy tube drainage in the treatment of pediatric parapneumonic collections? J Ped Surg 2005;40:838-41

[60] Margenthaler JA, Weber TR, Keller TS. Predictors of surgical outcome for complicated pneumonia in children: impact of bacterial virulence. World J Surg 2004;28:87-91

[61] Crawford SE, Daum RS. Bacterial pneumonia, Lung Abscess and Empyema. In: Taussig LM, Landau LI. Pediatric respiratory medicine, Mosby Elsevier. Philadelphia 2008:501-553

[62] Patradoon-Ho P, Fitzgerald DA. Lung abscess in children. Pediatr Resp Rev 2007;8:77-84

[63] Leonardi S, del Giudice MM, Spicuzza L, Saporito M, Nipitella G, La Rossa M. Lung abscess in a child with Mycoplasma pneumoniae infection. Eur J Pediatr 2010;169:1413-1415

[64] Sawicki GS, Lu FL, Valim C, Cleveland RH, Colin AA. Necrotising pneumonia is an increasingly detected complication of pneumonia in children. Eur Respir J 2008;31:1285-1291

[65] Hacimustafaoglu M, Celebi S, Sarimehmet H, Gurpinar A, Ercan I. Necrotizing pneumonia in children. Acta Paediatr 2004;93:1172-1177

[66] Bender JM, Ampofo K, Korgenski K, Daly J, Pavia AT, Mason EO, Byington CL. Pneumococcal necrotizing pneumonia in Utah: Does serotype matter? Clin Infect Dis 2008;46:1346-52

[67] Hsieh Y-C, Hsiao C-H, Tsao P-N, Wang J-Y, Hsueh P-R, Chiang B-L, Lee W-S, Huang L-M. Necrotizing pneumococcal pneumonia in children: the role of pulmonary gangrene. Pediatr Pulmonol 2006;41:623-629

[68] American Academy of Pediatrics. Policy statement – modified recommendations for use of palivizumab for prevention of respiratory syncytial virus infections

[69] American Academy of Pediatrics. Policy statement – Recommendations for the prevention of Streptococcus pneumoniae Infections in Infants and Children: Use of 13-Valent Pneumococcal Conjugate Vaccine (PCV13) and Pneumococcal Polysaccharide Vaccine (PPSV23). Pediatrics DOI: 10.1542/peds.2010-1280

[70] Ruckinger S, von Kries R, Siedler A, van der Linden M. Association of serotype of Streptococcus pneumonia with risk of severe and fatal outcome. Pediatr Infect Dis J 2009;28:118-122

[71] Tan TQ, Mason EO Jr, Wald ER, Barson WJ, Schutze GE, Bradley JS, Givner LB, Yogev R, Kim KS, Kaplan SL. Clinical characteristic of children with complicated pneumonia caused by Streptococcus pneumonia. Pediatrics 2002;110:1-6

[72] McCullers JA. Insights into the interaction between influenza virus and Pneumococcus. Clin Microb Rev 2006;19:571-582

[73] Prayle A, Atkinson M, Smyth A. Pneumonia in the developed world. Pediatr Resp Rev 2011:12;60-69

[74] Wexler ID, Knoll S, Picard E, Villa Y, Shoseyov D, Engelhard D, Kerem E. Clinical characteristics and outcome of complicated pneumococcal pneumonia in pediatric population. Pediatr Pulmon 2006;41:726-734

[75] Gonzalez BE, Hulten KG, Dishop MK, Lamberth LB, Hammerman WA, Mason EO Jr, Kaplan SL. Pulmonary manifestations in children with invasive community acquired Staphylococcus aureus infection. Clin Infect Dis 2005;41:583-90

[76] Defres S, Marwick C, Nathwani D. MRSA as a cause of lung infection including airway infection, community-acquired pneumonia and hospital acquired pneumonia. Eur Resp J 2009;34:1470-1476

[77] Shilo N, Quach C. Pulmonary infections and community associated methicillin resistant Staphylococcus aureus: A dangerous mix? Pediatr Respir Rev 2011;12:182-189

[78] Creech CB, Kernodle DS, Alsentzer A, Wilson C, Edwards KM. Increasing rates of nasal carriage of methicillin-resistant Staphylococcus aureus in healthy children. Pediatr Infect Dis J 2005;24:617-621

[79] Holmes A, Ganner M, McGuane S, Pitt TL, Cookson BD, Kearns AM. Staphylococcus aureus isolates carrying Panton – Valentine leukocidin genes in England and Wales: frequency, characterization and association with clinical disease. J Clin Microbiol 2005;43:2384-90

[80] Wallin TR, Hern G, Frazee BW. Community – associated methicillin resistant Staphylococcus aureus. Emerg Med Clin North Am. 2008;26:431-55

[81] Shehab ZM. Mycoplasma Infections. In: Taussig LM, Landau LI. Pediatric respiratory medicine, Mosby Elsevier. Philadelphia 2008:615-620

[82] Tamura A, Matsubara K, Tanaka T, Nigami H, Yura K, Fukuya T. Methylprednisolone pulse therapy for refractory Mycoplasma pneumoniae pneumonia in children. J Infect 2008;57:223-228

[83] American Thoracic Society Documents. An official statement of the American Thoracic Society and the Infectious Diseases Society of America. Guidelines for the management of Adults with hospital – acquired, ventilator associated and healthcare – associated pneumonia. Am J Respir Crit Care Med 2005;171:388-416

[84] Rotstein C, Evans G, Born A, Grossman R, Light RB, Magder S, McTaggart B, Weiss K, Zhanel GG. Clinical practice guidelines for hospital – acquired pneumonia and ventilator-associated pneumonia in adults. Can J Infect Dis Med Microbiol 2008;19:19-53

[85] Zar HJ, Cotton MF. Nosocomial pneumonia in pediatric patients. Practical problems and rational solutions. Pediatr Drugs 2002;4:73-83

[86] Bigham MT, Amato R, Bondurrant P, Fridriksson J, Krawczeski CD, Raake J, Ryckman S, Schwartz S, Shaw J, Wells D, Brill RJ. Ventilator – associated pneumonia in the pediatric intensive care unit: characterizing the problem and implementing a sustainable solution. J Pediatr 2009;154:582-7

[87] Foglia E, Meier MD, Elward A. Ventilator – associated pneumonia in neonatal and pediatric intensive care unit patients. Cil Microbiol Rev 2007;20:409-425

[88] Srinivasan R, Asselin J, Gildengorin G, Wiener-Kronish J, Flori HR. A prospective study of ventilator – associated pneumonia. Pediatrics 2009;123:1108-1115

[89] Raymond J, Aujard Y. European Study Group. Nosocomial infections in pediatric patients: a European, multicenter prospective study. Infect Control Hosp Epidemiol 2000;21:260-263

[90] Richards MJ, Edwards JR, Culver DH, Gaynes RP. Nosocomial infections in pediatric intensive care units in the United States. National Nosocomial Infections Surveillance System. Pediatrics 1999;103:E39

[91] Elward AM, Warren DK, Fraser VJ. Ventilator-associated pneumonia in pediatric intensive care unit patients: risk factors and outcomes. Pediatrics 2002;109:758-764

[92] Horan TC, Andrus M, Dudeck MA. CDC/NHS surveillance definition of health care –associated infection and criteria for specific types of infections in the acute care setting. Am J Infect Control 2008;36:309-32

[93] Gauvin F, Dassa C, Chaibou M, Proulx F, Farrel CA, Lacroix J. Ventilator-associated pneumonia in intubated children: comparison of different diagnostic methods. Pediatr Crit Care Med 2003;4:437-443

[94] Toltzis P, Hoyen C, Spinner – Block S, Salvator AE, Rice LB. Factors that predict preexisting colonization with antibiotic – resistant gram – negative bacilli in patients admitted to a pediatric intensive care unit. Pediatrics 1999;103:719-723

[95] Labenne M, Poyart C, Rambaud C, Goldfarb B, Pron B, Jouvet P, Delamare C, Sebag G, Hubert P. Blind protected specimen brush and bronchoalveolar lavage in ventilated children. Crit Care Med 1999; 27:2537-2543

[96] Masterton RG, Galloway A, French G, Street M, Armstrong J, Brown E, Cleverley J, Dilworth P, Fry C, Gascoigne AD, Knox A, Nathwanii D, Spencer R, Wilcox M. Guidelines for the management of hospital acquired pneumonia in the UK: report of the working party on hospital – acquired pneumonia of the British Society of Antimicrobial Chemotherapy. J Antimicrob Ther 2008;62:5-34

Chapter 7

Cystic Fibrosis Pulmonary Exacerbation – Natural History, Causative Factors and Management

Iara Maria Sequeiros and Nabil Jarad

Additional information is available at the end of the chapter

http://dx.doi.org/10.5772/54336

1. Introduction

Cystic Fibrosis (CF) is the most common life-threatening inherited disease in the United Kingdom, affecting over 9,000 people, 56% of which are 16 years or older (UK CF Registry Annual Data Report 2009). Life expectancy currently remains well below the general population, but with improvement of care most CF patients born after 1980 are expected to reach adulthood. Much of the morbidity and mortality associated with CF are related to the respiratory system (Goss & Burns, 2007).

Recurrent acute infective pulmonary exacerbations are one of the most important features of CF. Pulmonary exacerbations are common events throughout the lifetime of a patient with CF. Frequent exacerbations are associated with impaired quality of life and accelerated decline in lung function (Marshall, 2004; Britto et al., 2002; Liou et al., 2001; Ramsey, 1996). Statistical models have demonstrated that frequent pulmonary exacerbations are also associated with premature mortality (Liou et al., 2001).

Preventing and treating pulmonary exacerbations promptly and appropriately are therefore key therapeutic goals of the CF community that clinicians endeavour to employ in the effort to positively impact on long term outcomes, survival and quality of life of CF patients.

2. The pathophysiology of CF lung disease

Despite CF being one of the most studied and understood genetic diseases, the exact pathophysiology of recurrent CF pulmonary exacerbations is still not completely understood. The most accepted hypothesis to explain how the primary defect in CF, the mutations in the cystic fibrosis transmembrane conductance regulator gene (CFTR), leads to the colonisation of the airways by bacteria, chronic infection and inflammation and ultimately airway injury is the "low volume hypothesis" (Boucher, 2004).

The airways are covered by airway surface liquid, composed by two separate fluid layers, a superficial mucus layer and an underlying lubricating pericellular environment near the cell surface. A thin layer of surfactant separates the mucus and the periciliary fluid layer (figure 1).

The mucus layer is produced by goblet cells and submucosal glands and is composed of water, carbohydrates, proteins and lipids, extending from the intermediate airways to the upper airways. It normally is composed of a network of mucous glycoproteins or mucin. Its adhesive characteristic means that the mucus layer binds and traps deposited particles and its viscoelastic properties facilitate cilia movement into transporting mucus and also its clearance by cough. Mucus containing cellular debris and possible trapped microorganisms is transported from the lower respiratory tract to the pharynx by mucociliary clearance and air flow (Rubin, 2002). Mucus clearance is considered a most important innate airway defence mechanism (Randell & Boucher, 2006; Knowles & Boucher, 2002), and disruption of the normal mucus secretion and mucociliary clearance impairs lung defence and increases the risk of infection.

The periciliary fluid provides a watery environment that enables the cilia to beat and propel the mucus away towards the upper airways. Appropriate clearance and hygiene maintenance of the respiratory tract requires coordinated interaction of the mucus and periciliary layers and for this to be effective, adequate hydration of the near-cell airway surface is critical.

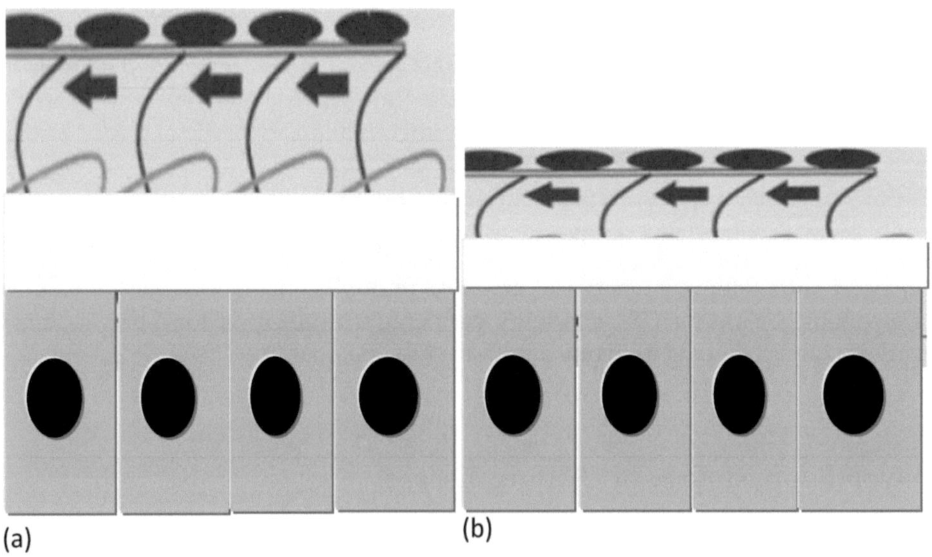

Figure 1. The fluid surface area in normal patients (a) and in patients with CF (b). The epithelial cells are covered by two layers of fluid – a serous layer (white band) and a mucous layer (grey area). In CF patients and due to the disease process, both layers shrink and the shape of the cilia and its movement are adversely affected.

The volume of the periciliary airway surface fluid is normally precisely regulated and is critical for efficient mucus flow and elimination. In the normal airway epithelium, the amount of fluid is determined by a combination of ion channels that promote the secretion of salt and water, such as the CFTR and alternative anion channels, and others that promote absorption of sodium and fluid, such as epithelial sodium channels (ENaC) in the apical cell membrane. The CFTR also acts as a conductance regulator, influencing and down regulating the latter.

In the CF epithelium, in consequence of the CFTR mutations, the CFTR gene product is faulty, whilst in normal conditions it is a transmembrane protein that functions as a chloride channel. The CFTR down regulatory function of ENaC activity is absent or compromised, resulting in abnormal ion transport properties due to the combined defects of accelerated sodium transport and failure to secrete chloride, resulting in overall increased absorption of sodium and fluid from the airway surface and consequently reduced, low volume of the airway surface liquid (Guggino & Guggino, 2000).

The loss of functional height of the periciliary layer in which the cilia beat, defined by the length of extended cilia, interferes with cilia motion and causes impaired ciliary function, resulting in slower mucociliary clearance with accumulation of mucus with trapped debris, microorganisms and airway secretory products, such as cytokines (e.g., interleukin-8), neutrophil proteases and growth factors that promote airway inflammation and mucus cell hyperplasia. In consequence of increased number of mucus secreting goblet cells, there is persistent mucin secretion, which generates high volume of thick, inspissated mucus, which adheres to and obstructs the airways and is resistant to cough clearance and is an ideal site and reservoir for bacterial growth. The poor liquid content and hypoxic environment in these thick mucus plaques promote biofilm bacterial formation and bacterial overgrowth.

Mucus stasis and the presence of accumulated secretory products and bacteria triggers the recruitment of neutrophils to the airways and the release of pro-inflammatory cytokines, which lead to a vicious cycle of inflammation, airway obstruction, chronic infection, repeated pulmonary exacerbations and resultant airway tissue damage and loss of lung function (Frizzell & Pilewski, 2004).

3. Microbiology in the CF lung disease and relationship with pulmonary exacerbations

Pulmonary exacerbations in CF are caused by recognised typical pathogens that are acquired following a characteristic age-dependent pattern (figure 2). Whilst still very young, CF patients suffer their first infections most frequently caused by *Staphylococcus aureus* and *Haemophilus influenzae*. *S. aureus* is often the first organism isolated from children with CF, but the role of this bacteria in the pathogenesis of CF remains under debate as studies reveal conflicting results in regards to clinical benefits from anti-staphylococcal therapy (Smyth & Walters, 2003; Lyczak et al., 2002). Non-typeable *H. influenzae* is also commonly cultured from CF children as early as in their first year of life, but although it can cause exacerbations in patients with non-CF bronchiectasis (Barker, 2002), its role in CF is still unclear (Goss & Burns, 2007).

Other relevant pathogens in CF usually cultured later in the course of the disease include *Burkholderia cepacia* complex, *Stenotrophomonas maltophilia* and *Achromobacter xylosoxidans*. The *B. cepacia* complex has at least 10 distinct genomovars and is related with rapid clinical deterioration. The most virulent and transmissible form is the genomovar III, B. cenocepacia, due to its well recognised association with severe necrotising pneumonia and death first described over 20 years ago (Isles et al., 1984). *S. maltophilia* and *A. xylosoxidans* are more prevalent than the *B. cepacia* complex, but seem to be less virulent, although their role in the pathogenesis of the CF lung is not yet completely understood (Goss et al., 2002).

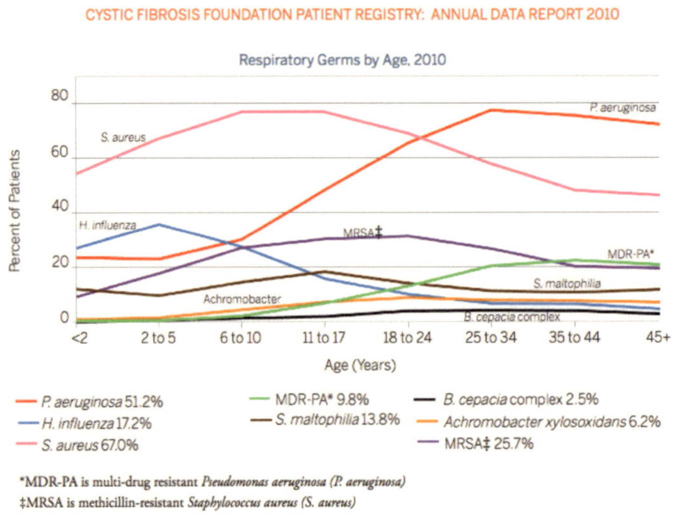

Figure 2. Prevalence of respiratory pathogens according to patient's age. Data from Cystic Fibrosis Foundation Patient Registry, 2010 Annual Data Report.

Pseudomonas aeruginosa is considered to be the most important pathogen in CF. By the time patients reach adulthood, up to 80% of them become infected with *P. aeruginosa*. The transformation of *P. aeruginosa* from the non-mucoid to the mucoid strains, which often occurs during adolescence years (figure 3a), is pivotal and is known to be associated with clinical (figure 3b) and radiological deterioration (figure 3c) (Li et al., 2005). At initial colonisation, *P. aeruginosa* presents a phenotype similar to environmental strains, but this changes dramatically with time and prolonged infection as *P. aeruginosa* has the potent ability of quorum sensing which leads to biofilm formation (Drenkard & Ausubel, 2002). Biofilm is a matrix of proteins, carbohydrate and collagen and muco-polysaccharide within which the bacteria reside. This layer is often called alginate formation. The formation of alginate biofilm has 3 important consequences:

1. The bacteria are protected from antibiotics, which increases the minimal-inhibitory concentration.
2. The film reduces the activity of aminoglycosides and beta-lactam antibiotics by changing the pH of the respiratory mucosa and by production of beta-lactamase – ironically,

http://dx.doi.org/10.5772/54336

mucoid *P. aeruginosa* tend to exhibit greater in vivo sensitivity to antibiotics than non-mucoid strains in the same patient.

3. The biofilm formation is highly immunogenic and tends to accelerate structural lung damage leading to significant histological and radiological changes.

The incidence and clinical impact of mucoid *P. aeruginosa* (figure 3a) in the sputum of a cohort of patients with CF according to age. The emergence of these bacteria is associated with decline in FEV1 (figure 3b) and worsening of radiograph appearance (figure 3c). (Adapted from Li et al., 2005).

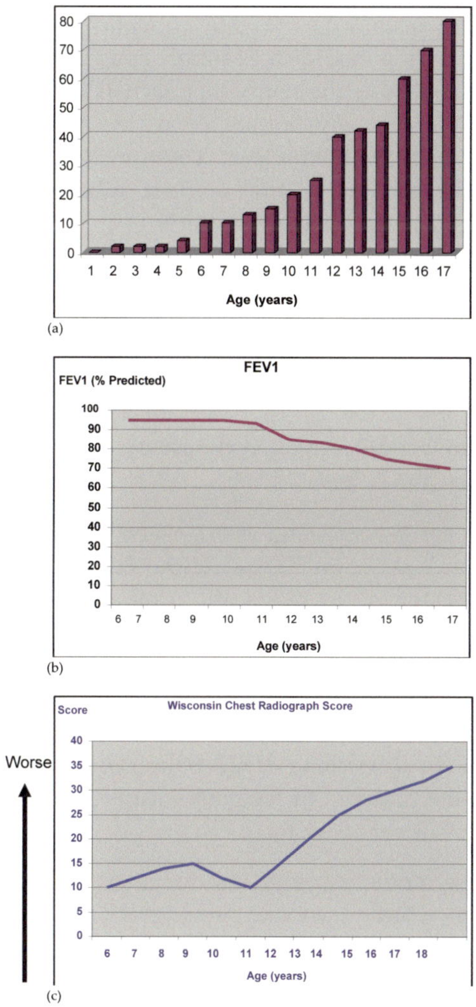

Figure 3. (a): Proportion (%) of *P. aeruginosa* with mucoid strains per age group. (b): Change in FEV1 for the same CF group as in 3a. (c): Change in the chest radiograph appearance in the same CF group as in 3a

4. Acute pulmonary exacerbations in CF

Pulmonary exacerbations in CF are an important feature of the disease. Frequency of pulmonary exacerbations is associated with accelerated decline in lung function tests, impaired quality of life and premature mortality. Nevertheless, defining what constitutes a pulmonary exacerbation remains controversial.

To date there is not yet a consensus or a standardised diagnostic criteria as to what clinically characterises pulmonary exacerbations in CF (Abbot et al., 2009; Dakin et al., 2001), but all descriptions point to that patients present with a combination of symptoms. Although, not stated clearly, the implication is that symptoms during exacerbations are greater than symptoms during 'disease stability'.

Pulmonary exacerbations are usually described by patients in subjective terms as an increase in one or more respiratory symptoms, such as cough, sputum volume, viscosity and colour change, breathlessness; altered systemic symptoms, such as increased fatigue, decreased appetite and energy levels. This is usually, but not always associated with an increase in objective clinical signs and changes in biomarkers. These included: weight loss, tachypnoea, tachycardia, decreased lung function parameters, chest radiographic changes and raised serum inflammatory markers (Ramsey et al., 1999; Fuchs et al., 1994).

The lack of a standardised definition is also present when it comes to classifying pulmonary exacerbations according to their severity. Pulmonary exacerbations are broadly divided into: a) mild exacerbations requiring treatment with oral antibiotics and b) severe exacerbations needing treatment with intravenous (IV) antibiotics. It also remains unclear if mild exacerbations are the originators of severe infections, if they are earlier milder versions of severe pulmonary exacerbations or in fact differentiated clinical episodes with no correlation between mild and severe infections (Goss & Burns, 2007).

Despite the lack of agreement, several diagnostic systems are described in the literature and used in CF clinical trials, such as the Fuchs et al. (1994) Pulmozyme® study and the Ramsey et al. (1999) inhaled Tobramycin study diagnostic criteria, and the consensus document by the US CF Foundation, 1994 (tables 1, 2 and 3).

These definitions, often called "symptom-related definitions", although widely used, have 3 shortcomings:

1. They do not account for differences of CF pulmonary exacerbations in children and adults. For example, the presence of fever and acute changes in chest radiographs are often seen in children, but not in adults.
2. They do not quantify symptom severity and do not give allowance for increased severity of a single symptom, which may make patients seek medical consultation and receive treatment. For example, marked increase in breathlessness, significant increase in cough production of viscous sputum or increased lethargy alone could be a single symptom that may constitute an exacerbation requiring treatment with antibiotics.
3. The above definitions do not stipulate that increase in symptoms should be sustained and should be beyond the natural fluctuation of symptoms encountered in most CF patients.

http://dx.doi.org/10.5772/54336

- Increased cough
- Dyspnoea or increased respiratory rate
- Change in appearance of sputum (i.e. consistency, increased purulence or volume)
- Lassitude and decreased exercise tolerance
- Decreased appetite
- Absenteeism from work or place of education
- Fever (>38°C)
- Progressive physical findings (crackles or wheeze) on chest auscultation
- New infiltrate on the chest X-ray
- Deterioration of 10% or more of the highest FEV1 measured in the last 6 months

Table 1. Signs and symptoms of pulmonary exacerbations as agreed by the consensus document of the US Cystic Fibrosis Foundation, 1994. Typically a combination of 3 or more signs and symptoms represent a pulmonary exacerbation.

- Change in sputum
- New or increased haemoptysis
- Increased cough
- Increased dyspnoea
- Malaise, fatigue, or lethargy
- Temperature above 38°C
- Anorexia or weight loss
- Sinus pain or tenderness
- Change in sinus discharge
- Change in physical examination of the chest
- Decrease in pulmonary function by 10% or more from a previously recorded value
- Radiographic changes indicative of pulmonary infection

Table 2. Fuchs et al. (1994) Pulmozyme Study: "Exacerbation of respiratory symptoms": a patient treated with parenteral antibiotics for any 4 of the following 12 signs or symptoms:

- Fever (oral temperature >38°C)
- More frequent coughing (increase of 50%)
- Increased sputum volume (increase of 50%)
- Loss of appetite
- Weight loss of at least 1 kg
- Absence from school or work (at least 3 or preceding 7 days) due to illness
- Symptoms of upper respiratory tract infection
- These symptoms had to have been associated with at least 1 of the following 3 additional criteria:
- Decrease in FVC of at least 10%
- An increase in respiratory rate of at least 10 breaths/min
- A peripheral blood neutrophil count of 15,000/mm3

Table 3. Ramsey et al. (1999) Inhaled Tobramycin Study: Pulmonary exacerbation indicated by at least 2 of the following 7 symptoms during the study.

In a retrospective analysis of 77 pulmonary exacerbations in 88 adult patients, the authors found that IV antibiotics were given to 18 patients (24.4%) whose symptoms did not meet the US CF criteria (table 1) (Jeffcote et al., 2004). This would suggest that nearly one quarter of patients presented with sufficiently severe symptoms to warrant treatment with IV antibiotics, although the combination of factors did not meet the pre-designed criteria.

For this reason, we explored another definition of pulmonary exacerbations, which resembled the internationally accepted definition of exacerbation in chronic obstructive pulmonary disease (COPD). In such patients, pulmonary exacerbations are defined as "an event in the course of the disease in which there is a sustained worsening of the patient's respiratory symptoms from the stable state that is beyond normal day-to-day variations, that is acute in onset and necessitates escalation of treatment". This is often termed as "an action-definition" in which an exacerbation is regarded to be present when the following 3 criteria are met:

1. The increase in respiratory symptoms is sustained (lasting 2-3 days).
2. The symptoms are subjectively more than the patient's own baseline symptoms – enough so that the patient seeks medical treatment.
3. The symptoms are objectively compelling to the physicians as to be deemed to require escalation of treatment with antibiotics.

This definition has its problems too. Patients have different thresholds for seeking medical care and therefore some may present more frequently than others, despite similar severity of symptoms. Another problem is that in countries where patients have to pay for their treatment, financial restraint may prevent patients from seeking medical treatment for exacerbation of symptoms.

To try to resolve this issue, Sarfaraz et al. (2010) conducted a study using electronic remote daily telemonitoring of symptoms in a cohort of adult CF patients. The study highlighted several issues in the management of CF exacerbations. Out of the 51 patients enrolled in the study, 32 (63%) patients were subsequently excluded as their recordings were not frequent enough to form a baseline data or insufficient to look into the natural history of the disease (Figure 4). Furthermore, for the remaining 19 patients who completed the study, an average of only 60% of the total number of study days was recorded.

Despite these significant deficiencies, there were enough CF pulmonary exacerbations for analyses. The authors noticed that 75% of all CF exacerbations had a "prodromal" phase in which one or more than one symptom increased in the 2 weeks prior to exacerbations (Figure 5).

In order to examine whether the problem with daily recording was related to the introduction of a modern system, a parallel study in COPD patients was carried out (Sund et al., 2009). A systematic comparison between the 2 groups was later published (Jarad & Sund, 2011). The comparison revealed that the dropout rate was much smaller for COPD patients, who recorded daily data in 77% of the total number of study days (figure 6). In accordance with the higher recording rate by COPD patients, the number of early exacerbations diagnosed was higher than that in CF patients and the number of hospitalisation was much reduced in COPD patients (but not in CF patients) compared to a similar period without daily monitoring the year prior to the study.

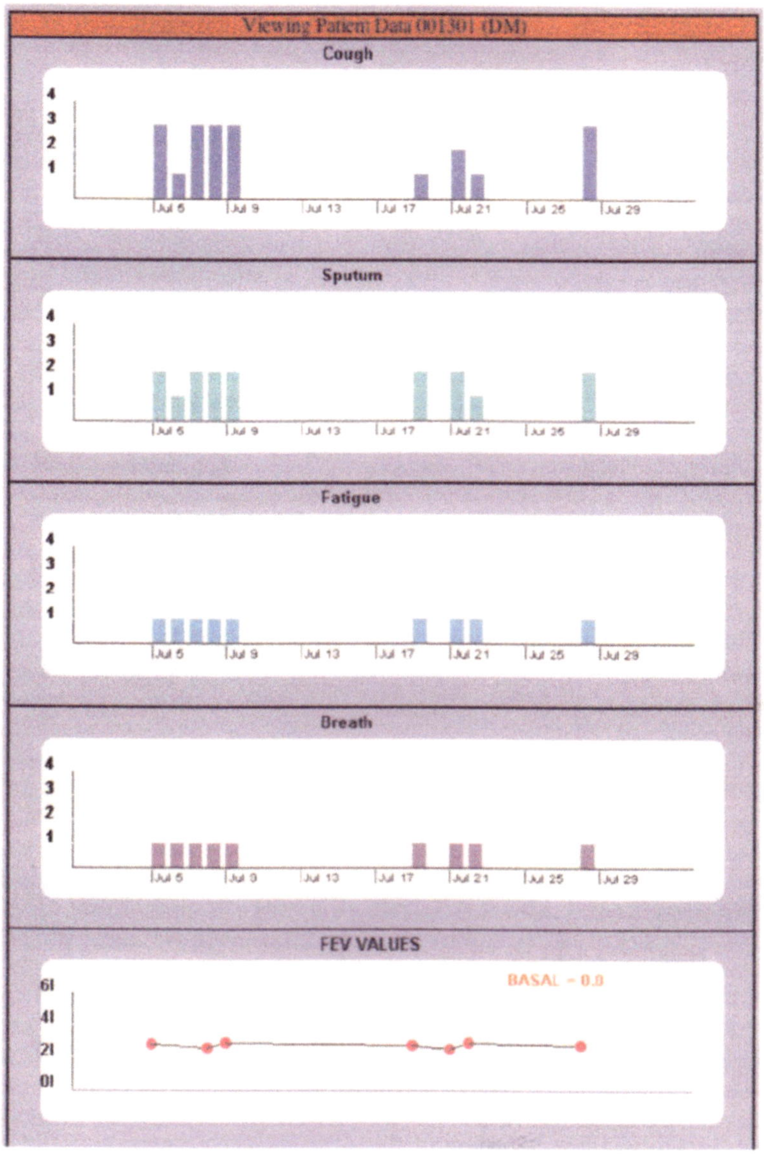

Figure 4. An example of the daily recording of a 23 male CF patient. The Y axis is the score of each symptom (cough, sputum, breathlessness and fatigue). For FEV1, the Y axis is the value in litres. The time line on the X axis is divided in weeks. Note that only 9 days were recorded by the patients out of possible 49 days (7 weeks). This patient was withdrawn from the study.

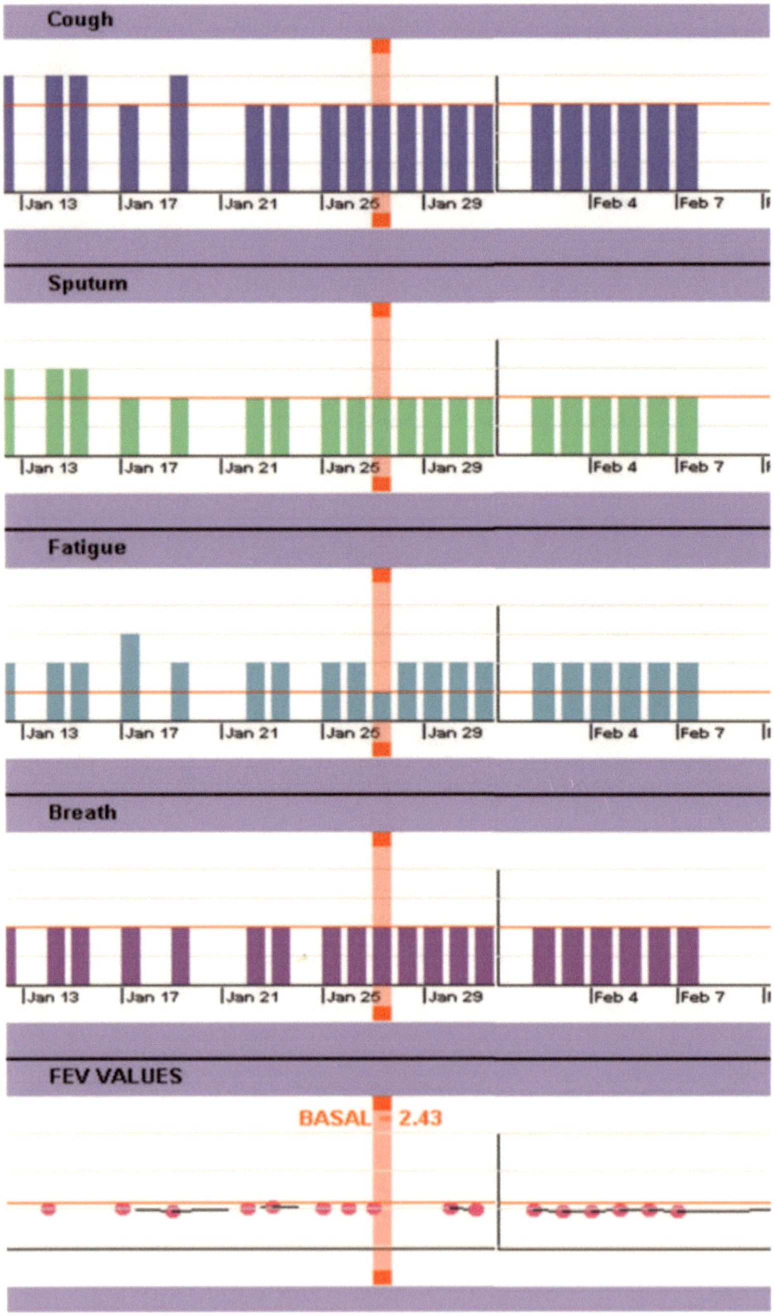

Figure 5. A 24 year old female CF patient who had a pulmonary exacerbation (marked with the red vertical line) defined by the decline in FEV_1. Note that there was a "prodromal phase" manifested by increase in cough and fatigue within the 2 weeks prior to the exacerbation.

http://dx.doi.org/10.5772/54336

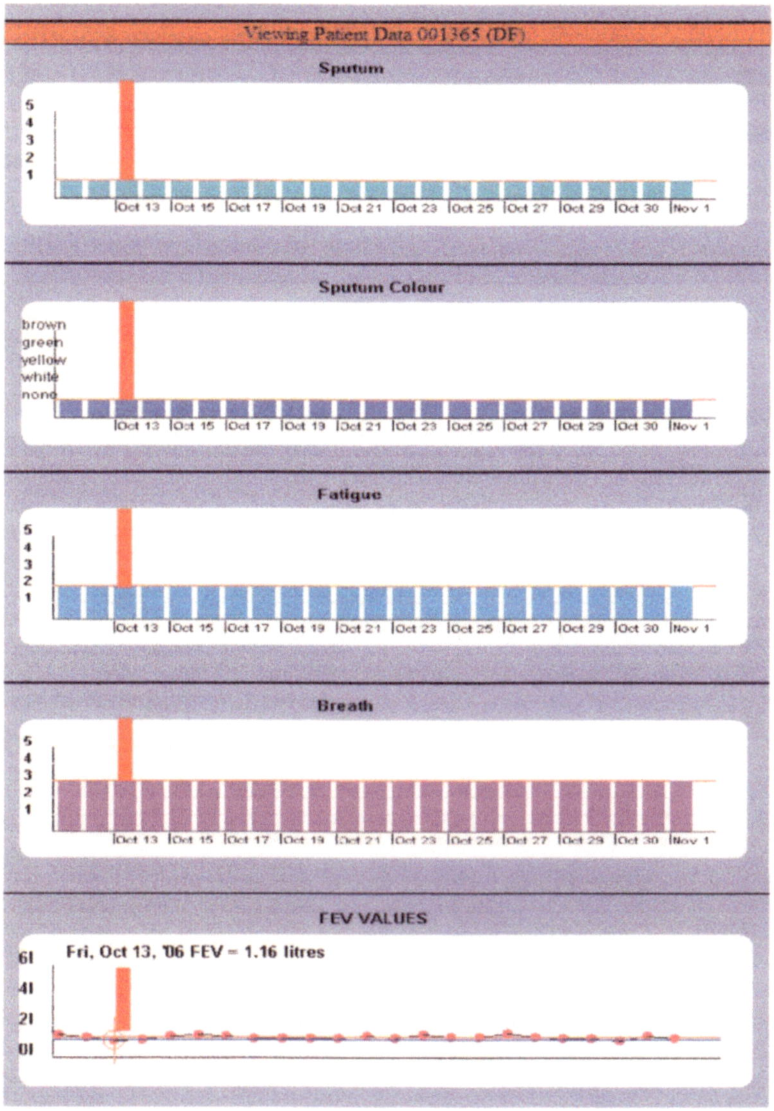

Figure 6. A recording from a patient with COPD. The red line represents an exacerbation defined as 15% decline in FEV1 below the baseline. Note the patient performed a daily recording without interruption allowing a proper identification of acute exacerbation.

Differences between the two groups may not only reflect differences in disease processes and age groups. They may also disclose the differences in the system of care for CF patients who tend to have a privileged access to hospital care through direct contact with a CF multidisciplinary team. This is not available to COPD patients, whose contact with healthcare takes place through a general practitioner.

5. Causes of pulmonary exacerbations

Whilst still not completely understood, causes of pulmonary exacerbations are most likely multi-factorial, and may differ amongst patients.

Nevertheless, CF pulmonary exacerbations are probably a consequence of a loss of equilibrium between host defence mechanisms and the airway microorganisms. It is believed that viruses, including respiratory syncytial virus, have a role in pulmonary exacerbations (Hiatt et al., 1999), and whilst these have also been associated with the acquisition of new organisms, for the majority of adult CF patients a new pulmonary exacerbations seems to be caused much more commonly by a clonal expansion of already present colonising bacteria (Aaron et al., 2004).

Only rarely are pulmonary exacerbations a consequence of newly acquired bacteria. The increase in bacterial load in conjunction with an inflammatory response of the airways result in a local influx of polymorphonucleocytes and the release of inflammatory mediators such as interleukins – (IL) 8, 6, 1β, tumour necrosis factor alpha (TNF-α), leukotriene B4 and free neutrophil elastase.

Treatment with antimicrobial agents is associated with decreased levels of inflammatory mediators and bacterial density and improvement of symptoms and lung function parameters (Colombo et al., 2005; Ordonez et al., 2003; Sagel et al., 2001; Bonfield et al., 1995; Konstan et al., 1994; Konstan et al., 1993). This suggests that the increased density of microbes plays an important role in pulmonary exacerbations. What remains unclear is the lack of ability of powerful antibiotics given at great doses in eradicating pulmonary microbes in CF patients. Rather it would seem that the role of antibiotics is akin to cutting the grass in a front garden lawn, only for the grass to grow again.

6. Epidemiology and risk factors

CF pulmonary exacerbations are common and the impact they have on patient care, especially in terms of labour intensiveness, is the main reason for the establishment of CF centres and teams. In addition, treatment of pulmonary exacerbations accounts for a significant part of the cost of CF care.

In a cross sectional study on adult CF patients in the South West of England, Jarad & Giles (2008) found that a significant number of patients did not suffer from any pulmonary exacerbation. Many patients, however, suffered from at least one exacerbation every year (figure 7). When examining risk factors of exacerbations, reduced FEV1 (figure 8), infection with *P. aeruginosa* (figure 9) and cystic fibrosis related diabetes (CFRD) were correlated with increased rate of exacerbations (figure 10) (adapted from Jarad & Giles, 2008). Remarkably, genetic profile, diagnostic sweat chloride, body mass index, age and gender did not correlate with frequency of pulmonary exacerbations.

In addition, this study concords with previous studies that have demonstrated factors associated with pulmonary exacerbations, such as young age, female gender, lower FEV1, CFRD and previous history of multiple exacerbations (Block et al., 2006; Marshall et al., 2005).

Conversely inhaled antibiotics such as aminoglycosides, oral macrolides, mucolytics and inhaled hypertonic saline have been shown to reduce the rate of pulmonary exacerbations (Gibson et al., 2003; Saiman et al., 2003; Ramsey et al. 1999; Fuchs et al., 1994), presumably by reducing the bacterial load and inflammation and clearing the airways, reducing the volume of retained secretions.

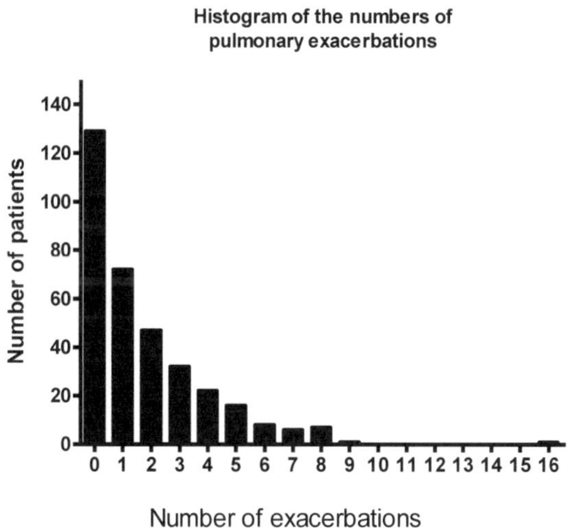

Figure 7. A histogram of the number of exacerbations experienced in one year by 680 patients in the South West of England.

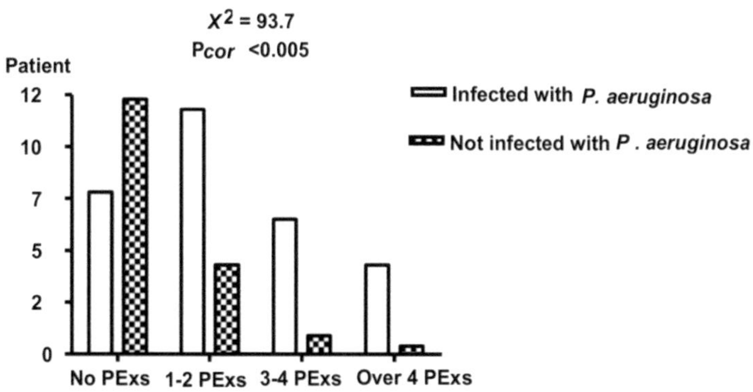

Figure 8. Patients with and without chronic infection with *P. aeruginosa* in 4 annual exacerbations category. Note that the proportion of those who are infected is greater with increased frequency of annual exacerbations. PExs = number of pulmonary exacerbations per year.

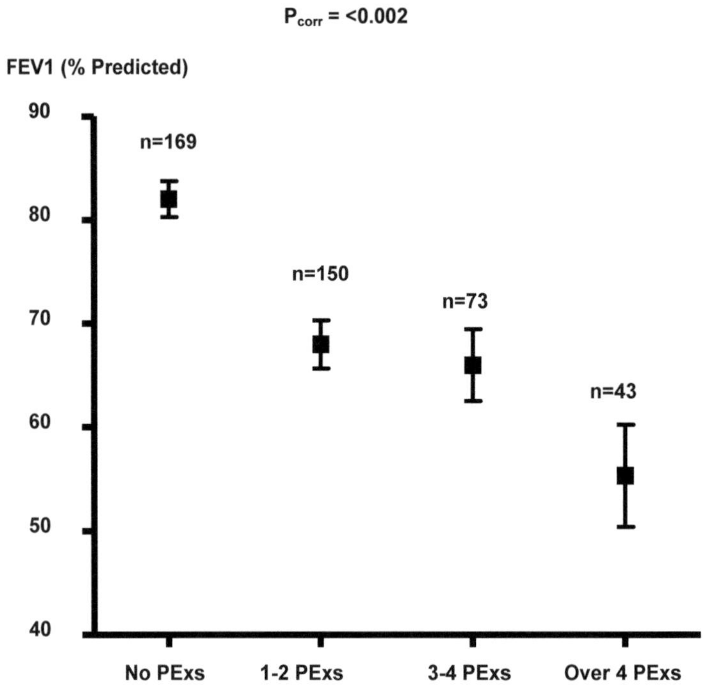

Figure 9. Annual exacerbation frequency increases in patients with lower FEV1. N = number of patients per group. PExs = number of pulmonary exacerbations per year.

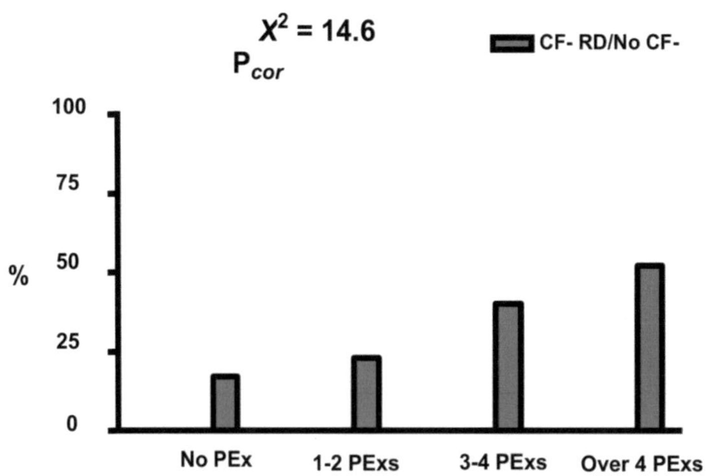

Figure 10. Proportion of patients with CFRD and without CFRD according to annual exacerbation frequency. PExs = number of pulmonary exacerbations per year.

7. What affects the time until the subsequent CF pulmonary exacerbations?

Time from the end of one pulmonary exacerbation until the subsequent exacerbation (time until the next exacerbation) is a significant health outcome and one of the significant end points in many CF clinical trials. Shorter periods until the following exacerbation is a marker of increased impact of disease on patients. In a prospective study on 170 exacerbations in 58 adult CF patients, (Sequeiros & Jarad, 2012), the median time until subsequent exacerbations was 112 days, although this varied considerably (figure 11).

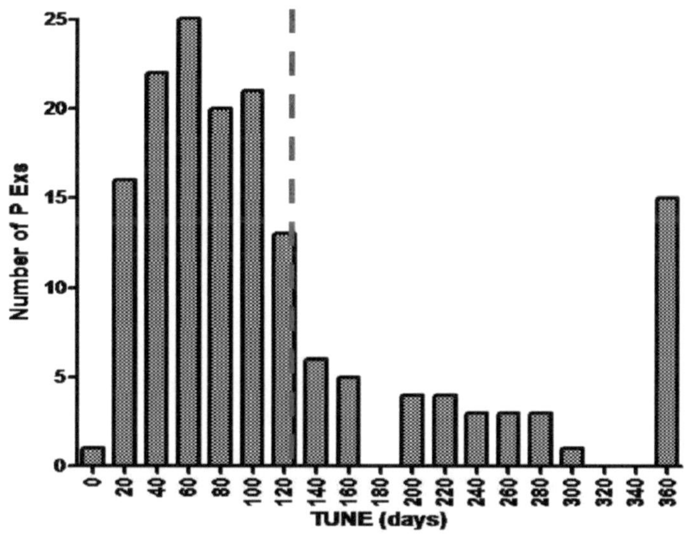

Figure 11. A histogram of time until the next exacerbation on the X axis. Median time (red vertical line) was 121 days, although this varied considerably. Those patients who did not have an exacerbation during the subsequent year after the first pulmonary exacerbation were regarded to have a time until the next exacerbation of 360 days (adapted from Sequeiros & Jarad, 2012).

Factors affecting shorter periods until the following pulmonary exacerbation were examined, including age, lung disease severity, CF related complications (CFRD, allergic broncho-pulmonary aspergillosis (ABPA)), chronic infection with *P. aeruginosa* and site of administration of antibiotics – either home or in hospital. In addition, symptom scores, lung function tests and inflammatory biomarkers at the end of the IV treatment were examined.

When analysing individual variables, patients with lower FEV1, greater symptom scores and higher C-reactive protein (CRP) at the end of the exacerbation treatment were associated with shorter time until the next exacerbation. Also patients with ABPA and CFRD had a shorter time until the next exacerbations than those without. After adjustments to confounding factors, however, older CF patients and those with lower FEV1 at the end of course of treatment were found to be the two independent risk factors.

8. Management of pulmonary exacerbations

The mainstay of treatment of pulmonary exacerbations is administration of antibiotics. For mild exacerbations oral antibiotics are usually administered – mainly quinolones. This approach is based on little evidence, since a large proportion of patient have quinolone resistant *P. aeruginosa*.

More severe exacerbations are prescribed IV antibiotics. As most patients with frequent exacerbations commonly grow *P. aeruginosa* in their sputum, CF physicians prescribe two antibiotics aiming to effectively decrease the bacterial load and reduce the probability of developing antibiotic resistance. The choice of antibiotic class range would often include an aminoglycoside (tobramycin, gentamycin and amikacin) and a beta-lactam (ceftazidime, aztreonam, pipracillin or ticarcillin) or a quinolone (ciprofloxacin). In more recent years, carbopenims (imipenim or meropenim) are being more frequently used. Occasionally IV colistine is prescribed in cases of bacterial resistance. The duration of treatment is often 2 weeks.

The doses of antibiotics given for CF patients are often larger than those given to other respiratory and non-respiratory infections. This is, theoretically, thought to be necessary due the high bacterial load in the damaged and inflamed lungs and the difficulty of antibiotics penetrating the thick layer of inspissated sputum to reach the bacteria – in particular when mucoid *P. aeruginosa* is present.

Lack of evidence of how to optimally manage CF pulmonary exacerbations is, in part, due to the fact that the determinants of the successful outcome of treatment of an exacerbation have not yet been clearly identified. In most CF centres improvement in general clinical status and in lung function tests are accepted to determine the 'end' of the exacerbation. For those patients who do not show sufficient improvement in the opinion of the treating physicians, the course of antibiotics is either extended or the combination of antibiotics is changed. Despite its shortcomings, this approach has been endorsed in a consensus document published by the UK CF Trust (UK CF Trust Antibiotic Guidelines 2008).

For pulmonary exacerbations treated with IV antibiotics, the combination of choice is often determined on arbitrary grounds. Previous *in vitro* sensitivity and previous clinical response normally determine the choice of antibiotics. However, several retrospective and prospective studies found that the concordance of *in vitro* sensitivity did not affect any of the outcomes of the CF exacerbations, including lung function tests and the time until the subsequent pulmonary exacerbation (Jarad et al., 2007; Foweraker et al., 2005).

Frequent and longer courses of IV treatment, particularly with aminoglycosides, have been shown to be associated with renal impairment (Smyth et al., 2008; Al Aloul et al., 2005) and ototoxicity (Mulheran et al., 2001; Scott et al., 2001), as well as increased rate of antibiotic allergy (Moss et al., 1984). In addition, extension of duration of IV antibiotic treatment is associated with added volume of work to patients and CF staff and in incremental cost pressure of CF care.

Two retrospective studies (Sanders et al., 2010; Rosenberg & Scharamm, 1993) found that administration of antibiotics for 14 days in adolescent and young adult CF patients resulted in clinical recovery in 72% and 75% of patients respectively. A recent guideline committee for treatment of CF pulmonary exacerbations that studied the literature of management of exacerbations found no evidence for the optimal duration of treatment of CF pulmonary exacerbations (Flume et al., 2009). The committee recommended that future studies should examine short and long term subjective and objective outcomes of management of exacerbations according to duration of treatment.

Risk factors and efficacy of extending the course of antibiotics have been prospectively examined (Sequeiros & Jarad, 2012). As in previous studies, nearly 23% of 168 pulmonary exacerbations in 58 adult CF patients did not recover after 2 weeks of IV antibiotic treatment, needing extension of duration of treatment. For those prescribed extended courses, most patients required additional 7 days of treatment, but some needed doubling of the duration of treatment (figure 12). Unlike previous studies, a validated symptom score was used and biomarkers measured at the end of treatment were examined.

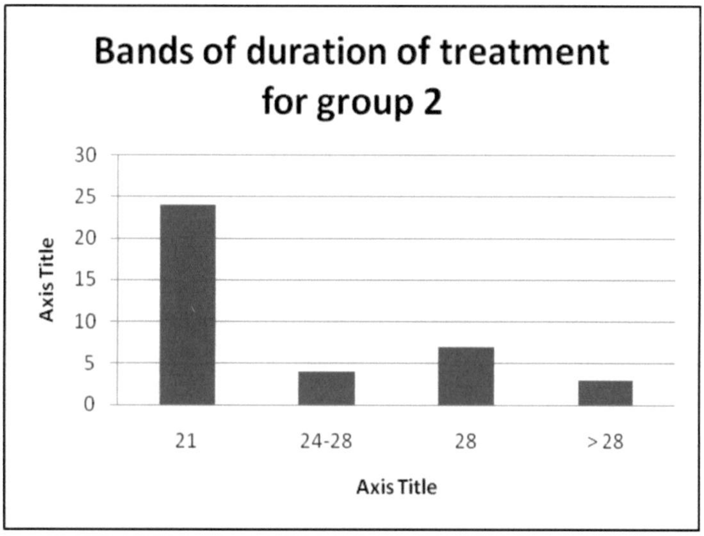

Figure 12. A histogram of the number of patients (Y axis) and duration of treatment for exacerbations for patients needing extension of IV treatment (X axis). Most patients needed additional 7 days, but some needed at least doubling the duration of treatment (Adapted from Sequeiros & Jarad, 2012).

Risk factors for extending the IV course were found to be more severe lung disease and persistent respiratory symptoms and systemic inflammation as assessed by CRP at the end of treatment. The extension of treatment beyond 14 days resulted in improvement of symptoms, but not of FEV1. Extension of treatment did not result in increased time to the next exacerbation.

9. What measurements determine the outcome of CF pulmonary exacerbations?

The aim of management of CF pulmonary exacerbations is to restore patients to pre-exacerbation clinical status. In most CF centres, determining the end of an exacerbation is done arbitrarily during clinical consultation.

Sequeiros et al. (2009) examined several clinical parameters throughout the duration of treatment of exacerbations with IV antibiotics to assess which one best correlated with the patient's clinical picture. These included spirometry, airway calibre and airway resistance assessed by high frequency test. A novel symptom scoring system was also used, which has been more recently validated (Jarad & Sequeiros, 2012).

The symptom score was the parameter that changed most frequently at the end of treatment of exacerbations, more so than FEV1 and FVC (figure 13). As for airway calibre and resistance, these did not significantly change at the end of exacerbations. Changes in symptom score correlated with changes in FEV1 and FVC. The authors concluded that the novel symptom scoring system is sensitive to change with treatment and can be a useful tool for the assessment of treatment of pulmonary exacerbations.

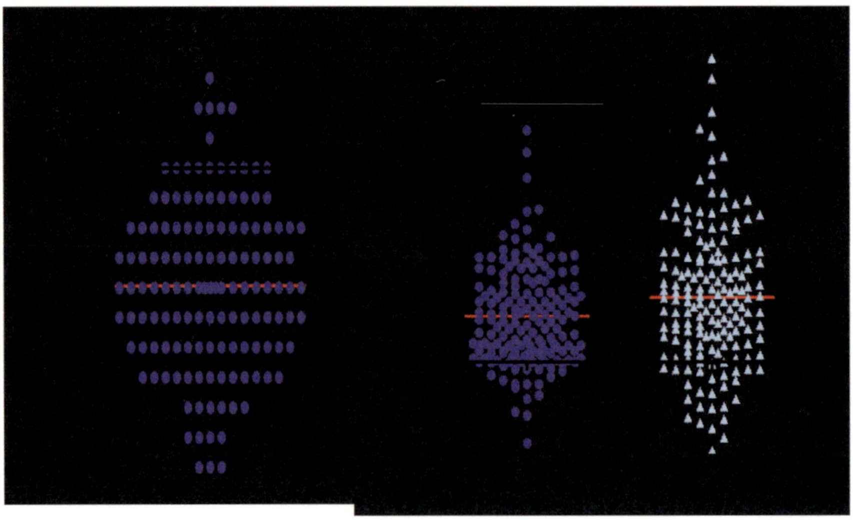

Figure 13. Change after 14 days of IV antibiotics in symptom score (lower score is better health status), FEV1 and FVC in a cohort of adult CF patients treated for acute pulmonary exacerbations. The symptom score improved in a higher proportion of patients in comparison with FEV1 and FVC.

http://dx.doi.org/10.5772/54336

10. Oral corticosteroids as an adjuvant to antibiotics

As discussed above, in addition to excessive bacterial growth, exuberant local lung inflammation is considered to play an important role in CF pulmonary exacerbations. In this context, using corticosteroids in addition to antibiotics during the treatment of exacerbations would be thought to be a logical approach.

Managing exacerbations with corticosteroids and antibiotics is the norm in patients with COPD. In a prospective study on inpatients with severe COPD who were hospitalised due to acute exacerbations, Davies et al. (1999) found that adding 30mg prednisolone for 14 days to usual treatment resulted in improvement of FEV1 and shortening of length of hospital stay compared with placebo-treated patients.

For CF patients, an open label study found that adding oral corticosteroids resulted in an improvement of FEV1 in a small cohort of adult CF patients (Dovey et al., 2007). Furthermore, a national UK survey performed in the authors' unit, found that all UK CF physicians had used adjuvant corticosteroids to different extents in managing CF pulmonary exacerbations (Hester et al., 2007).

This is important because of the increased propensity of CF patients to develop diabetes and osteoporosis by virtue of the CF disease process. Corticosteroids are bound to adversely affect the likelihood of these two complications, (increase the incidence and severity), as a significant negative side effect of the drug. To date there are no large trials to answer the question of whether adding corticosteroids to antibiotics improves outcome of treatment of CF exacerbations, and the issue remains contentious.

11. Elective courses of antibiotics versus symptomatic treatments

Elective regular administration of IV antibiotics several times per year has been a practice adopted by many CF teams to improve symptoms and reduce decline in lung function tests. In a national UK survey of CF centres (Higgs & Jarad, 2005), the authors found that greater proportion of paediatric patients received regular (elective) courses of IV antibiotics compared to adult CF patients (figure 14).

This is despite the fact that a previous study showed no differences in spirometry improvement in patients who received elective 3 monthly anti-pseudomonal antibiotic treatment compared to those who received conventional symptomatic treatment, triggered by increased symptoms. The elective group received an average of 4 courses of antibiotics per year, compared with an average of 3 courses per year in the symptomatic group (Elborn et al., 2000).

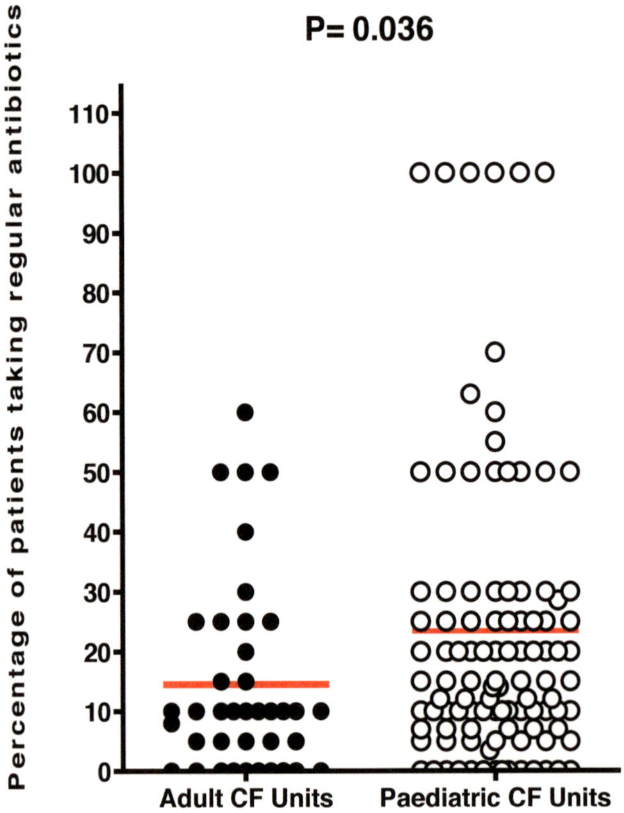

Figure 14. Larger proportion of paediatric CF patients received elective IV antibiotics in comparison to adult CF patients (Higgs & Jarad, 2005).

12. Self-administration of IV antibiotics

Delivery of healthcare for CF patients has changed significantly over the past 20 years. Previously all patients were managed in hospital, but there has been a drive for the management of chronic conditions at home. Although not specifically suggested, management of acute exacerbations of clinical conditions such as COPD, bronchiectasis and CF is also frequently being done at home.

CF patients with pulmonary exacerbations requiring IV antibiotics place a great strain on the capacity of hospitals in terms of the available number of beds, on their manpower and other financial resources with repeated admissions. Accommodation and boarding for patients and, sometimes, members of their families account for the largest fraction of hospital costs for inpatients. Equipment and drugs make up the largest proportion of home therapy costs (Wolter et al., 1997).

http://dx.doi.org/10.5772/54336

Self-administration of antibiotics was first introduced 30 years ago. This practice has been facilitated by improvement in technology and increased familiarity of patients and CF teams with antibiotics.

For patients with available peripheral venous access and infrequent exacerbations, antibiotics are administered via a peripherally inserted central catheter (PIC line) (figure 15). If such lines are inserted in the non-dominant arm, patients can self-administer their antibiotics.

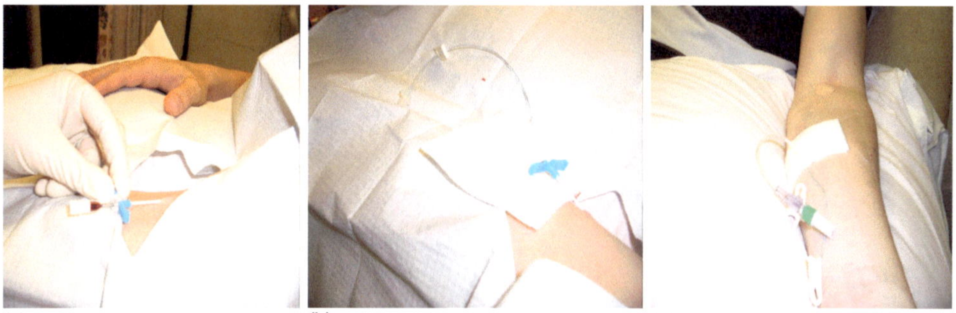

(a) (b) (c)

Figure 15. Insertion of a PIC line in the left arm of a right handed CF patient. The patient is able to self-administer antibiotics using his right hand.

Over the years, venous access frequently becomes more difficult to attain due to repeated use and occlusion of peripheral veins. In such patients, placement of a long-term totally implantable venous access system is an option. One of these methods, a port-a-cath, consists of a reservoir surgically inserted under the skin in the upper chest or arm, with the use of sedation or general anaesthesia. The reservoir is covered by a silicone mesh and appears as a bump under the skin. It leads to a long venous catheter, which is inserted into a central vein, usually a subclavian vein, and terminates in the superior vena cava. It is completely internal, so bathing and swimming are not a problem, although contact sports are contra-indicated due to risk of trauma and dislodgement of the device (figure 16).

Ports and peripherally inserted lines have their own complications and require specific care, such anti-septic manipulation and monthly local anticoagulation to prevent blockage from blot clots. Despite careful maintenance, infection and blockage are not uncommon. Irreversible occlusion of ports almost inevitably necessitates complete replacement.

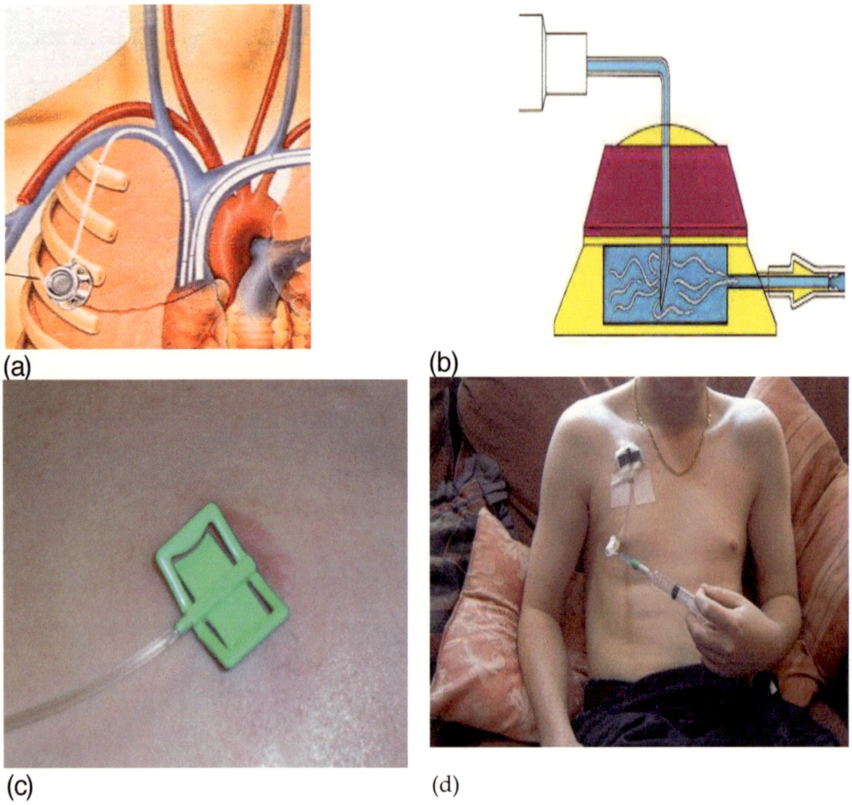

Figure 16. The port-a-cath. (a): schematic representation of the position of a port-a-cath. (b): accessing the device chamber by a specifically designed needle. (c) and (d): a needle is inserted into the port-a-cath chamber and a patient self-administering IV antibiotic via his port-a-cath.

13. Managing cystic fibrosis pulmonary exacerbations at home versus in hospital

Home therapy is becoming a preferred treatment option for patients with CF suffering from pulmonary exacerbations in the UK and other parts of the world. With the widespread practice of home based IV antibiotic therapy, concern has been expressed by CF healthcare workers about whether the outcome of care for those treated at home by self-administering IV antibiotics might be inferior to that of patients treated in hospital.

Hospital management is not favoured by most CF patients, who prefer home therapy (Thornton et al., 2005; Pond et al., 1994; Strandvik et al., 1992; Donati et al., 1987). Hospital treatment is probably disruptive to patients and their families, taking patients away from school or work commitments and social activities for considerable amounts of time. There are also financial strains on patients due to earning losses as a result of time off from work and travelling to hospital expenses, especially if the treatment centre/hospital is at a considerable distance from the patient's home. After numerous admissions throughout their lives, patients and their families become acquainted with many aspects of IV drug administration and often want to start self-administration of these medications, avoiding hospital admissions (Gilbert et al., 1988). Reasons for patients' preference for home treatment are outlined in table 4.

- Less interruption to education and career
- Reduced earning losses and travelling expenses
- Tastier food
- More facilities to exercise
- Less disruption to sleep
- More convenient timing of drug administration
- Improved quality of life
- Reduced risk of cross infection
- Lack of hospital beds

Table 4. Reasons why patients prefer home IV antibiotic treatment.

The superior outcome of hospital management over home treatment has been attributed to closer supervision and direct input by the multidisciplinary team, including physiotherapists, dieticians and nursing staff, throughout the period of hospital stay (Thornton et al., 2004; Pond et al., 1994), ensuring increased adherence to treatment. Albeit unproven, bed rest during exacerbations has also been widely regarded as another reason for the favourable outcome of hospital treatment.

Conversely, there are numerous reasons why home treatment could be clinically less effective in treating exacerbations in CF patients (table 5). Considerable commitment is required from patients who are on home based treatment, as, in addition to their treatment schedules, they may wish to maintain their domestic routines and social lives, as well as fulfil educational and work commitments. Continuing with normal life and not taking time off work or school would mean maintaining higher general activity levels. These patients are probably not getting the amount of rest they need as part of their treatment (Thornton et al., 2005). Self-performed physiotherapy may not be as effective during exacerbations compared to the treatment provided by a professional physiotherapist and calorie intake may suffer without daily encouragement (Pond et al., 1994).

- Reduced medical input
- Reduced input from physiotherapists and dieticians
- Reliance on patients to diagnose own complications
- Possible lack of compliance with the IV treatment
- Lack of rest

Table 5. Reasons why healthcare professionals are concerned about the practice of home IV treatment.

Some antibiotic regimens for home treatment are adapted to make administration more convenient and more compatible with work and school hours (Pond et al., 1994). This includes twice daily beta-lactam antibiotics versus the recommended thrice-daily regime.

Another important issue is adherence, which is recognised as being potentially poor in CF (Dodd & Webb, 2000) and may be worse in some patients on home IV treatment. Although assessed by the multidisciplinary team for competency in terms of self-administration of drugs, the level of adherence of patients to treatment is not truly known. This is a widely anecdotally known phenomenon, often revealed when considerable amounts of unused antibiotics and other drugs are returned by patients and their families to the caring CF centre.

The conflict between patients' preference for home treatment and health providers' concern to achieve a favourable outcome of care during stages of clinical instability in CF is ongoing. This is currently handled in variable ways by different CF centres. Most centres feel that they have to offer some kind of home treatment, although a small number do not. Others prefer a happy medium of starting treatment in hospital and then discharging patients a few days later to complete the antibiotic course at home. Some CF centres prefer not to treat patients at home for two successive exacerbations.

More recently, Collaco et al. (2010) published a large retrospective study with a total of 834 treated exacerbations in both paediatric and adult patients in the United States. They conclude that similar decline in long term FEV1 was observed regardless whether antibiotics were administered in hospital or at home, with equivalence also found in regards to interval duration in between successive exacerbation episodes. Interestingly though, subjects treated in hospital had a statistically significant greater improvement of lung function immediately after treatment (immediate recovery) in comparison to the home treated group, despite similar pre-treatment spirometry. Also, patients treated in hospital had shorter total number of days of IV antibiotic treatment, implying that patients overcame their exacerbations quicker when treated in hospital (12.7 days versus 18.9 days), which of course impacts on quality of life, drug toxicity, antibiotic resistance and healthcare costs.

Given the controversy around this subject, Sequeiros & Jarad (2010) prospectively examined the effect of home treatment with intensive assistance from CF nurses, physiotherapists and dieticians on patient outcomes. The authors compared outcomes of this intensive intervention with outcomes of exacerbations treated at home without intensive assistance and in hospital.

The study showed that, unlike previous studies, those who were treated in hospital had initially poorer quality of life and were underweight compared to those who were treated at, but these recuperated to match post treatment levels similar to home based patients. The research also showed that, despite intensive home intervention, outcomes did not differ from standard home treatment and were inferior to those treated in hospital. The study has been published in abstract form (Sequeiros & Jarad, 2010) and is presently being prepared as a full manuscript for publication (figure 17).

Ideally, outcome of care for home treatment should be at least equal to outcome for hospital treatment and clinical improvement not sacrificed on the basis of economic considerations

http://dx.doi.org/10.5772/54336

and convenience (Pond et al., 1994). Selection of patients that are considered competent and safe for self-administered home treatment should be made carefully. A hygienic environment and adequate knowledge of preparation and administration of antibiotics should be ensured, as well as regular physiotherapy, rest and suitable nutrition, which are crucial for the successful treatment of CF exacerbations. Better still is the availability of support from family and friends, who are familiar with home treatment methods, as well as from the CF multidisciplinary team.

Patients need to be aware of the perceived reasons for an inferior outcome of home treatment and the CF community should definitively address these.

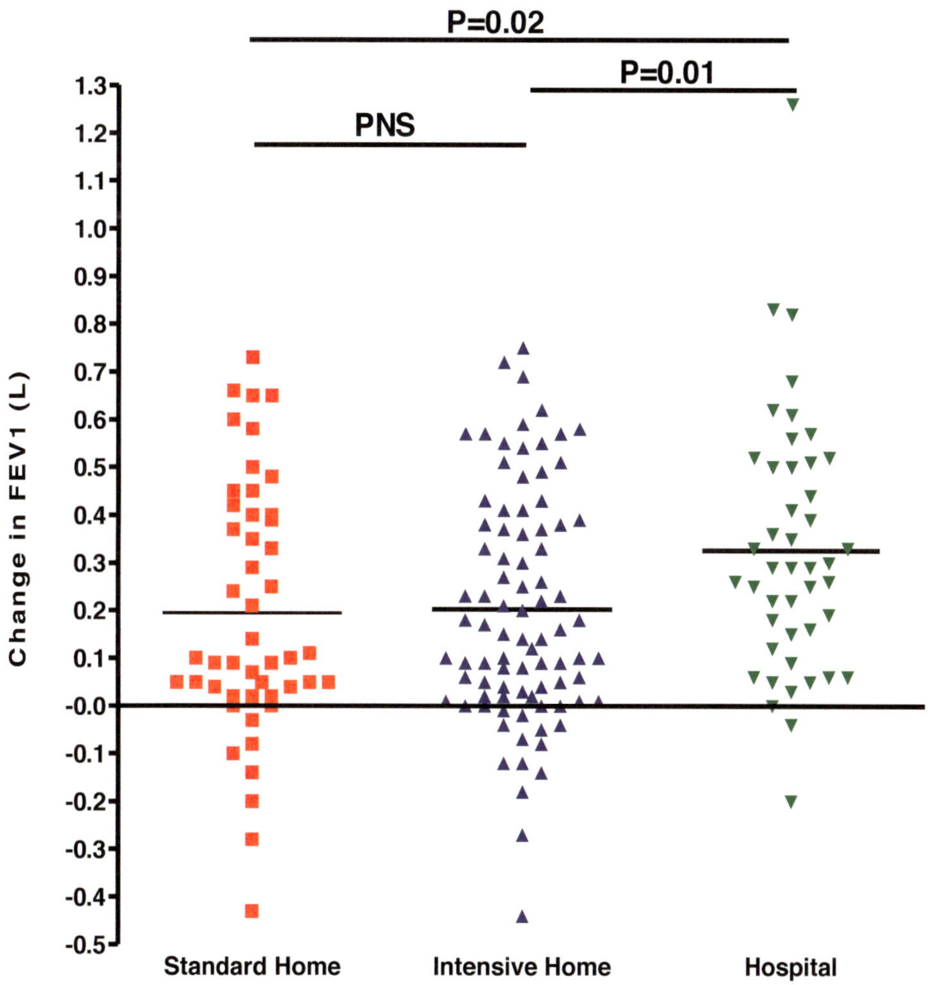

Figure 17. Changes in FEV1 with treatment of exacerbations treated at home with and without intensive assistance and in hospital. Best outcome is seen in the hospital treatment group (Sequeiros & Jarad, 2010).

14. Conclusion

CF exacerbations are complex and still not completely understood. However, they remain an important part of the CF lung disease due to their great negative impact on quality of life, resultant decline in lung function and mortality.

This chapter addresses the natural history, causes and aspects of management, and prognosis of CF exacerbations pertinent mainly to adult CF patients. Until introduction of more effective and disease modifying treatments for CF, better understanding and management of CF exacerbations remain an important goal for the CF community.

Prevention, accurate identification and treatment of pulmonary exacerbations are key to the improved survival and quality of life of CF patients. Efforts should be made to standardize treatments and ensure high standards of care throughout different CF centres worldwide.

Author details

Iara Maria Sequeiros and Nabil Jarad

University Hospitals Bristol NHS Foundation Trust , United Kingdom

References

[1] Aaron SD, Ramotar K, Ferris W, Vandemheen K, Saginur R, Tullis E, Haase D, Kottachchi D, St. Denis M, Chan F. (2004) Adult cystic fibrosis exacerbations and new strains of Pseudomonas aeruginosa. *American Journal of Respiratory and Critical Care Medicine*, 169:811-815.

[2] Abbot J, Holt A, Hart A, Morton AM, MacDougall L, Pogson M, Milne G, Rodgers HC, Conway SP. (2009) What defines a pulmonary exacerbation? The perceptions of adults with cystic fibrosis. *Journal of Cystic Fibrosis*, 8(5):356-359.

[3] Al Aloul M, Miller H, Alapati S, Stockton PA, Ledson MJ, Walshaw MJ. (2005) Renal impairment in cystic fibrosis patients due to repeated intravenous aminoglycoside use. *Pediatric Pulmonology*, 39:15-20.

[4] Barker AF. (2002) Bronchiectasis. *New England Journal of Medicine*, 346:1383-1393.

[5] Block JK, Vandemheen KL, Tullis E, Fergusson D, Doucette S, Haase D, Berthiaume Y, Brown N, Wilcox P, Bye P, Bell S, Noseworthy M, Pedder L, Freitag A, Paterson N, Aaron SD. (2006) Predictors of pulmonary exacerbations in patients with cystic fibrosis infected with multi-resistant bacteria. *Thorax*, 61:969-974.

[6] Bonfield TL, Panuska JR, Konstan MW, Hilliard KA, Hilliard JB, Ghnaim H, Berger M. (1995) Inflammatory cytokines in cystic fibrosis lungs. *American Journal of Respiratory and Critical Care Medicine*, 152:2111-2118.

[7] Boucher RC. (2004) New concepts of the pathogenesis of cystic fibrosis lung disease. *European Respiratory Journal*, 23:146-158.

[8] Britto MT, Kotagal UR, Hornung RW, Atherton HD, Tsevat J, Wilmott RW. (2002) Impact of recent pulmonary exacerbations on quality of life in patients with cystic fibrosis. *Chest*, 121:64-72.

[9] Collaco JM, Green DM, Cutting GR, Naughton KM, Mogayzel, Jr PJ. (2010) Location and duration of treatment of cystic fibrosis respiratory exacerbations do not affect outcomes. *American Journal of Respiratory and Critical Care Medicine*, 182(9):1137-1143.

[10] Colombo C, Constantini D, Rocchi A, Cariani L, Garlaschi ML, Tirelli S, Calori G, Copreni E, Conese M. (2005) Cytokine levels in sputum of cystic fibrosis patients before and after antibiotic therapy. *Pediatric Pulmonology*, 40(1):15-21.

[11] Cystic Fibrosis Trust Website. (2012) UK CF Registry Annual Data Report 2009. Available at: www.cftrust.org.uk/aboutcf/publications/cfregistryreports/

[12] Cystic Fibrosis Foundation. (2011) Cystic Fibrosis Patient Registry 2010 Annual Data Report, Bethesda, Maryland. Available at: http://www.cff.org

[13] Cystic Fibrosis Foundation. (1994) Consensus Conferences: Concepts in Care, vol. 5, section 1, Bethesda, Maryland.

[14] Davies L, Angus RM, Calverley PM. (1999) Oral corticosteroids in patients admitted to hospital with exacerbations of chronic obstructive pulmonary disease: a prospective randomised controlled trial. Lancet, 7;354(9177):456-60.

[15] Dakin C, Henry RL, Field P, Morton J. (2001) Defining an exacerbation of pulmonary disease in cystic fibrosis. *Pediatric Pulmonology*, 31(6):436-442.

[16] Dodd ME, Webb AK. (2000) Understanding non-compliance with treatment in adults with cystic fibrosis. *Journal of the Royal Society of Medicine*, 93(S38):2-8.

[17] Donati MA, Guenette G, Auerbaeh H. (1987) Prospective controlled study of home and hospital therapy of cystic fibrosis pulmonary disease. *Journal of Paediatrics*, 111:28-33.

[18] Dovey M, Aitken ML, Emerson J, McNamara S, Waltz DA, Gibson RL. (2007) Oral corticosteroid therapy in cystic fibrosis patients hospitalized for pulmonary exacerbation: a pilot study. *Chest*, 132(4):1212-1218.

[19] Drenkard E, Ausubel FM. (2002) Pseudomonas biofilm formation and antibiotic resistance are linked to phenotypic variation. *Nature*, 416:740-743.

[20] Elborn JS, Prescott RJ, Stack BHR, Goodchild MC, Bates J, Pantin C, Ali N, Shale DJ, Crane M. (2000) Elective versus symptomatic antibiotic treatment in cystic fibrosis patients with chronic Pseudomonas infection of the lungs. *Thorax*, 55:355-358.

[21] Flume PA, Mogayazel PJ, Robinson KA, et al. (2009) Cystic fibrosis pulmonary guidelines-treatment of pulmonary exacerbations. *American Journal of Respiratory and Critical Care Medicine*, 180:802-808.

[22] Foweraker J, Laughton C, Brown D, Bilton D. (2005) Phenotypic variability of Pseudomonas aeruginosa in sputa from patients with acute infective exacerbation of cystic fibrosis and its impact on the validity of antimicrobial susceptibility testing. *Journal Antimicrobiol. Chemo*, 55:921-927.

[23] Frizzell RA, Pilewski JM. (2004) Finally, mice with CF lung disease. *Nature Medicine*, 10:452-454.

[24] Fuchs HJ, Borowitz DS, Christiansen DH, Morris EM, Nash ML, Ramsey BW, Rosenstein BJ, Smith AL, Wohl ME. The Pulmozyme Study Group. (1994) Effect of aerosolized recombinant human DNase on exacerbations of respiratory symptoms and on pulmonary function in patients with cystic fibrosis. *New England Journal of Medicine*, 331(10):637-642.

[25] Gibson RL, Emerson J, McNamara S, Burns JL, Rosenfeld M, Yunker A, Hamblett N, Accurso F, Dovey M, Hiatt P, Konstan MW, Moss R, Retsch-Bogart G, Wagener J, Waltz D, Wilmott R, Zeitlin PL, Ramsey B. The Cystic Fibrosis Therapeutics Development Network Study Group. (2003) Significant microbiological effect of inhaled tobramycin in young children with cystic fibrosis. *American Journal of Respiratory and Critical Care Medicine*, 167:841-849.

[26] Gilbert J, Robinson T, Littlewood JM. (1988) Home intravenous antibiotic treatment in cystic fibrosis. *Archives of Disease in Childhood*, 63(5):512-517.

[27] Goss CH, Burns JL. (2007) Exacerbations in cystic fibrosis 1: Epidemiology and pathogenesis. *Thorax*, 62:360-367.

[28] Goss CH, Otto K, Aitken ML, Rubenfeld GD. (2002) Detecting Stenotrophomonas maltophilia does not reduce survival of patients with cystic fibrosis. *American Journal of Respiratory and Critical Care Medicine*, 166:356-361.

[29] Guggino WB, Guggino SE. (2000) Amiloride-sensitive sodium channels contribute to the woes of the flu. *Proceedings of the National Academy of Science*, 97(18):9827-9829.

[30] Hester KLM, Powell T, Downey DG, Elborn SJ, Jarad NA. (2007) Glucocorticoids as an adjuvant treatment to intravenous antibiotics for cystic fibrosis pulmonary exacerbations: a UK survey. *Journal of Cystic Fibrosis*, 6:311-313.

[31] Hiatt PW, Grace SC, Kozinetz Ca, Raboudi SH, Treece DG, Taber LH, Piedra PA. (1999) Effects of viral lower respiratory tract infection on lung function in infants with cystic fibrosis. *Pediatrics*, 103(3):619-626.

[32] Higgs S, Jarad NA. (2005) National United Kingdom survey of cystic fibrosis pulmonary exacerbations: management variation amongst paediatric and adult physicians. *Thorax*, 60:94.

[33] Isles A, Maclusky I, Corey M, Gold R, Prober C, Fleming P, Levison H. (1984) Pseudomonas cepacia infection in cystic fibrosis: an emerging problem. *Journal of Pediatrics*, 104:206-210.

[34] Jarad NA, Sequeiros IM. (2012) A novel respiratory symptom scoring system for cystic fibrosis pulmonary exacerbations. *Quarterly Journal of Medicine*, 105(2):137-143.

[35] Jarad NA, Sund ZM. (2011) Telemonitoring in chronic obstructive airway disease and adult patients with cystic fibrosis. *Journal of Telemedicine and Telecare*, 17(3):127-132.

[36] Jarad NA, Giles K. (2008) Risk factors for increased need for intravenous antibiotics for pulmonary exacerbations in adult patients with cystic fibrosis. *Chronic Respiratory Disease*, 5(1):29-33.

[37] Jarad NA, Stanley C, Gunasekera W, Webster S. (2007) Concordance between intravenous antibiotics and in vitro susceptibility of sputum bacteria does not influence the outcome of pulmonary exacerbations in adults with cystic fibrosis patients. *Journal of Cystic Fibrosis*, 6(S1) S33.

[38] Jeffcote T, Lentaigne J, Price M, Wathen K, Jarad NA. (2204) Does the diagnosis of pulmonary exacerbation meet the USCF criteria? *Journal of Cystic Fibrosis*, 3: S214.

[39] Knowles MR, Boucher RC. (2002) Mucus clearance as a primary innate defence mechanism for mammalian airways. *Journal of Clinical Investigation*, 109(5):571-577.

[40] Konstan MW, Hilliard KA, Norvell TM, Berger M. (1994) Bronchoalveolar lavage findings in cystic fibrosis patients with stable, clinically mild lung disease suggest ongoing infection and inflammation. *American Journal of Respiratory and Critical Care Medicine*, 150(2):448-454.

[41] Konstan MW, Walenga RW, Hilliard KA, Hilliard JB. (1993) Leukotriene B4 markedly elevated in the epithelial lining fluid of patients with cystic fibrosis. *American Review of Respiratory Disease*, 148:896-901.

[42] Li Z, Kosorok MR, Farrell PM, Laxova A, West SEH, Green CG, Collins J, Rock MJ, Splaingard ML. (2005) Longitudinal development of mucoid Pseudomonas aeruginosa infection and lung disease progression in children with cystic fibrosis. *The Journal of the American Medical Association*, 293:581-588.

[43] Liou TG, Adler FR, Fitzsimmons SC, Cahill BC, Hibbs JR, Marshall BC. (2001) Predictive 5-year survivorship model of cystic fibrosis. *American Journal of Epidemiology*, 153:345-352.

[44] Lyczak JB, Cannon CL, Pier GB. (2002) Lung infections associated with cystic fibrosis. *Clinical Microbiology Reviews*, 15:194-222.

[45] Marshall BC, Butler SM, Stoddard M, Moran AM, Liou TG, Morgan WJ. (2005) Epidemiology of cystic fibrosis related diabetes. *Journal of Pediatrics*, 146(5):681-687.

[46] Marshall BC. (2004) Pulmonary exacerbation in cystic fibrosis. It's time to be explicit. *American Journal of Respiratory and Critical Care Medicine*, 169:781-782.

[47] Moss RB, Babin S, Hsu YP, Blessing-Moore J, Lewiston NJ. (1984) Allergy to semi synthetic penicillins in cystic fibrosis. *Journal Pediatrics*, 104:460-466.

[48] Mulheran M, Degg C, Burr S, Morgan DW, Stableforth DE. (2001) Occurrence and risk of cochleotoxicity in cystic fibrosis patients receiving repeated high-dose aminoglycoside therapy. *Antimicrobial Agents Chemotherapy*, 45: 2502-2509.

[49] Ordonez CL, Henig NR, Mayer-Hamblett N, Accurso FJ, Burns JL, Chmiel JF, Daines CL, Gibson RL, McNamara S, Retsch-Bogart GZ, Zeitlin PL, Aitken ML. (2003) Inflammatory and microbiologic markers in induced sputum after intravenous antibiotics in cystic fibrosis *American Journal of Respiratory and Critical Care Medicine*, 168:1471-1475.

[50] Pond NM, Newport M, Joanes D, Conway S. (1994) Home versus hospital intravenous antibiotic therapy in the treatment of young adults with cystic fibrosis. *European Respiratory Journal*, 7:1640-1644.

[51] Ramsey BW, Pepe MS, Quan JM, Otto KL, Montgomery AB, Williams-Warren J, Vasiljev-K M, Borowitz D, Bowman CM, Marshall BC, Marshall S, Smith AL. The Cystic Fibrosis Inhaled Tobramycin Study Group. (1999) Intermittent administration of inhaled tobramycin in patients with cystic fibrosis. *New England Journal of Medicine*, 340:23-30.

[52] Ramsey BW. (1996) Management of pulmonary disease in patients with cystic fibrosis. *New England Journal of Medicine*, 335:179-188.

[53] Randell SH, Boucher RC. (2006) Effective mucus clearance is essential for respiratory health. *American Journal of Respiratory Cell and Molecular Biology*, 35:20-28.

[54] Rosenberg SM & Scharamm CM. (1993) Predictive value of pulmonary function testing during pulmonary exacerbation in cystic fibrosis. *Paediatric Pulmonology*, 4:227-235.

[55] Rubin BK. (2002) Physiology of airway mucus clearance. *Respiratory Care*, 47(7): 761-768.

[56] Sagel SD, Kapsner R, Osberg I, Sontag MK, Accurso FJ. (2001) Airway inflammation in children with cystic fibrosis and healthy children assessed by sputum induction. *American Journal of Respiratory and Critical Care Medicine*, 164(8):1425-1431.

[57] Saiman L, Marshall BC, Mayer-Hamblett N, Burns JL, Quittner AL, Cibene DA, Coquillette S, Fieberg AY, Accurso FJ, Campbell PW 3rd. The Macrolide Study Group. (2003) Azithromycin in patients with cystic fibrosis chronically infected with Pseudo-

monas aeruginosa: a randomized controlled trial. *Journal of the American Medical Association*, 290(13):1749-1756.

[58] Sanders DB, Bittner RC, Rosenfield M, Hoffman LR, Redding GJ, Goss CH. (2010) Failure to recover to baseline pulmonary function after cystic fibrosis pulmonary exacerbation. *American Journal of Respiratory and Critical Care Medicine*, 182(5):627-632.

[59] Sarfaraz S, Sund Z, Jarad NA. (2010) Real-time, once-daily monitoring of symptoms and FEV in cystic fibrosis patients - a feasibility study using a novel device. *Clinical Respiratory Journal*, 4(2):74-82.

[60] Scott CS, Retsch-Bogart GZ, Henry MM. (2001) Renal failure and vestibular toxicity in an adolescent with cystic fibrosis receiving gentamicin and standard-dose ibuprofen. *Pediatric Pulmonology*, 31:314-316.

[61] Sequeiros IM, Jarad NA. (2012) Extending the course of intravenous antibiotics in adult patients with cystic fibrosis with acute pulmonary exacerbations. *In press Chronic Respiratory Disease*.

[62] Sequeiros IM, NA Jarad. (2010) Outcome of care for home management with intensive input in adult CF patients during pulmonary exacerbations – a comparative prospective study with hospital care. *Journal of Cystic Fibrosis*, 9:S1(P223).

[63] Sequeiros I, Hester K, Kendrick AH, Jarad NA. (2009) Which quantitative measurement of lung function correlates best with clinical picture during treatment of pulmonary exacerbations in CF? *Journal of Cystic Fibrosis*, 8:S62(247).

[64] Smyth AR, Walters S. (2003) Prophylactic anti-staphylococcal antibiotics for cystic fibrosis. *Cochrane Database of Systematic Reviews*, (3):CD001912.

[65] Smyth A, Lewis S, Bertenshaw C, Choonara I, McGaw J and Watson A. (2008) A case control study of acute renal failure in cystic fibrosis patients in the United Kingdom. *Thorax*, 63:532-535.

[66] Strandvik B, Hjelte L, Malmborg AS, Widen B. (1992) Home intravenous antibiotic treatment of patients with cystic fibrosis. *Acta Paediatrica*, 81(4):340-344.

[67] Sund ZM, Powell T, Greenwood R, Jarad NA. (2009) Remote daily real-time monitoring in patients with COPD – a feasibility study using a novel device. *Respiratory Medicine*, 103(9):1320-1328.

[68] Thornton J, Elliot RA, Tully MP, Dodd M, Webb AK. (2005) Clinical and economic choices in the treatment of respiratory infections in cystic fibrosis: Comparing hospital and home care. *Journal of Cystic Fibrosis*, 4(4):239-247.

[69] Thornton J, Elliott R, Tully MP, Dodd M, Webb AK. (2004) Long term clinical outcome of home and hospital intravenous antibiotic treatment in adults with cystic fibrosis. *Thorax*, 59:242-246.

[70] Wolter JM, Bowler SD, Nolan PJ, McCormack JG. (1997) Home intravenous therapy in cystic fibrosis: a prospective randomized trial of examining clinical, quality of life and cost aspects. *European Respiratory Journal*, 10:896-900.

Section 3

Helminthic Infections of Lung

Chapter 8

Helminthic Infections and Asthma: Still a Challenge for Developing Countries

Isabel Hagel, Maira Cabrera and
Maria Cristina Di Prisco

Additional information is available at the end of the chapter

http://dx.doi.org/10.5772/54690

1. Introduction

Asthma is one of the most common chronic diseases in the world. It is estimated that around 300 million people in the world currently have asthma [1]. Asthma has become more common in both children and adults around the world in recent decades. The increase in the prevalence of this disease has been associated with an increase in atopic sensitization, and is paralleled by similar increases in other allergic disorders such as eczema and rhinitis [1]. The rate of asthma increases as communities adopt western lifestyles and become urbanized. With the projected increase in the proportion of the world's population that is urban from 45% to 59% in 2025, there is likely to be a marked increase in the number of asthmatics worldwide over the next two decades [2]. Nevertheless the prevalence of asthma in rural developing countries has been under estimated for many years [3]. In many areas of the world persons with asthma do not have access to basic asthma medications or medical care and are not included in any statistical survey [4]. Increasing the economic wealth and improving the distribution of resources between and within countries represent important priorities to enable better health care to be provided. The burden of asthma in many countries is of sufficient magnitude to warrant its recognition as a priority disorder in government health strategies. Particular resources need to be provided to improve the care of disadvantaged groups with high morbidity. Resources also need to be provided to address preventable factors [1, 2]. It is estimated that asthma accounts for about 1 in every 250 deaths worldwide. Many of the deaths are preventable, being due to suboptimal long-term medical care and delay in obtaining help during the final attack. The economic cost of asthma is considerable both in terms of direct medical costs (such as hospital admissions and cost of pharmaceuticals) and indirect medical costs (such as time lost from work and premature death) [1]. Therefore there is a greater understanding of the factors that cause asthma which may lead to novel public health and pharmacological measures to reduce the prevalence of asthma seems to be a worldwide priority.

Among the many factors influencing the prevalence of asthma in developing countries from the tropics are geo-helminthic infections [3], including those caused by *Ascaris lumbricoides*, *Trichuris trichiura* and hookworm (*Ancylostoma duodenale* and *Necator americanus*). These infections have a worldwide distribution being present in almost all geographic and climatic regions. The prevalence of these infections tends to be highest in warm, moist climates; also they are closely correlated with poor environmental hygiene and lack of access to health services [5, 6]. The estimated global prevalence of *A. lumbricoides*, *T. trichiura* and hookworm are 1.5 billion, 1.3 billion and 900 million, respectively, and greater than 2 billion humans are infected with at least one of these parasites [5, 6]. Hookworm is transmitted through skin contact with free-living larvae in the soil, whereas *A. lumbricoides* and *T. trichiura* are transmitted through ingestion of embryonated eggs from the environment. *A. lumbricoides* and hookworm undergo a phase of larval migration through the lungs, whereas *T. trichiura* has a purely enteric life cycle. Infections with *A. lumbricoides* and *T. trichiura* peak in prevalence and intensity between 5 and 15 years of age in endemic areas and there is a decline in both epidemiological parameters in adulthood [5, 6]. Morbidity, including important effects on growth, nutrition and mental development in childhood tends to be greatest in heavily infected children and vulnerable adults (e.g. women of child-bearing age) with long exposure histories [6]. Epidemiological observations have provided evidence that geo-helminthic infections can influence the development of allergic diseases such as asthma. Different studies carried out mostly in rural areas from different countries have shown that infection by intestinal helminths stimulates the risk of asthma [7, 8, 9], whereas other studies in similar populations, have shown an inverse association between asthma and the infection of these parasites [10]. Whether helminthic infections increase or decrease the risk of asthma may depend on environmental factors determining time of exposure and the prevalence and intensity of the infection [3]. On the other hand the individual capacity of the immune system to recognize certain allergenic components of the many molecules involved in host parasite interactions as well as the possible role of parasite mediators to inhibit inflammatory processes may be important aspects in the modulation of the pathogenesis of asthma by these parasites.

2. Immunological aspects of asthma

It is well accepted that asthma is a chronic inflammatory disorder of the bronchial mucosa [11]. The symptoms include chest tightness, wheeze, and cough, and often variable obstruction of airflow through the bronchi. The clinical manifestation of asthma is the result of three events within the airways: reversible obstruction, airway hyper-reactivity and inflammation. Among these factors, airway inflammation is believed to play a major role in the development of the disease [11].

The bronchial inflammation process of asthma is stimulated by cells of the innate immune system (dendritic cells, mast cells, eosinophils, neutrophils, macrophages and NK-cells) and of the adaptive immune system (CD4 + T-lymphocytes, and antigen-specific IgE secreting B-lymphocytes). The innate and adaptive cells are of Th2 class, secreting the cytokines IL-13 and IL-4 prominently or responding to these cytokines through their transduction molecule STAT6 [12, 13]. Thus, the input of these cells into the bronchus and the release or secretion of many mediators (e.g. heparin, reactive lipids or eicosanoids, and enzymes including tryptase and chitinase) lead to increased permeability of blood vessels and consequent edema, increased mucus production, and exaggerated smooth muscle contraction [13] causing airflow obstruction and the symptoms described above. Also, continued inflammation results in remodeling of the airway in which it is thought that TGF-β cytokine may drive the metaplasia of the epithelium, increased vascularity, thickening of the basement membrane, and muscular hypertrophy, leading to lasting airflow obstruction and breathlessness [14, 15].

The induction of adaptive immunity requires antigen-presenting cells (APCs). It is well known that dendritic cells (DCs) are the main type of APC involved in the induction of Th2 responses to allergens in asthma [16]. In the lung, DCs can be found throughout the conducting airways, interstitium, vasculature and pleura and in bronchial lymph nodes. Lung DCs express many receptors, including Toll-like receptors, Nod-like receptors and C-type lectin receptors up regulate the expression of several co-stimulatory molecules (such as CD80 and CD86) and chemokines (such as CCL17 and CCL22) that attract T cells, eosinophils and basophils into the lungs[16-19]. In humans, monocyte-derived conventional DCs promote Th2 responses by secreting pro-inflammatory cytokines and up-regulating the expression of co-stimulatory molecules after antigen stimulation[20] suggesting that lung DCs are necessary for Th2 cell stimulation during airway inflammation.

As mentioned above, various inflammatory cells, such as basophils, eosinophils and mast cells are recruited to airways after allergen challenge. Although the main focus in asthma has been on their roles as inflammatory cells, increasing data suggest that these cells also function as APCs to initiate or enhance Th2 responses. Basophils, which are circulating granulocytes that express the high-affinity IgE receptor FcεRI, amplify immediate hypersensitivity responses by releasing histamine-containing granules and by producing large quantities of IL-4 [13]. Moreover, several studies have highlighted a crucial previously unknown role for basophils as APCs that drive Th2 responses through their expression of major histocompatibility complex (MHC) class II and co stimulatory molecules [21]. Also it has been proposed that MHC class II- dependent interactions between basophils, which are prominent at sites of allergic inflammation, and CD4+ T cells may have an important role in the induction of Th2-mediated inflammation [22, 23]. Another circulating granulocyte that is prominent at sites of allergic inflammation is the eosinophil. After being stimulated, eosinophils have an important pro-inflammatory role by producing leukotrienes, as well as Th1 cytokines (interferon-γ and IL-2) and Th2 cytokines (IL-4, IL-5, IL-10, IL-13 and TNF-α which contribute to airway inflammation [11]. In addition, eosinophils, like basophils, can also function as APCs [24]. Other relevant components of airway inflammation are the mast cells which express FcεRI and c-Kit and reside in tissues near mucosal surfaces and blood vessels. Mast cells can initiate immediate hypersensitivity reactions by de-granulating in response to both adaptive (IgE-mediated) and innate immune signals. For example, mast cells can be activated through cross-linking of antigen-specific IgE bound to FcεRI [25] or in response to Toll-like receptor agonists, or to cytokines such as IL-33 [26]. In addition to producing histamine and leukotrienes, mast cells produce cytokines (IL-1, IL-3, IL-4, IL-5, IL-6, IL-8, IL-10, IL-13, IL-16, tumor necrosis factor and transforming growth factor-β) and chemokines (such as IL-8, lymphotactin, CCL1 (TCA-3), CCL5 (RANTES), CCL2 (MCP-1) and CCL3 (MIP1-α)[27].

An important mediator of airway inflammation is Nitric Oxide (NO) which it is a diffusible gas that can activate biochemical process either on the same cell that produced it or on neighboring cells [28]. NO is synthesized from L-arginine by enzyme nitric oxide synthase (NOS), of which there are three isoforms : NOS I or neuronal NOS (nNOS) was originally isolated from rat and porcine cerebellum; NOS II or inducible NOS (iNOS) from activated macrophages; NOS III or endothelial NOS (eNOS) from endothelial cells [28]. High NO levels could be harmful for asthmatic patients because at elevated concentrations, NO lead to the formation of reactive nitrogen species (RNS) and subsequent oxidation and nitration of proteins, which negatively affect protein functions that are biologically relevant to chronic inflammation in the asthmatic bronchial tissues [28,29]. In asthmatic patients, NO is mainly produced by iNOS expressed in bronchial epithelial cells and some inflammatory cells [30]. NO is also produced by neutrophils and macrophages in response to IFN-γ and a second signal provided by a PAMP ligand or TNF-α. iNOS expression is induced by these signals, this enzyme promotes the oxidation of the guadino nitrogen of L-arginine, resulting in the production of NO and citruline [31]. In addition, other mechanisms have been associated with NO production. It has been demonstrated that the ligation of CD23 (low affinity receptor for IgE FcεRII) on human macrophages is a strong inducer of NO [32]. Indeed, the cross-linking of CD23 by IgE, (IgE - immune complexes or by specific monoclonal antibodies) induces pro-inflammatory response, including NO production [33]. Therefore, allergic sensitization inside the lower airways may account for NO production. In this context, it has been reported that aeroallergen sensitization correlated with exhaled NO (eNO) in mild to moderated asthmatic subjects [34]. Also, the late-phase influx of eosinophils may contribute to NO production at the respiratory mucosa.

3. Stimulation of airway inflammation by helminths parasites

It is important to point out that there are close similarities between the allergic inflammatory responses stimulated in the host by environmental allergens (described above) with the immune responses elicited by parasite antigens. Gut inflammation stimulated by intestinal nematode also include innate (mastocytes, basophils and eosinophils) and adaptive cells of Th2 class which secret preferentially IL-13 and IL-4 cytokines. Pro- inflammatory cells like mastocytes and eosinophils stimulated by these cytokines may release many mediators (heparin, reactive lipids or eicosanoids, and enzymes including tryptase and chitinase) leading to increased permeability of blood vessels, increased mucus production and smooth muscle contraction [35]. Also, inflammation induced by most helminths in the host is associated with NO production through somatic and excretory-secretory antigens of adult worm and larvae [36-40]. These mechanisms may contribute to make a hostile microenvironment in the gut for the parasites promoting worm expulsion.

The capacity of helminths, to stimulate inflammatory responses has been well documented and they are probably related to the complex lifecycle and the antigenic composition of this nematode. For example, there is evidence that after penetration of the intestinal mucosa *A. suum* larvae migrate to the liver, inducing the formation of granulomas, extensive inflammation and tissue injury [41]. Surviving larvae reach the lungs and generate an inflammatory infiltrate in the airways dominated by severe per-alveolar eosinophilia [41, 42]. Pulmonary eosinophilia due to the passage of helminth larvae through the lungs is referred to as Loeffler's syndrome [43]. Eosinophilic pulmonary infiltrates and respiratory symptoms due to *A. lumbricoides or A. suum* are generally part of a self-limited process due to the transient nature of larval passage through the lungs in the *Ascaris* life cycle [44]. The majority of patients remain asymptomatic, however 8 to 15% of infected individuals display morbidity, with respiratory symptoms occurring 9 to 12 days after the ingestion of eggs and lasting 5 to 10 days [45, 46]. Symptoms may include cough, dyspnea, wheeze, and hemoptysis and may progress to frank respiratory distress [43]. Peripheral eosinophilia is often present at the onset of symptoms, but the peak level of eosinophilia will have a delay of several days from presentation [47, 48]. Also, *Strongyloides stercoralis* may cause pulmonary symptoms and infiltrates as a manifestation of chronic infection or as a result of hyper-infection in immune-compromised hosts [49]. The unique life cycle of *S. stercoralis* allows a chronic infection of extended duration to occur due to the ability of new filariform larvae to continuously infect the human host through the perianal skin or bowel mucosa [50]. Patients with chronic infection may have repeated episodes of fever and pneumonitis that may be mistaken for recurrent bacterial pneumonias [51]. Eosinophilia, though often absent during the acute episodes, may occur during the intervening period between episodes [51]. Pulmonary involvement of strongyloidiasis has been reported as an asthma mimic.

The mechanisms by which these parasites induce airway inflammation are still not well elucidated. High levels of polyclonal and specific IgE against adult stages of the parasite are a characteristic of *A. lumbricoides* infection [52]. It has been shown that *Ascaris* can induce allergic sensitization in animal models [42] and in human beings, including immediate cutaneus hyperreactivity [52] and airway response after aerosol challenge with parasite extracts [53] suggesting the presence of an allergenic component on the stimulation of the respiratory symptoms by these parasites. Helminths harbor an arsenal of many pro- allergenic molecules which may be involved in airway inflammatory processes. One of the most studied is the *A. lumbricoides* body fluid antigen -1 (ABA-1) [54-57] which constitutes the most important of the group of antigens of the denominated family of nematode polyprotein allergens (NPA) for its capacity to stimulate strong IgE responses [58]. Recognition of ABA-1 may have a genetic basis [59, 60]. For example, evidences from studies carried out in Colombian endemic areas have shown that polymorphisms of LIG4 and TNFSF13B of the 13q33 region are associated with high levels of specific IgE to ABA-1 in *A. lumbricoides* infected children [60, 61]. However, the possible role of this allergen in airway inflammation remains unclear. Another important allergenic component of helminths is tropomyosin, which is a microfilament associated protein present in all eukaryotic cells, essential in the process of muscle work, proper action of the movement apparatus and the basic functionality of filaments within the cytoskeleton [62]. There is a high degree of homology among tropomyosins even of phylogenetically distant species of invertebrates, but not with vertebrate tropomyosins [62]. Invertebrate tropomyosins induce IgE antibodies and are potent allergens for humans whereas vertebrate ones were reported to be non-allergenic [62, 63]. Tropomyosin from *A. lumbricoides* presents a high degree of sequence identity to those from other invertebrates, including cockroach, mites, and shrimp [64]. It is expressed in high levels in the third stage larvae (L3), which is the stage of pulmonary passage of the parasite and stimulates strongly the production of IgE [64], high positivity to skin prick tests and histamine release from basophils[64, 65]. *A.lumbricoides* tropomyosin cross-reacts with other invertebrate tropomyosins [64] thus enhancing the allergic response to other environmental allergens containing tropomyosin (cockroach, mites, and shrimp) [64, 65] which are known to induce airway inflammation and asthma [65]. Other important nematode allergens are chitins, an important component for egg shell integrity and for the structure of the rigid pharynx, including the buccal cavity and grinder, a specialized cuticle that is shed and re-synthesized during molting [66]. There is evidence that chitins are involved in Th2 type inflammation. For example, experimental models of asthma using mice have shown that the intranasal administration of chitin induced an accumulation of eosinophils and basophils [67]. Exposure to chitin also stimulated the alternative activation of macrophages as indicated by the presence of arginase-expressing cells in the lungs as early as 6 h post intranasal administration of chitin [67]. The recruitment of innate immune cells has shown to be dependent both upon expression of the high affinity receptor for leucotriene B4, BLT1 and upon the presence of macrophages [68] suggesting a possible role of chitin in innate immune cell recruitment, leading to preferential Th2 type responses. In humans, The non-chitinolytic chitinase YKL-40 has been linked to allergic inflammation. YKL-40 levels are elevated in the serum and bronchoalveolar lavage (BAL) fluid of asthmatics [69]. Furthermore, increased YKL-40 levels correlated with asthma severity and are elevated in response to allergen challenge. Nematode proteases which constitute a group of highly evolutionary conserved molecules may exhibit allergenic properties such as other proteases like house dust mite-derived *Der p 1*, domestic cats- derived *Fel d1*, and fungal allergens [70, 71]. These allergens most often gain access to host tissues at mucosal sites and in some individuals elicit potent Th2 cytokine responses, reflecting the hallmarks of the immune response to helminthic infection including eosinophilia, goblet cell hyperplasia and elevated serum IgE levels as explained above. Basophils which are innate immune cells able to rapidly secrete IL-4 *in vitro* following stimulation with anti-IgE [72] as well as in response to allergens and helminth products [73], would be involved in the innate sensing of these products which may lead to the initiation of adaptive Th2 cytokine responses to parasite and/or environmental allergens. For example, immunization of mice with the cysteine protease allergen, papain, resulted in the transient recruitment of basophils to lymph nodes that peaked 1 day prior to the peak of IL-4 producing CD4+ T cells [74]. These papain-elicited basophils within the lymph node were shown to express thymic stromal lymphopoietin (TSLP), an IL-7-like cytokine produced predominantly by epithelial cells and implicated in CD4+ Th2 cell differentiation [74]. Given their multiple roles in regulating inflammation, cellular trafficking and epithelial barrier function members of the protease-activated receptor (PAR) family [75] would be potential molecular targets for helminth proteases.

Regardless of the intrinsic allergenic potential of these parasites, there are evidences that active infection can potentiate the allergic response to non-related antigens. For example, it has been shown that antigenic extracts of *A. suum* potentiate allergic responses to ovalbumin in pigs (76, 77). It has been also reported that co-administration of hen egg lysozyme with the excretory / secretory products of *N. brasiliensis* in mice results in the generation of egg-lysozyme-specific lymphocyte proliferation, IL-4 release and IgG1 antibody responses [78]. Furthermore, it has been shown that unidentified components in the body fluid of *A. suum* promotes a Th2 response and are adjuvant for specific IgE synthesis to some parasitic allergens like ABA-1 [79]. Because, in addition to this allergen, *A. lumbricoides* extract has at least 11 human-IgE-binding components, the adjuvant effect may be more generalized in humans beings, and because of co-exposure with other environmental allergens, this could happen for cross-reactive and non-cross-reactive mite allergens [61].These observations are consistent with early studies carried out in atopic Venezuelan children in which an elevated percentage of skin positivity as well as high levels of specific serum IgE toward aero-allergens, were found among children infected with *A. lumbricoides* compared to their non parasitized counterparts [80].

4. Epidemiological studies showing a positive association between helminthic infections and asthma

Human immune response to infections with helminths parasites may differ according to the profile of the infection. As mentioned above, acute or seasonal infections may include primary infections and repeated or intermittent infections without long period of continuous infections and may result from infrequent short exposures or intermittent exposure after treatment in endemic areas [3, 5]. It has been proposed that mild, seasonal helminthic infections stimulate preferentially inflammatory Th2 type immune responses among parasitized populations [3, 81] characterized by the production of high levels of serum specific IgE and allergic reactivity toward parasite soluble antigens [82] which may lead to the development of bronchial hyper reactivity and asthma [83, 84] particularly among atopic individuals [85]. This situation may be reflected on the increased prevalence of asthma and allergic diseases observed in many low and middle-income countries [86, 87] undergoing parasite eradication programs [5, 6]. For example, epidemiological studies carried out in different rural communities in China, have shown a strong association between Ascaris lumbricoides infection and the development of asthma [88]. These early results are consistent with a meta-analysis of many of studies investigating the association between the presence of geohelminth eggs in stool samples and asthma providing some evidence for parasite-specific effects [7]. In this work in which thirty-three studies were taken in account, *Ascaris lumbricoides* was associated with significantly increased odds of asthma (OR, 1.34; 95% CI, 1.05–1.71; 20 studies. Further studies carried out in urban Brazil have shown positive associations between Ascaris lumbricoides infection with recent wheeze [9] which in turn have been associated to allergic sensitization toward A. lumbricoides antigens [9]. Other studies carried out in Costa Rica have shown a relationship between sensitization (defined as a positive IgE) to A. lumbricoides and measures of asthma morbidity and severity in a population with low prevalence of parasitic infection but high prevalence of parasitic exposure [89]. In this work, a cross-sectional study of 439 children (ages 6 to 14 years) with asthma was carried out and linear regression and logistic regression were used for the multivariate statistical analysis. Sensitization to A. lumbricoides was associated with having at least 1 positive skin test to allergens (odds ratio, 5.15; 95% CI, 2.36-11.21; $P < .0001$), increased total serum IgE and eosinophils in peripheral blood, reductions in FEV (1) and FEV (1)/forced vital capacity, increased airway responsiveness and bronchodilator responsiveness, and hospitalizations for asthma in the previous year (odds ratio, 3.08; 95% CI, 1.23-7.68; $P = 0.02$). Similarly, it has been also reported that sensitization to A. lumbricoides is associated with increased severity of asthma among Romanian children [90]. This association was mediated by a high degree of atopy among the asthmatic children sensitized to A. lumbricoides and belonging to a population with a low prevalence of helminthiasis. In according to these findings, studies carried out in Venezuela have shown strong associations between A. Lumbricoides infection and bronchial hyper-reactivity [84]. In this work, 470 school children from different rural and urban communities were evaluated. It was found that in rural children, bronchial hyper reactivity was associated with increased specific levels of anti- IgE ($p<0.0001$) and skin test positivity toward A lumbricoides antigens ($p<0.0001$). The percentage of FVE1 predictive values correlated inversely ($p<0.0001$) with anti-A lumbricoides IgE levels. Elevated numbers of circulating CD3+CD4+ and CD20+CD23+ cells were found in rural children with bronchial hyper reactivity compared to their asymptomatic counterparts. They correlated positively with anti-A lumbricoides IgE levels ($p<0.005$ and $p<0.0001$ respectively). In contrast, in urban children, bronchial hyper reactivity was associated with elevated anti-D pteronissinus IgE levels (p=0, 0089), skin hyper reactivity towards this aero allergen (p=0,003) and to an increase in the number of CD3+CD8+ ($p<0.0001$). These results were consistent with previous work showing that monthly treatments of parasitized asthmatic children with anti-helminthic drugs in Venezuela may reduce BHR, symptoms of wheeze and the need for asthma medications [2]. Taking together these findings suggest the importance of the atopic condition on the airway inflammatory response stimulated by these parasites [91]. On the other hand, studies performed in slum children from endemic areas have shown that parasitized non-asthmatic children can significant respond to bronchodilator inhalation, and that this response can be reversed by anti-helminthic treatment suggesting that these parasites cause bronchoconstriction [92]. Moreover, in a more recent study it was shown that infestation with *Ascaris lumbricoides* in Brazilian children increased the risk of non-atopic asthma [8] such that children with high load infestation (≥100 eggs/g) have been found to be five times more likely to have BHR than children with low load or no infestation [8]. Thus, regardless the atopic status of the individuals, the link between helminth infestation and non-atopic asthma could be mediated by the stimulation of transient inflammatory responses by parasite antigens in the pulmonary phase of the helminth life cycle such as those described according to the Loeffler's syndrome.

5. The other side of the coin: Chronic helminthic infection may suppress allergic manifestation and the development of asthma

Because parasites are in constant attack by a range of effective immune mechanisms, they have developed effective evasion mechanisms which may vary from simple avoidance to a more active modulation of the immune response in order to establish a non inflammatory environment that allows the parasite to survive. Nematode parasites may enhance survival by directing the immune response to that of a less appropriate type. For example interference with the Th1/-Th2 response balance, the production of high levels of regulatory cytokines such as IL-10 and TGF- β which may lead to a general suppression of T and B cell responses and also mimicry of host proteins which direct the immune response to tolerance have been reported [93]. It has been proposed that because these suppressing mechanisms are not parasite- specific, they may affect the development of allergic reactions in chronically exposed populations [94, 95]. It has been proposed that the effect of geo-helminths on the suppression of atopy is more important early in life causing a deviated Th2 immune phenotype that is not changed later in life, after elimination of the infection [96]. Moreover, there is evidence that maternal helminthic infections could affect infant immunity [97, 98] raising the possibility that the immunologic effects of infection start in the fetus. Further, the inverse association between chronic helminthic infections and allergic disorders among school children from different rural populations from Venezuela, Gambia, Ethiopia, Taiwan, Ecuador and Ghana has been well documented [99].

The exact mechanisms by which these parasites dampen allergic responses are probably multiple. Chronic helminthic infections may protect against allergic disease because of their profound suppression of the host immune system, leading to a general T-cell hypo responsiveness that is facilitated by the activity of regulatory T (Treg) and B cells and the modulation effects of innate immune cells such as macrophages, dendritic cells (DCs) and local stromal cells, resulting in an anti-inflammatory environment characterized by increased levels of interleukin (IL)-10 and transforming growth factor (TGF)-β [100]. In humans, several studies have shown that Treg cell activity (both by natural CD4+CD25+FoxP3+ and adaptive CD4+IL10+ Tr1 cells) protects against allergic disease [100,101, 102]. Indeed, successful allergen specific immunotherapy in humans which leads to a reduction in allergic symptoms has been associated with the emergence of IL-10–producing Treg cells which may be involved in the increase in IgG4 and IgA responses and a simultaneous decrease in IgE [103]. Several studies carried out in distinct experimental models have revealed a number of active molecules in extracts of helminths that can modulate the immune system of the host. Early work conducted by Itami et al [104] have demonstrated that high molecular weight components purified by gel filtration chromatography from an *A. suum* adult worm extract were able to suppress the murine antibody production to a bystander antigen. This effect was attributed to a 200 KD a protein component called PAS-1. The protein was affinity purified using a monoclonal antibody (MAIP-1) produced against high molecular weight suppressive components. Pas-1 was shown to be capable of down regulating antibody production Th2 secretion; eosinophils recruitment and airway hyper-responsiveness induced by *A. suum* allergens [105]. This effect was mediated by the stimulating capacity of Pas-1 on the production of regulatory cytokines such as IL-10. Probably the best-characterized groups of helminth immunomodulators are the cystatins (cysteine protease inhibitors) [106] which can inhibit antigen processing and presentation [107], interfering with antigen-specific T cell responses and the proliferation of T and B cells. They can also modulate cytokine responses. Particularly they are involved in the up regulation of IL-10 that leads to the down regulation of co-stimulatory surface molecules of macrophages [108]. These properties contribute to induction of an anti-inflammatory environment, concomitant with a strong inhibition of cellular proliferation. Also, carbohydrates linked to proteins and lipids of nematodes, particularly those of phosphorylcholine (PC)-modified carbohydrates [109] have attracted significant attention in the past years due to their immunogenic and immunomodulatory properties. Structural features of glycolipids including oligosaccharide backbone, substitution with PC, and ceramide composition are shared between all the parasitic nematode species with widespread anatomical location in the worm [109] suggesting the importance of these components in host parasite interactions. The secreted filarial nematode glycoprotein ES-62 constitutes a suitable example. Through PC modifications, ES-62 can inhibit the proliferation of CD4+ T cells and conventional B2 cells *in vivo*, and reduces CD4+ cell IL-4 and IFN-γ production [110]. Conversely, ES-62 promotes proliferation and IL-10 production by peritoneal B1 cells [111]. It has been proposed that inhibition of proinflammatory Th1 responses occurs as ES-62 interacts with toll-like receptor (TLR) 4 through its PC residues [112], also in mast cells the interaction of TLR 4 with ES-62 results in the inhibition of degranulation and release of inflammatory mediators [113]. On the other hand, like proteins, glycolipids can be target of antibody responses. In the case of helminths antibody reactivity to lipids has been described in schistosomiasis [114] and more recently in *A. lumbricoides* infection [115]. Epidemiological studies using *Ascaris* derived glicolipids have shown that children carrying heavy infections show highest IgG reactivity glycolipids compared to lightly or non-infected children [115]. In the same study IgG antibody reactivity to both glyco proteins and glycolipids were directed to the PC moiety as determined by either removal of this group or a competition assay suggesting that *A. lumbricoides* specific glycolipids have antigenic properties. The mechanism by which glycolipids can stimulate IgE and IgG responses is not clear. It is possible that antibodies could develop directly to glycolipids through activation of CD1d which is a non classical MHC lipid presenting molecule. Nevertheless, cross reactivity between glycolipids and PC present on proteins may also occur [115]. The immunomodulatory effects exhibited by PC- substituted molecules can be seen as a contribution to equilibrium in host -parasite interactions in which expanding of TH2 type responses enables the parasite to survive preventing harmful pro-inflammatory mechanisms in the host. Since PC substituted molecules from nematode differ clearly from those from the host, they would be a suitable target for the development of new anti inflammatory drugs.

6. Future challenges and research perspectives

As mentioned above, the prevalence of asthma in rural developing countries has been under estimated for many years and in many areas of the world in which persons with asthma do not have access to basic asthma medications or medical care and are not included in any statistical survey. Thus adequate control of asthma in developing countries would require improvements in health care and the development of technologies to obtain the information needed to identify high-risk groups (disease mapping) [3]. This goal would be difficult to achieve if countries do not allocate resources to enable better health care. On the other hand, since many years several global efforts have been made to address the health effects of human parasitism by helminths which results from poverty and exert a well known detrimental impact on the health status of children continuously exposed to these parasites. The World Health Assembly (WHA) has adopted several resolutions calling for the control or elimination of these diseases, and for the implementation of a number of large-scale control and elimination programs. However, despite such WHA/WHO resolutions, the control of morbidity and the elimination of these infections are still a big challenge for global health programs. Some of the identified obstacles include the current scarcity of tools for updated disease mapping, the development of new anthelmintic drugs and vaccines, the improvement of sensitive diagnostic tools and the monitoring of the progress of control interventions and quantification of changes in incidence of infection and disease [116]. However and according to the WHA/WHO resolution, mass chemotherapy have been widely implemented in rural areas of many developing countries in which sanitary limitations are far to be overcome [6]. Under these conditions, this approach would reduce worm burdens without elimination of the infection in endemic areas, which gradually will change the profile of the infection from a chronic pattern, with moderate to heavy worm burdens [5] to a more mild and seasonal pattern [5], thereby disrupting the regulatory, anti-inflammatory effect of chronic infections on the immune response, allowing allergic sensitization in atopic parasitized individuals [117, 118]. Thus, the development of diagnosis protocols facilitating rapid identification of atopic individuals among rural populations is an immediate challenge to achieve control of parasites without affecting the health status of a significant proportion of these populations. On the other hand, the presence of respiratory symptoms as a consequence of inflammation due to the parasite migratory phase in non atopic individuals [8] must also be considered. For these purposes, large birth cohort studies designed according to specific epidemiological objectives and based on results from cross-sectional studies, small longitudinal and pilot intervention studies would help to elucidate the role of the many parameters involved in host- parasite interactions contributing to the pathogenesis of asthma. Also, the identification of conserved features of helminth products that interact with innate immune cells to co-ordinate adaptive anti-parasite responses as well as of potent parasite derived allergens is a key challenge to improve the technology used in the diagnosis and monitoring of allergic diseases in the tropics. Noteworthy is the cross-reactivity of helminth antigens with environmental allergens which may explain the high prevalence of IgE sensitization to invertebrate allergens leading to the development of asthma and other allergic diseases [61]. Finally, the identification and characterization of individual helminth-derived immunomodulatory molecules that selectively induce regulatory immune responses will provide potential candidates for immunotherapy [119] and must be the subject for future research programs.

This work has been supported by the Central University of Venezuela through the project: CDCH, PG: 09-7946-2010/1.

Author details

Isabel Hagel, Maira Cabrera and Maria Cristina Di Prisco

*Address all correspondence to: isabelhagel@yahoo.com

Institute of Biomedicine, Faculty of medicine, Central University of Venezuela, Venezuela

References

[1] Akinbami, L. J, Moorman, J. E, Bailey, C, & Liu, X. Trends in asthma prevalence, health care use, and mortality in the United States, NCHS data brief, Hyattsville, MD: National Center for Health Statistics. 2012.(94), 2001-2010.

[2] National HeartLung, and Blood Institute, National Institutes of Health. National Asthma Education and Prevention Program. Expert Panel Report 3: Guidelines for the diagnosis and management of asthma. NIH Publication (2007). (07-4051), 07-4051.

[3] Cooper, P. J, Rodrigues, L. C, Cruz, A. A, & Barreto, M. L. Asthma in Latin America: a public health challenge and research opportunity. Allergy (2009). , 64, 5-17.

[4] Akinbami, L J, & Schoendorf, K C. Trends in Childhood Asthma: Prevalence, Health Care Utilization, and Mortality, Pediatrics (2002).

[5] Brooker, S, & Hotez, P. J. Bundy DAP. The Global Atlas of Helminth Infection: Mapping the Way Forward in Neglected Tropical Disease Control, (2010). PLoS Negle Trop Dis; 4: e779.

[6] Brooker, S. Clements ACA, Bundy DAP ((2006). Global epidemiology, ecology and control of soil-transmitted helminth infections. Adv Parasitol 2006; , 62, 221-261.

[7] Leonardi-bee, J, Pritchard, D, & Britton, J. Asthma and current intestinal parasite infection: systematic review and meta-analysis. Am J Respir Crit Care Med (2006). , 174, 514-523.

[8] Pereira, M. U, Sly, P. D, & Pitrez, P. M. Nonatopic asthma is associated with helminth infections and bronchiolitis in poor children. Eur Respir J (2007). , 29, 1154-1160.

[9] da SilvaER, Sly, PD, de Pereira, MU. Intestinal helminth infestation is associated with increased bronchial responsiveness in children. Pediatr Pulmonol (2008). , 43, 662-665.

[10] Scrivener, S, Yemaneberhan, H, Zebenigus, M, Tilahun, D, Girma, S, & Ali, S. (2001). Independent effects of intestinal parasite infection and domestic allergen exposure on the risk of wheeze in Ethiopia: a nested case-control study. Lancet, , 358, 1493-1499.

[11] Holgate, S. T. Pathogenesis of asthma. Clin Exp Allergy (2008). , 38, 872-897.

[12] Webb, D. C, Cai, Y, Matthaei, K. I, & Foster, P. S. Comparative roles of IL-4, IL-13, and IL-4R in dendritic cell maturation and CD4+ Th2 cell function. J Immunol (2007). , 178, 219-227.

[13] Bloemen, K, & Verstraelen, S. Van Den Heuvel R, Witters H, Nelissen I & Schoeters G. The allergic cascade: review of the most important molecules in the asthmatic lung. Immunol Lett (2007). , 113, 6-18.

[14] James, A. L, Maxwell, P. S, & Pearce-pinto, G. Elliot JG & Carroll NG. The relationship of reticular basement membrane thickness to airway wall remodeling in asthma. Am J Respir Crit Care Med (2002). , 166, 1590-1595.

[15] Puxeddu, I, Pang, Y. Y, & Harvey, A. The soluble form of a disintegrin and metalloprotease 33 promotes angiogenesis: implications for airway remodeling in asthma. J Allergy Clin Immunol (2008). , 121, 1400-6.

[16] Lambrecht, B. N, & Hammad, H. Biology of lung dendritic cells at the origin of asthma. Immunity (2009). , 31, 412-424.

[17] Van Rijt, L. S, Jung, S, Kleinjan, A, Vos, N, Willart, M, Duez, C, Hoogsteden, H. C, & Lambrecht, B. N. In vivo depletion of lung CD11c+ dendritic cells during allergen challenge abrogates the characteristic features of asthma. J Exp Med (2005). , 201, 981-991.

[18] Lambrecht, B. N, Salomon, B, Klatzmann, D, & Pauwels, R. A. Dendritic cells are required for the development of chronic eosinophilic airway inflammation in response to inhaled antigen in sensitized mice. J Immunol (1998). , 160, 4090-4097.

[19] Lambrecht, B. N, De Veerman, M, Coyle, A. J, Gutierrez-ramos, J. C, Thielemans, K, & Pauwels, R. A. Myeloid dendritic cells induce TH2 responses to inhaled antigen, leading to eosinophilic airway inflammation. J Clin Invest (2000). , 106, 551-559.

[20] Robays, L. J, Maes, T, Joos, G. F, & Vermaelen, K. Y. Between a cough and a wheeze: dendritic cells at the nexus of tobacco smoke-induced allergic airway sensitization. Mucosal Immunol (2009). , 2, 206-219.

[21] Sokol, C. L, Barton, G. M, Farr, A. G, & Medzhitov, R. A. A mechanism for the initiation of allergen-induced T helper type 2 responses. Nat. Immunol. (2008). , 9, 310-8.

[22] Perrigoue, J. G, Saenz, S. A, Siracusa, M. C, Allenspach, E. J, Taylor, B. C, Giacomin, P. R, Nair, M. G, Du, Y, Zaph, C, Van Rooijen, N, Comeau, M. R, Pearce, E. J, Laufer, T. M, & Artis, D. MHC class II-dependent basophil-CD4+ T cell interactions promote TH2 cytokine-dependent immunity. Nat Immunol. (2009). , 10, 697-705.

[23] [23]Yoshimoto, T, Yasuda, K, Tanaka, H, Nakahira, M, Imai, Y, Fujimori, Y, & Nakanishi, K. Basophils contribute to TH2-IgE responses in vivo via IL-4 production and presentation of peptide-MHC class II complexes to CD4+ T cells. Nat Immunol. (2009). , 10, 706-712.

[24] Akuthota, P, Wang, H. B, Spencer, L. A, & Weller, P. F. Immunoregulatory roles of eosinophils: a new look at a familiar cell. Clin Exp Allergy. (2008). , 38, 1254-1263.

[25] Prussin, C, Metcalfe, DD, & Ig, . , mast cells, basophils, and eosinophils. J Allergy Clin Immunol 2006; 117:S450-S456.

[26] Silver, M. R, Margulis, A, Wood, N, Goldman, S. J, Kasaian, M, & Chaudhary, D. IL-33 synergizes with IgE-dependent and IgE-independent agents to promote mast cell and basophil activation. Inflamm Res (2010). , 59, 207-218.

[27] Taube, C, Wei, X, Swasey, C. H, Joetham, A, Zarini, S, Lively, T, Takeda, K, Loader, J, Miyahara, N, Kodama, T, Shultz, L. D, Donaldson, D. D, Hamelmann, E. H, Dakhama, A, & Gelfand, E. W. Mast cells, FcεRI, and IL-13 are required for development of airway

hyperresponsiveness after aerosolized allergen exposure in the absence of adjuvant. J Immunol (2004). , 172, 6398-6406.

[28] Ghosh, S, & Erzurum, S. C. Nitric oxide metabolishm in asthma pathophysiology. Bioch Biophys Acta (2011). , 1810, 1008-16.

[29] Cieslewicz, G, Tomkinson, A, Adler, A, Duez, C, Schwarze, J, Takeda, K, Larson, K. A, Lee, J. J, Irvin, C. G, & Gelfand, E. W. The late, but not early, asthmatic response is dependent on IL-5 and correlates with eosinophil infiltration. J Clin Invest (1999). , 104, 301-308.

[30] Hamid, Q, Springall, D. R, Riveros-moreno, V, Chanez, P, Howarth, P, Redington, A, Bousquet, J, Godard, P, Holgate, S, & Polak, J. M. Induction of nitric oxide synthase in asthma. Lancet. (1993). , 342, 1510-3.

[31] Nathan, C, & Shiloh, M. U. Reactive oxygen and nitrogen intermediated in the relationship between mammalian hosts and the microbial pathogens. Proc Natl Acad Sci USA (2000).

[32] Mossayi, P. E, Sarfati, D, Yamaoka, K, Aubry, J. P, Bonnefoy, J. Y, Dugas, B, & Kolb, J. P. Evidence for a role of Fc epsilon RII/CD23 in the IL-4 induce nitric oxide production by normal human mononuclear phagocytes. Cell Immunol (1995).

[33] Mossalayi, M. D, Arock, M, & Debré, P. CD23/FcεRII:signaling and clinical implication.Int Rev Immunol.(1997). , 16, 129-46.

[34] [34]Craig, T. J, & King, T. S. Lemanske RF Jr, Wecjsler ME, Icitovic M,Zimmerman RR Jr, Wasserman S. Aeroallergen sensitization correlates with PC(20) and exhaled nitric oxide in subjects with mild to moderated asthma. J Allergy Clin Immunol (2008). , 121, 671-7.

[35] Hopkin, J. Immune and genetic aspects of asthma, allergy and parasitic worm infections: evolutionary links. Parasite Immunology (2009).

[36] Nahrevanian, H. Involvement of Nitric Oxide and Its Up/Down Stream Molecules in the immunity against parasitic Infections. Brazilian J Infect Dis (2009). , 13, 440-448.

[37] Nacher, M, Singhasivanon, P, Traore, B, Vannaphan, S, Gay, F, Chindanond, D, Franetich, J. F, Mazier, D, & Looareesuwan, S. Helminth infections are associated with protection from cerebral malaria and increased nitrogen derivatives concentrations in Thailand. Am J Trop Med Hyg (2002). , 66, 304-9.

[38] Ait Aissa SAmri M, Bouteldja R, Wietzerbin J, Touil-Boukoffa C. Alterations in interferon-gamma and nitric oxide levels in human echinococcosis. Cell Mol Biol (Noisy-le-grand) (2006). , 52, 65-70.

[39] Touil-boukoffa, C, Bauvois, B, Sancéau, J, Hamrioui, B, & Wietzerbin, J. Production of nitric oxide (NO) in human hydatidosis: relationship between nitrite production and interferon-gamma levels. Biochimie (1998). , 80, 739-44.

[40] Bascal, Z. A, Cunningham, J. M, Holden-dye, L, Shea, O, & Walker, M. RJ. Characterization of a putative nitric oxide synthase in the neuromuscular system of the parasitic nematode, Ascaris suum. Parasitology (2001)., 122(2), 219-31.

[41] Enobe, C. S, Araffljo, C. A, Perini, A, & Martins, M. A. Macedo MS & Macedo-Soares MF. Early stages of Ascaris suum induce airway inflammation and hyperreactivity in a mouse model. Parasite Immunol (2006)., 28, 453-461.

[42] Phills, J. A, & Harrold, A. J. Whiteman GV & Perelmutter L. Pulmonary infiltrates, asthma and eosinophilia due to Ascaris suum infestation in man. N Engl J Med (1972)., 286, 965-970.

[43] Loeffler, W. (1956). Transient lung infiltrations with blood eosinophilia. Int Arch Allergy Appl Immunol 1956;, 8, 54-59.

[44] Diemert, D. J. Ascariasis. In Guerrant RL, Walker DH, Weller PF (ed), Tropical infectious diseases: principles, pathogens & practice, 3rd ed. Churchill Livingstone, Philadelphia, PA., (2011)., 794-798.

[45] Dold, C. Holland CV Ascaris and ascariasis. Microbes Infect (2011)., 13, 632-637.

[46] Wilson, M. E, & Weller, P. F. Eosinophilia,. In Guerrant RL, Walker DH, Weller PF (ed), Tropical infectious diseases: principles, pathogens & practice, 3rd ed. Churchill Livingstone, Philadelphia, PA.. (2011)., 939-949.

[47] Weller, P. F, & Bubley, G. J. The idiopathic hypereosinophilic syndrome. Blood (1994)., 1994, 83-2759.

[48] Phills, J. A, Harrold, A. J, Whiteman, G. V, & Perelmutter, L. Pulmonary,infiltrates, asthma and eosinophilia due to Ascaris suum infestation in man. N Engl J Med (1972)., 1972, 286-965.

[49] Weller, P. F. (1994). Parasitic pneumonias. In Pennington J (ed), Respiratory infections: diagnosis and management, 3rd ed. Raven Press, New York, NY, 1994;, 695-714.

[50] Siddiqui, A. A, Genta, R. M, Maguilnik, I, & Berk, S. L. Strongyloidiasis. In Guerrant RL, Walker DH, Weller PF (ed), Tropical infectious diseases: principles, pathogens&practice, 3rd ed. Churchill Livingstone Philadelphia, PA., (2011)., 805-812.

[51] Praveen, A, & Weller, P. F. Eosinophilic Pneumonias. Clin Microbiol Rev (2012).

[52] Hagel, I, & Lynch, N. R. Di Prisco MC, Lopez RI, Garcia N. Allergic reactivity of children of different socioeconomic levels in tropical populations. Int Archs Allergy Immunol (1993)., 101, 209-214.

[53] Lynch, N. R, Isturiz, G, & Sanchez, Y. Di prisco MC. Bronchial challenge of tropical asthmatics with Ascaris lumbricoides. J Invest Allergol Clin Immunol (1992)., 2, 97-105.

[54] Mcdermott, L, Cooper, A, & Kennedy, M W. Novel classes of fatty acid and retinol binding proteins from nematodes. Biochem. J, (1999)., 192, 69-77.

[55] Xia, Y, Spence, H J, Moore, J, Heaney, N, Mcdermott, L, Cooper, A, Watson, D G, Mei, B, Komuniecki, R, & Kennedy, M W. The ABA-1 allergen of Ascaris lumbricoides: sequence polymorphism, stage and tissue-specific expression, lipid binding function, and protein biophysical properties. Parasitology (2000).

[56] Moore, J, Mcdermott, L, Price, N. C, Kelly, S. M, Cooper, A, & Kennedy, M. W. Sequence-divergent units of the ABA-1 polyprotein array of the nematode Ascaris suum have similar fatty-acid- and retinol-binding properties but different binding-site environments. Biochem J (1999). , 340, 337-343.

[57] Kennedy, M. W. The polyprotein lipid binding proteins of nematodes. Biochim Byophis Acta (2000).

[58] Turner, J. D, Faulkner, H, Kamgno, J, Kennedy, M W, Behnke, J, Boussinesq, M, & Bradley, J E. Allergen-specific IgE and IgG4 are markers of resistance and susceptibility in a human intestinal nematode infection. Microbes Infect (2005). , 2005(7), 990-996.

[59] Kennedy, M. W, Tomlinson, L. A, Fraser, E. M, & Christie, J. F. The specificity of the antibody response to internal antigens of Ascaris: Heterogeneity in infected human and MHC (H-2) control of the repertoire in mice. Clin Exp Immunol (1990). , 80, 219-224.

[60] Acevedo, N, Mercado, D, Vergara, C, Sánchez, J, Kennedy, M W, Jiménez, S, Fernández, A. M, Gutiérrez, M, Puerta, L, & Caraballo, L. Association between total immunoglobulin E and antibody responses to naturally acquired Ascaris lumbricoides infection and polymorphisms of immune system-related LIG4, TNFSF13B and IRS2 genes. Clin Exp Immunol (2009). , 157, 282-290.

[61] Acevedo, N, Sánchez, J, Erler, A, Mercado, D, Briza, P, Kennedy, M, Fernandez, A, Gutierrez, M, Chua, K. Y, Cheong, N, Jiménez, S, Puerta, L, & Caraballo, L. IgE cross-reactivity between Ascaris and domestic mite allergens: the role of tropomyosin and the nematode polyprotein ABA-1. Allergy (2009). , 64, 1635-1643.

[62] Reese, G, Ayuso, R, & Lehrer, S. B. Tropomyosin: an invertebrate pan-allergen. Int Arch Immunol (1999). , 119, 247-258.

[63] Arruda, L. K, & Santos, A. B. Immunologic responses to common antigens in helminthic infections and allergic disease. Curr Opin Allergy Clin Immunol (2005). , 5, 399-402.

[64] Santos, A. B, Rocha, G. M, Oliver, C, Ferriani, V. P, Lima, R. C, Palma, M. S, Sales, V. S, Alberse, R C, Chapman, M. D, & Arruda, L. K. Cross-reactive IgE antibody responses to tropomyosins from Ascaris lumbricoides and cockroach. J Allergy Clin Immunol (2008). , 121, 1040-1046.

[65] Sereda, M. J, Hartmann, S, & Lucius, R. Helminths and allergy: the example of tropomyosin. Trends parasitol (2008). , 24, 272-278.

[66] Arnold, K, Brydon, L. J, Chappell, L. H, & Gooday, G. W. Chitinolytic activities in Heligmosomoides polygyrus and their role in egg hatching. Mol Biochem Parasitol (1993).

[67] Reese, T. A, & Liang, H. E. Tager ANM, Luster AD, Rooijen N, Voehringer D, Locksley RM. Chitin Induces Tissue Accumulation of Innate Immune Cells Associated with Allergy. Nature, (2007). , 447, 92-96.

[68] Lee, C. G. Chitin, chitinases and chitinase-like proteins in allergic inflammation and tissue remodeling Yonsei Med J (2009). , 28, 22-30.

[69] Kuepper, M, Bratke, K, & Virchow, J. C. Chitinase-like protein and asthma. N Engl J Med (2008). , 358, 1073-1075.

[70] Trap, C, & Boireau, P. Proteases in helminthic parasites. Vet Res (2000). , 31, 461-471.

[71] Falcone, F. H, Loukas, A, Quinnell, R. J, & Pritchard, D. I. The innate allergenicity of helminth parasites. Clin Rev Allergy Immunol (2004). , 26, 61-72.

[72] Gessner, A, Mohrs, K, & Mohrs, M. Mast cells, basophils, and eosinophils acquire constitutive IL-4 and IL-13 transcripts during lineage differentiation that are sufficient for rapid cytokine production. J Immunol (2005). , 174, 1063-1072.

[73] Phillips, C, Coward, W. R, Pritchard, D. I, & Hewitt, C. R. Basophils express a type 2 cytokine profile on exposure to proteases from helminths and house dust mites. J Leukoc Biol (2003). , 73, 165-171.

[74] Sokol, C. L, Barton, G. M, Farr, A. G, & Medzhitov, R. A mechanism for the initiation of allergen-induced T helper type 2 responses. Nat Immunol (2008). , 9, 310-318.

[75] Amadesi, S, & Bunnett, N. Protease-activated receptors: protease signaling in the gastrointestinal tract. Curr Opin Pharmacol (2004). , 4, 551-556.

[76] Stromberg, B. E. Potentiation of the reaginic (IgE) antibody response to ovalbumin in the guinea pig with a soluble metabolic product from Ascaris suum. J Immunol (1980). , 125, 833-836.

[77] Marretta, J, & Casey, F. B. Effect of Ascaris suum and other adjuvants on the potentiation of the IgE response in guinea-pigs. Immunology (1979). , 37, 609-613.

[78] Holland, M. J, & Harcus, Y. M. Riches PL & Maizels RM. Proteins secreted by the parasitic nematode Nippostrongylus brasiliensis act as adjuvants for Th2 responses. Eur J Immunol 2000; (1977). , 30, 1977-1987.

[79] Paterson, J. C, & Garside, P. Kennedy MW & Lawrence CE. Modulation of a heterologous immune response by the products of Ascaris suum. Infect Immun (2002). , 70, 6058-6067.

[80] Hagel, I, Lynch, N. R, & Perez, M. Di Prisco MC, Lopez R, Rojas E. Modulation of the allergic reactivity of slum children by helminthic infection. Paras Immunol (1993). , 15, 311-315.

[81] Cooper, P. J, Barreto, M. L, & Rodrigues, L. C. Human allergy and geohelminth infections: a review of the literature and a proposed conceptual model to guide the investigation of possible causal associations. British Medical Bulletin (2006). and , 80, 203-218.

[82] Hagel, I, & Lynch, N. R. Di Prisco MC, Lopez RI, Garcia N. Allergic reactivity of children of different socioeconomic levels in tropical populations. Int Archs Allergy Immunol (1993). , 101, 209-214.

[83] Lynch, N. R, & Hagel, I. Di Priso MC. Asthma in the tropics: the importance of parasitic infection. In "Asthma: a link between environment, immunology and the airways." H. Neffen, C. Baena-Cagnani, L. Fabbri, S. Holgate, P. O'Byrne (eds). Hogrefe & Huber, Gottingen, (1999). , 74-77.

[84] Hagel, I, Cabrera, M, Hurtado, M. A, et al. Infection by Ascaris lumbricoides and bronchial hyper-reactivity: an outstanding association in Venezuelan school children from endemic areas. Acta Trop (2007). , 103, 231-241.

[85] Lynch, N. R, Hagel, I, & Palenque, M. E. Di Prisco MC, Escudero JE, Corao LA, Sandia JA, Ferreira LJ, Botto C, Perez M, Le Souef PN. Relationship between helminthic infection and IgE response in atopic and non-atopic children in a tropical environment. J Allergy Clin Immunol (1998).

[86] Asher, M. I, Montefort, S, Björkstén, B, Lai, C. K, Strachan, D. P, & Weiland, S. K. Williams H; ISAAC Phase Three Study Group. Worldwide time trends in the prevalence of symptoms of asthma, allergic rhinoconjunctivitis, and eczema in childhood: ISAAC Phases One and Three repeat multi country cross-sectional surveys. Lancet (2006). , 368, 733-743.

[87] Pearce, N, Aït-khaled, N, Beasley, R, Mallol, J, Keil, U, Mitchell, E, & Robertson, C. and the ISAAC Phase Three Study Group. Worldwide trends in the prevalence of asthma symptoms: phase III of the International Study of Asthma and Allergies in Childhood (ISAAC). Thorax (2007). , 62, 758-766.

[88] Palmer, L, Celedón, J. C, Weiss, S. T, Wang, B, Fang, Z, & Xu, X. Ascaris lumbricoides Infection Is Associated with Increased Risk of Childhood Asthma and Atopy in Rural China.Am. J. Respir Crit Care Med (2002). , 165, 1489-1493.

[89] Hunninghake, G. M, Soto-quiros, M. E, Avila, L, Ly, N. P, Liang, C, Sylvia, J. S, Klanderman, B. J, Silverman, E. K, Celedón, J. C, et al. Sensitization to Ascaris lumbricoides and severity of childhood asthma in Costa Rica. J Allergy Clin Immunol (2007). , 119, 654-661.

[90] Rîpa, C, Bahnea, R. G, Cojocaru, I, Luca, M. C, Leon, M, & Luca, M. Sensitization to Ascaris lumbricoides and asthma severity in children. Rev Med Chir Soc Med Nat Iasi (2011). , 115, 387-91.

[91] Lynch, N. R, Palenque, M, & Hagel, I. Di Prisco MC, Clinical improvement of asthma after anthelminthic treatment in a tropical situation. Am J Respir Crit Care Med (1997). , 156, 50-57.

[92] Lynch, N. R, Hagel, I, & Perez, M. Di Prisco M, Alvarez N, Rojas E.. Bronchoconstriction in helminthic infection. Int. Arch Allergy Immunol (1992). , 98, 77-79.

[93] Allen, J. E, & Maizels, R. M. Immunology of human helminth infection. Int. Arch. Allergy Immunol (1996). , 109, 3-10.

[94] Matera, G, Giancotti, A, Scalise, S, Pulicari, M. C, Maselli, R, Piizzi, C, Pelaia, G, Tancrè, V, Muto, V, Doldo, P, Cosco, V, Cosimo, P, Capicotto, R, Quirino, A, Scalzo, R, Liberto, M. C, Parlato, G, & Focà, A. Ascaris lumbricoides-induced suppression of total and specific IgE responses in atopic subjects is interleukin independent and associated with an increase of CD25(+) cells. Diagn Microbiol Infect Dis. (2008). , 10.

[95] Bradley, J. E, & Jackson, J. A Immunity, immunoregulation and the ecology of trichuriasis and ascariasis. Parasite Immunol (2004). , 26, 429-441.

[96] Rodrigues, L. C, Newcombe, P. J, Cunha, S. S, Alcantara-neves, N. M, Genser, B, Cruz, A. A, Simoes, S. M, Fiaccone, R, Amorim, L, & Cooper, P. J. Barreto ML; Social Change, Asthma and Allergy in Latin America.: Early infection with Trichuris trichiura and allergen skin test reactivity in later childhood. Clin Exp Allergy (2008).

[97] Guadalupe, I, Mitre, E, Benitez, S, Chico, M. E, & Nutman, T. B. Cooper PJ: Evidence for in utero sensitization to Ascaris lumbricoides in newborns of mothers with ascariasis. J Infect Dis (2009).

[98] Djuardi, Y, Wibowo, H, Supali, T, Ariawan, I, Bredius, R. G, Yazdanbakhsh, M, Rodrigues, L. C, & Sartono, E. Determinants of the relationship between cytokine production in pregnant women and their infants. PLoS One (2009). e7711.

[99] Smits, H. H. Yazdanbakhsh M: Chronic helminth infections modulate allergen-specific immune responses: protection against development of allergic disorders? Ann Med (2007).

[100] Akdis, M. Immune tolerance in allergy. Curr Opin Immunol (2009).

[101] Satoguina, J. Mempel M Larbi J, Badusche M,Loliger C, Adjei A, Gachelin G, Fleischer B, Hoerauf A, regulatory-1 cells are associated with immunosuppression in a chronic helminth infection (onchocerciasis). Microbes Infect (2002).

[102] Doetze, A, Satoguina, J, Burchard, G, Rau, T, Löliger, C, Fleischer, B, & Hoerauf, A. Antigen-specific cellular hyporesponsiveness in a chronic human helminth infection is mediated by T(h)3/T(r)type cytokines IL-10 and transforming growth factor-beta but not by a T(h)1 to T(h)2 shift. Int Immunol (2000). , 1.

[103] Aalberse, R. The role of IgG antibodies in allergy and immunotherapy. Allergy (2011). , 66, 28-30.

[104] ItamiDM Oshiro, TM, Araujo CA, Perini A, Martins MA, Macedo MS, Macedo-Soares, MF. Modulation of murine experimental asthma by Ascaris suum components. Clin Exp Allergy (2005). , 35, 873-879.

[105] Oshiro, T. M, Enobe, C. S, Araújo, C. A, Macedo, M. S, & Macedo-soares, M. F. PAS-1, a protein affinity purified from Ascaris suum worms, maintains the ability to modulate the immune response to a bystander antigen. Immunol Cell Biol (2006). , 84, 138-144.

[106] [106]Knox, D. P. Proteinase inhibitors and helminth parasite infection. Parasite Immunol (2007). , 29, 57-71.

[107] Hartmann, S, & Lucius, R. Modulation of host immune responses by nematode cystatins. Int. J Parasitol. (2003). , 33, 1291-1302.

[108] Manoury, B, Gregory, W. F, Maizels, R. M, & Watts, C. Bm-CPI-2, a cystatin homolog secreted by the filarial parasite Brugia malayi, inhibits class II MHC-restricted antigen processing. Curr Biol (2001).

[109] Lochnit, G, Dennis, R. D, & Geyer, R. Phosphorylcholine substituents in nematodes: structures, occurrence and biological implications. Biol Chem (2000). , 381, 839-847.

[110] Goodridge, H. S, Wilson, E. H, Harnett, W, Campbell, C. C, Harnett, M. M, & Liew, F. Y. Modulation of macrophage cytokine production by ES-62, a secreted product of the filarial nematode Acanthocheilonema viteae. J Immunol (2001). , 167, 940-945.

[111] Wilson, E. H, Deehan, M. R, Katz, E, Brown, K. S, Houston, K. M, Grady, O, Harnett, J, & Harnett, M. M. W. Hyporesponsiveness of murine B lymphocytes exposed to the filarial nematode secreted product ES-62 in vivo. Immunology (2003). , 109, 238-245.

[112] Harnett, W, & Harnett, M. M. Modulation of the host immune system by phosphorylcholine-containing glycoproteins secreted by parasitic filarial nematodes. Biochim Biophys Acta (2001). , 1539, 7-15.

[113] Melendez, A. J, Harnett, M. M, Pushparaj, P. N, Wong, W. S, Tay, H. K, Mc Sharyy, C. P, & Harnett, W. Inhibition of Fc epsilon RI-mediated mast cell responses by ES-62, A product of parasitic filarial nematodes. Nat Med (2007). , 13, 1375-1381.

[114] Van Der Kleij, D, Tielens, A. G, & Yazdanbakhsh, M. Recognition of schistosome glycolipids by immunoglobulin E: possible role in immunity. Recognition of schistosome glycolipids by immunoglobulin E: possible role in immunity. Infect Immun (1999). , 67, 5946-5950.

[115] Van Riet, E, Wuhrer, M, Wahyuni, S, Retra, K, Deelder, A. M, Tielens, A. G, Van Der Kleij, D, & Yazdanbakhsh, M. Antibody responses to Ascaris-derived proteins and glycolipids: the role of phosphorylcholine. Parasite Immunol (2006). , 28, 363-371.

[116] Lustigman, S, Prichard, R. K, Gazzinelli, A, Grant, W. N, Boatin, B. A, Mc Carthy, J, & Basanez, M. G. A Research Agenda for Helminth Diseases of Humans: The Problem of Helminthiases. PLoS Negl Trop Dis (2012). e1582. doi:10.1371/journal.pntd.0001582.

[117] van den Bigelaar AHJvan Ree R, Rodrigues LC, Lell B, Deelder AM, Kremsner PG, Yazdanbakhsh M. Decreased atopy in children infected with Schistosoma hematobium: a role for parasite-induced interleukin-10. Lancet (2000). , 356, 1723-1727.

[118] Lynch, N. R, Hagel, I, & Perez, M. Di Prisco MC, Lopez R, Alvarez N. Effect of anthelmintic treatment on the allergic reactivity of children in a tropical slum. J Allergy Clin Immunol (1993). , 92, 404-411.

http://dx.doi.org/10.5772/54690

[119] Hagel, I, & Giusti, T. Ascaris lumbricoides: An overview of therapeutics targets. Infectious Disorders-Drug Targets (2010). , 10, 349-367.

Section 4

Smoking Cessation and Lung

Chapter 9

Psychological Approaches to Increase Tobacco Abstinence in Patients with Chronic Obstructive Pulmonary Disease: A Review

Jennifer Lira-Mandujano,
M. Carmen Míguez-Varela and Sara E. Cruz-Morales

Additional information is available at the end of the chapter

http://dx.doi.org/10.5772/53265

1. Introduction

In the last century, the definition of COPD was considered as a disease constituted by chronic bronchitis and pulmonary emphysema; however, nowadays these terms are in disuse. In the last decades emerged the Global Initiative for Chronic Obstructive Lung Disease (GOLD), a group formed by researches with the objective of count with a diagnostic guide to study this disease. According to the GOLD, the COPD is a common preventable and treatable disease, characterized by persistent airflow limitation that is usually progressive and associated with an enhanced chronic inflammatory response in the airways and the lung to noxious particles or gases, exacerbations and co-morbidities contribute to the overall severity in individual patients [1]. However, some of the parameters and the definition have been questioned [2-4].

The prevalence of COPD in developed countries ranges from 3 to 6% in subjects over 50 years of age. According to the National Center for Health Statistics (NCHS) in the United States, prevalence of COPD was stable from 1998 through 2009 and was significantly higher among women than in men, and the prevalence was higher in old groups. The prevalence was high among non-Hispanic white (5.7%) and Puerto Rican (6.9%) adults, Mexican-American adults had the lowest COPD prevalence (2.6%) [5]. The prevalence of COPD appears to be increasing not only in many developed countries, but also in Latin America. COPD occupies the fourth place in terms of mortality around the world, in Mexico is currently located between the sixth and the fourth. In 2005 there was more than 11 000 deaths in men, against just over 9 000 in women, recent studies show that the prevalence is equal between men and women [6]. According the European Federation of Allergies and Airways Diseases (EFA), in Europe the prevalence of COPD varies among the different countries, having in the extremes more than 10% Germany and 2% in Netherlands: with an annual mortality of 0.28 per 1000 in Germany and 0.30 per 1000 in Austria [7]. An important problem is that COPD prevalence varies across the world, mainly to the different definitions of the disease, leading to an over-diagnosis or under-diagnosis.

Smoking contributes too many health problems including cancer, cardiovascular disease, and lung diseases, among others. In respiratory illnesses smoking increase the probability of bronchitis, emphysema, chronic obstructive lung disease and pneumonia [8]. Diagnoses of these illnesses are more common in smokers than in non-smokers; in fact is the most important risk factor of COPD and their health complications [1,9]. Therefore, in a person with the diagnosis COPD, if it is smoking, the intervention plan should include the elimination of the tobacco, since it is the most effective measurement in the prevention of this illness, provoking a delay in the loss of the pulmonary function and improving the survival [10].

2. Pathophysiology

The exposure to noxious particles produces lung inflammation, this chronic inflammation produces several airways disease as obstructive bronchiolitis and parenchymal destruction (known as emphysema) and impair defense mechanisms, all these changes result in a progressive airflow limitation [1].

The main risk factors for COPD are tobacco smoking, occupational dusts and chemicals, indoor and outdoor air pollution. In countries as Mexico, Nepal, New Guinea and Colombia, exposure to wood smoke also cause COPD. Inhalation in the work environment of dusts, gases, fumes and chemicals are other risk factors. For example in United States 19% of patients with COPD had an occupational exposure.

The symptoms more frequently observed include dyspnea, chronic cough and excessive sputum production or expectoration. However, COPD is not just simply a "smoker's cough", but an under-diagnosed, life threatening lung disease that may progressively lead to death. Physical examination includes cyanosis of lips and fingers, breathing with pursed lips (more common in patients with emphysema), use of accessory muscles of respiration: scalene and sternocleidomastoid (in cases of severe COPD), engorgement jugular, decrease in respiratory or abolished (in severe stages of COPD) noise, vibrations reduced vowels (advanced stage), there may be wheezing.

The spirometry is a simple diagnostic test that confirms the presence of COPD, it measures the amount and speed of air inhaled and exhaled. Spirometry measures the forced expiratory volume in one second (FEV1), which is the greatest volume of air that can be breathed out in the first second of a large breath; also measures the forced vital capacity (FVC), which is the greatest volume of air that can be breathed out in a completely large breath (OMS). Normally, at least 70% of the FVC comes out in the first second (i.e. the FEV1/FVC ratio is

http://dx.doi.org/10.5772/53265

>70%). A ratio less than normal defines the patient as having COPD. The diagnosis of COPD is made when the FEV1/FVC ratio is <70%. The GOLD criteria also require that values be after bronchodilator medication has been given to make the diagnosis, and the NICE criteria require FEV1%. According to the ERS criteria, it is FEV1% predicted that defines when a patient has COPD, that is, when FEV1% predicted is < 88% for men, or < 89% for women [1].

At the beginning, the airflow obstruction first causes breathlessness that reduces the forced expiratory volume in one second (FEV1) to about 1 liter, which is less than half the normal value. Then, the condition progresses persistently over five or more years, with further loss of FEV, causing more and more distressing disability and, finally, death from respiratory failure [11]. The (FEV1) declines normally with aging by approximately 30 mL/yr, but in vulnerable smokers, the decline is greater (about 60 mL/yr), resulting in the development of COPD. Smoking cessation usually restores the normal or near-normal rate of FEV1 decline. Therefore, smoking cessation is a critical component for the prevention of COPD progression. FEV1 is an index in the definition of COPD and classification of its severity. FEV1 is a good predictor of exercise tolerance and correlates with survival and quality of life. More rapid FEV1 decline is also predictive of morbidity, mortality, and hospitalization rates [12].

3. Smoking cessation

With regard to lung diseases, COPD is which is more associated with cigarette smoking. Smoking cessation reduces the risk of COPD, improves the prognosis [11,13], prevents progression of the disease [14], and reduces exacerbations of COPD [15-17]. However, COPD patients find it difficult to quit smoking; in fact, the majority of new patients to the hospital for exacerbation of COPD continue smoking. COPD patients have a long smoking history, higher tobacco consumption, higher level of CO in the exhaled air, severe dependence to nicotine, and most have experienced numerous unsuccessful previous quit attempts [18,19]. This makes smoking cessation even more difficult for this group. Smoke quitting not only reduces the risk of COPD but also improve some symptoms like cough, coughing, shortness of breath and immune response, which leads to fewer respiratory infections to occur [20].

There are different drug treatments to quit smoking, however, when pharmacological treatments are combined with psychological techniques, the effectiveness increased significantly in patients with COPD [20-22]. Coronini-Cronberg et al. [21] pointed out that the main problems associated with the relapse of smoking in patients with COPD are the lack of motivation to quit smoking, poor communication with healthcare professionals, and the misleading information of the effects of smoking on health.

In patients with COPD, the comorbidity with anxiety and depression becomes more relevant. For that reason, it is important to review the available literature related to psychological techniques to quit smoking, specifically focused on psychological techniques to increase motivation, development of skills to deal with situations to prevent relapse, and the management of anxiety, depression, and stress. Therefore, the objective of this study was to conduct a review of the effectiveness of the treatments to quit smoking in patients with COPD, identifying the main difficulties to maintain abstinence and propose strategies to eliminate such obstacles.

4. Method

To perform this bibliographic review it was searched in the Cochrane Tobacco Addiction Group, as well as the databases MEDLINE, EMBASE, PsycINFO, PubMed, and SCOPUS from 2000 to 2012. We used the following keywords: smoking cessation, tobacco cessation, hospital, patient, medical setting, and chronic obstructive pulmonary disease. The inclusion criteria used in this review were: a) studies involving interventions for smoking cessation in smokers who have COPD, b) that smokers had 18 or more years; and c) that smokers submit voluntarily to interventions for smoking cessation.

5. Results

Ten reports were identified and grouped in three categories:

a. Studies with an experimental group with a psychological intervention (2)

b. Studies with an experimental group in which the treatment consisted of the combination of any pharmacological treatment with psychological intervention to quit smoking (6), and

c. Studies in which the intervention was done in hospitalized patients (2).

6. Psychological interventions for smoking cessation in patients with COPD

In a review on the effectiveness of interventions for smoking cessation, Lancaster and Stead [23] point out that psychological interventions that use behavioral and cognitive behavioral techniques are effective (e.g. control of stimuli, self-management, coping skills). In the same way, van der Meer et al. [24] reviewed the effectiveness of interventions for smoking cessation in people with COPD. The five studies included show the effectiveness of psychosocial interventions combined with pharmacological intervention: psychosocial interventions combined with NRT and a bronchodilator respect to any treatment with a 5-year follow-up (RD = 0.16, RR = 4, 0); psychosocial interventions combined with NRT and placebo with respect to any treatment with a 5-year follow-up (RD = 0.17, RR = 4.19). In addition the results demonstrated the effectiveness of various combinations of psychosocial and pharmacological interventions in the follow up at 6 months (RD = 0.07, RR = 1.74). The limitation of this review is that none of the included studies compared psychosocial interventions without pharmacotherapy. It is concluded that a combination of psychosocial and pharmacological interventions are superior to none apply any treatment. However, few studies have evaluated in the context of clinical trials the effectiveness of psychological interventions in patients with COPD (see table 1).

Hilberink, Jacobs, Bottema of Vries, and Grol [25] conducted in the Netherlands a randomized controlled trial in patients with COPD (392 smokers) to evaluate the type of intervention on smoking cessation rates, the interventions were a minimal intensity intervention for smoking cessation or the usual care. The intervention was educational and included patient support by health professionals. In the first visit, it was spoken of symptoms, health status and treatment, smoking behavior and motivational state for smoking cessation; also a brochure and a video designed for people with COPD were given. Based on the stages of change [26], the patients were assigned in three categories: 1) preparers (wanted to quit in the next month), 2) contemplators (wanted to quit in the next 6 months), and 3) precontemplators (not want to quit). According to these categories, smokers with no motivation to quit, just received information about the benefits of quitting (control group). Smokers motivated to quit received information to increase their self-efficacy from discussing how they could deal with barriers to quitting, and additionally, information on nicotine replacement therapies according to the level of nicotine dependence was given. After six months, the experimental group showed more attempts to quit smoking (44.9% vs. 36.5%), and quit smoking compared with control group (16.0% vs. 8.8%).

In a second study Wilson, Fitzsimons, Bradbury and Stuart [27] conducted a randomized controlled trial to evaluate the effectiveness of interventions to quit smoking based on the brief advise or brief advise accompanied by nurse support, either individually or in group; smoking status was biochemically validated at 2, 3, 6, 9 and 12 months. The sample consisted of 91 smokers with COPD from an Ireland hospital. All patients received a brief smoking cessation intervention from the physician (5-10 minutes); afterwards, smokers were randomly assigned to one of three groups: usual care, individual, or group support. The usual care group (n = 35) or control group, received only the brief advise; the intervention groups, individual support (n = 27) or group support (n = 29), underwent five weeks of support after the intervention; the nurses with approximately 6 hours of training carried out the interventions. Individual interventions consisted in providing self-help material and information about the personal benefits of quit smoking, discussion about the benefits of nicotine replacement therapy, to encourage setting a date to stop smoking and inform friends and family about the intent. In group interventions, patients were classified according to the phase of change [26] in order that nurses could adapt the intervention to the phase of each patient. In addition, the positive and negative aspects of smoking, particularly on health were discussed, as well as the previous efforts to quit smoking with the intention of to identify those factors that contributed to relapse. In addition, role play in risk situations was performed to increase their confidence to quitting smoking. Both interventions consisted of five sessions of 60 minutes, in which nicotine replacement therapy was given upon request. Twelve months after the intervention, no significant differences between the groups were observed. Abstinence in patients was of 6%

in control group and of 10% in intervention group, a significant reduction of their addiction to nicotine was observed in all groups. These data lead to the authors to conclude that patients with COPD were unable to quit smoking, regardless of the type of support they receive. Therefore, the reduction of tobacco consumption may be an alternative goal for these smokers.

7. Combination of pharmacological and psychological interventions for smoking cessation in patients with COPD

Pharmacologic therapies have as main function the relief of withdrawal symptoms produced by suppressing the consumption of tobacco and consequently help people quit smoking. Pharmacological therapies are classified in two categories, the nicotinic therapies such as nicotine gum, nicotine transdermal patch and inhaler, and non-nicotinic therapies such as bupropion, nortriptyline and varenicline [28]. A review of clinical trials to assess the effectiveness of nicotinic therapies to smokers without chronic disease, describes that all these types of treatments increase the probability of abstinence and is higher than placebo [29]. While with non-nicotinic drug therapy in smokers without the diagnosis of a chronic disease, varenicline and bupropion are most effective because the rate abstinence is higher than placebo or with any other treatment to stop smoking.

Several clinical trials had evaluated whether the efficacy of drug therapy increases when is combined with psychological intervention in patients with chronic diseases. For example, Molyneux et al. [30] compared NRT with placebo NRT or with no NRT. All subjects received a counseling intervention for smoking cessation. They found that counseling without NRT was equally effective. Another trial compared the effect of incorporating intensive cognitive-behavioral intervention or minimal counseling intervention combined with NRT [31]. The results showed that smoking cessation did not improve long-term quit rates with NRT interventions. The results are conflicting, some studies show that there is no increase in efficiency and others mention that it is indispensable the inclusion of a psychological intervention [24]. In the present review, we identified six studies (table 1) combining a psychological intervention with pharmacological therapy (bupropion, nortriptyline, varenicline or nicotine sublingual tablet).

In the first report [32] examined the effect of nicotine replacement therapy (NRT) in patients with COPD. In a double-blind, multicenter, placebo-controlled trial involving 370 patients the efficacy of sublingual tablets or placebo combined with two levels of behavioral support for smoking cessation in COPD patients who smoked on average 19.6 cigarettes per day was evaluated, 6 and 12 months after treatment.

Participants were assigned to one of four experimental conditions: 1) nicotine sublingual tablet with low behavioral support, 2) nicotine sublingual tablet with high behavioral support, 3) placebo sublingual tablet with low behavioral support or 4) placebo sublingual tablet with high behavioral support. The instructions given by nurses were to use nicotine tablets according to the number of cigarettes smoked per day. One or 2 tablets per hour

http://dx.doi.org/10.5772/53265

(minimum 10 tablets and maximum 40 tablets per day) for over 16 cigarettes; 1 tablet per hour (6 to 30 tablets per day) for 10 to 15 cigarettes and 1 tablet per hour (3 to 10 tablets per day) those who smoked 6 to 9 cigarettes. Abstinence rates were statistically significantly superior with nicotine sublingual tablets (low support 14% vs. high support 14%) compared to placebo (low support 5% vs. high support 6%).

No statistical differences were found between the different intensity of behavioral support. The main findings were sustained abstinence rates with nicotine sublingual tablet compared with placebo in a group of patients with mild, moderate and severe COPD. The authors point out the efficacy of NRT in combination with a smoking cessation program and suggest that NRT should be used for smoking cessation in smokers with COPD, regardless of the severity of the disease and the number of cigarettes smoked.

In the second report [33] the objective was to identify the factors detected in the initial assessment to predict abstinence in COPD patients when two different interventions were applied. The patients (N=225) with moderate to severe COPD were assigned to one of two interventions: 1) Minimal Intervention Strategy for Lung Patients (LMIS) of 180 min which consisted of individual counseling and telephone contacts and the use of pharmacological treatment was recommended if patients required or 2) Intensive Intervention [Smoke Stop Therapy (SST)] with 595 min of duration which consisted of group and individual counseling, telephone calls and support for the use of bupropion (available for the patients). In a one-year follow-up, the continuous abstinence rates (validated with cotinine in saliva) were 9% for LMIS and 19% for SST [RR = 2.22, 95% CI: 1.06-4.65]. Regarding variables identification to predict abstinence, the SST was no predictor for success; while for LMIS the attitude toward smoking cessation (OR: 11.8, 95% CI: 1.7-8.15, p =.013) and cotinine level (OR: 2.1, 95% CI: 1.08-3.93, p =.028) were significant predictors, 31% the variance in continuous abstinence was explained by these variables (p =.003). It is concluded that LMIS is suitable for COPD patients with a positive attitude to smoking cessation. SST may be an alternative for patients without such features.

Tashkin et al. [19] conducted a study to investigate the effect of bupropion in promoting abstinence from smoking in patients with COPD. Smokers (N=404) with mild or moderate COPD, who smoked 15 or more cigarettes per day, were assigned randomly to two groups receiving one of two treatments for 12 weeks: intervention group with bupropion (150 mg, twice daily) or placebo control. All patients received smoking cessation counseling by a nurse or doctor; each patient received telephone counseling to quit smoking for 3 days after discharge of the hospital and followed personally in each visit to the hospital. Medication was taking one week before patients attempted to quit. The objective was to obtain complete and continuous abstinence from week 4 until the end of week 7; there was a follow-up at 6 months. The abstinence rates were significantly higher in participants with bupropion compared with placebo (28% vs. 16%, p = 0.003). The abstinence rate between weeks 4 to 12 (18% vs. 10%) and between weeks 4 to 26 (16% vs. 9%) also were higher in participants receiving bupropion (p <0.05). The authors concluded that bupropion along with the counselling was an effective aid to smoke cessation in patients with COPD.

Wagena, Knipschild, Huibers, Wouters and van Schayck [34] explored the efficacy of bupropion and nortriptyline in smokers at risk of COPD versus smokers with COPD. In a randomized placebo-controlled, double blind trial, 255 adults at risk for COPD or with COPD were assigned to one of three groups that received different smoking cessation intervention: a) bupropion (15 mg twice daily), b) nortriptyline (75 mg once daily) for 12 weeks and c) placebo bupropion. All patients received advice to quit smoking. The main indicator of outcome was prolonged abstinence from smoking from 4 to 26 weeks after beginning the date of withdrawal. The results showed that bupropion (27.9%) and nortriptyline (25%) had high rates of prolonged abstinence at 26 weeks follow-up compared with placebo (14.6%), significant differences between bupropion and placebo were detected ($p = 0.03$), 13.1% [95% CI: -1.2% to 25.1%], and no differences for nortriptyline 10.2% [95% CI: 1.7% to 22.2%). In patients with COPD, bupropion (27.3%) and nortriptyline (21.2%) were equally effective in prolonged abstinence rates (differences with placebo 18.9% [95% CI: 3.6% -34.2%], for bupropion and 12.9% [95% CI: -0.8% to 26.4%] for nortriptyline). In subjects with COPD risk, no statistically significant differences were detected compared with placebo in prolonged abstinence rates (bupropion= 28.6% vs. nortriptyline= 32.1% vs. placebo = 22%). The authors conclude that bupropion combined with smoking cessation counselling is an effective treatment for smoking cessation in patients with COPD and nortriptyline is a useful alternative.

van Schayck, et al. [35] conducted a randomized, double-blind placebo-controlled trial to evaluate the efficacy of bupropion and nortriptyline in combination with behavioral cognitive intervention in smokers with COPD risk in Netherlands. Smokers (n=255) with COPD risk between 30-70 years, were counseled to quit smoking (three sessions of 20 minutes and 6 calls of 5 minutes). They were randomly allocated to one of three groups: bupropion, nortriptyline or placebo for 12 weeks. The results showed prolonged abstinence rate (defined by report of participants have not smoked in week 2 to 52 after the beginning of abstinence) for bupropion (20.9%), nortriptyline (20%) and placebo (13.5%). Significant differences were obtained between bupropion and placebo [relative risk (RR) = 1.6, 95%, confidence interval (CI) 0.8-3.0], in contrast, the differences between nortriptyline and placebo were not significant. The severity of the airway obstruction did not influence the significance of abstinence. The social costs were € 1368 with bupropion, € 1906 with nortriptyline and € 1212 with placebo. The authors concluded that bupropion and nortriptyline are equally effective, but bupropion was more cost effective compared with placebo and nortriptyline. One possible reason for the high cost of nortriptyline may be that participants who used nortriptyline experienced more side effects from treatment.

Finally, one study evaluated varenicline combined with psychological intervention. In 27 centers a randomized, controlled, double blind, trial in patients (N=504) with mild to moderate COPD the efficacy of varenicline was evaluated [36]. The intervention consisted in 12 weeks of varenicline with 40 weeks follow-up. All participants received an educational booklet on smoking cessation information and brief counseling sessions (10 minutes) at each telephone call or visit at the clinic. The primary endpoint to confirm the continuous abstinence rate with the carbon monoxide level was week 9 to 12. The secondary endpoint was week 9 to 52. The results showed that the rate of continuous abstinence from week 9-12 was significantly higher for patients in the varenicline group (42.3%) than for placebo patients (8.8%) (OR: 8.40, 95% CI: 4.99 -14.14, p <.0001). The continuous abstinence rate in patients treated with varenicline remained significantly higher than for those treated with placebo through week 9 to 52 (18.6% vs. 5.6%) (OR: 4.04, 95% CI: 2.13-7.67; p <.0001). Side effects commonly reported by patients in the varenicline group were nausea, nightmares, respiratory infection, and insomnia. The authors conclude that varenicline was more effective than placebo for smoking cessation in patients with mild and moderate COPD, and showed consistent with that observed in previous trials.

8. Interventions for smoking cessation in hospitalized patients with COPD

An additional component in treatments for smoking cessation in patients with COPD is hospitalization, which provides an excellent opportunity to help to stop smoking. Given that in this condition the perceived vulnerability of patients increase, as well the receptivity to the messages for the abandonment of smoking. In addition, access to health care allows patients to have direct contact with health professionals who can provide messages or interventions for smoking cessation, and smokers may find it easier to quit smoking in an environment smoke-free [37]. Despite this, in practice few hospitals provide this kind of help to their patients. Table 1 shows intervention for smoking cessation in patients hospitalized for COPD.

Regarding the above, a study [38] measured in successive discharged patients of the department of neumology of a university hospital, the percentage of smoking history and smoking cessation medical advice contained in 100 medical reports. They detected that most of the main diagnoses were smoking related diseases. From all reports, only 48% of patients had history related to tobacco, 14 were smokers and 11 had in the report a written advice to quit smoking. Only 36.7% of smokers received smoking advice. Of the patients who had no history, 16 were smokers and had not received advice. In addition, the first hospital admissions were 5.9% more likely to count with clinical history than readmissions (77.8% in first admission compared to 35.6% in readmissions). An interesting finding was that physicians who smoked where less likely record the smoking history than non-smoking physicians. The authors conclude that the interview related to tobacco and smoking advice should be improved.

Sundblad, Larsson and Nathell [39] designed a smoking cessation program in which patients were hospitalized for 11 days to develop their motivation to quit smoking through information, exercise the option to make a nicotine replace therapy, learning coping strategies and personal support. The results on smoking were evaluated after 1 and 3 years. The abstinence was compared in the patients with COPD who participated in the smoking cessation program (N = 247) and the ones receiving usual care (N = 231). Abstinence rates obtained in smoking cessation group at one year were 52% and 38% at follow-up to three years.

PSYCHOLOGICAL INTERVENTIONS

Author	Objetive	Patients	Interventions	Results	Validation
Hilberink et al. (2005)	To compare smoke cessation rates depending on the type of intervention.	392 smokers with COPD	IG: brief intervention (counsel+ self-help material) CG: usual care (counsel)	Attempts to stop the smoking at 6 months: IG: 44.9% vs. CG: 36.5%. Abstinence at 6 months: IG: 16.0% vs. CG: 8.8%.	Self-reports
Wilson et al. (2006)	Evaluate the effectiveness of interventions for smoking cessation based on brief counsel alone or with support from nurses (individual or group).	91 smokers with COPD IG 1=27 IG 2= 29 IG 3= 35	IG 1: individual support (briefings, self-help materials and telephone support 5 weeks). IG 2: group support by stage of change (group information sessions + 5 follow-up sessions after discharge). IG 3: usual care (brief counsel).	Abstinence at 12 months: IG 2: 10% vs CG: 6%. There were no significant differences between groups (p = 0.7).	Self-reports Carbon monoxide in expired air Cotinine in saliva

PHARMACOLOGICAL TREATMENT COMBINED WITH A PSYCHOLOGICAL INTERVENTION FOR SMOKING CESSATION

Author	Objetive	Patients	Interventions	Results	Validation
Tonnesen, Mikkelsen & Bremann (2006)	To identify predictors of abstinence	370 patients with COPD who smoke on average 19.6 cigarettes per day	IG1: sublingual tablet + low behavioral support IG2: sublingual tablet + high behavioral support CG1: sublingual tablet + placebo with low behavioral support CG2: placebo sublingual tablet + high behavioral support	Prolonged abstinence IG1: 14% vs.IG2: 14% CG1: 5% vs.CG2: 6% 12 months point prevalence IG1: 17% vs.IG2: 18% CG1: 6% vs.CG2: 13%	Self-reports Carbon monoxide in expired air
Christenhusz , Pieterse, Seydel & van der Palen (2007)	To evaluate the efficacy of sublingual tablets or placebo combined with two levels of behavioral support for smoking cessation in COPD patients after 6 and 12 months.	225 patients with moderate to severe COPD	CG: moderately intensive intervention: individual counseling + telephone contacts Total time: 180 minutes. IG: intensive intervention , group and individual counseling and support +phone calls + bupropion. Total time: 595 minutes.	Abstinence rates CG:9% IG:19%	Cotinine in saliva Self-reports
Tashkin et al. (2001)	To investigate the effect of bupropion promoting abstinence from smoking in patients with COPD	404 smokers with mild or moderate COPD who smoked 15 or more cigarettes / day.	IG: bupropion (150 mg twice daily) + counseling for smoking cessation CG: placebo for 12 weeks + counsel	Abstinence at 6 months: IG:28% vs. CG:16%. Abstinence between weeks 4 and 12: IG:18% vs. CG:10%. Abstinence between weeks 4 and 26: IG:16% vs. CG:9%.	Self-reports Carbon monoxide in expired air
Wagena et al.(2005)	Explore the efficacy of bupropion and nortriptyline in smokers with COPD risk compared with smokers with COPD.	255 adults at risk for COPD or with COPD	IG1:bupropion (15 mg twice daily) IG2: nortriptyline (75 mg once/day X 12 weeks) CG: bupropion placebo	Prolonged Abstinence 26 weeks: IG1:27.9% vs. IG2:25% vs. CG:14.6 %(p=0.03)	Self-reports Carbon monoxide in expired air

Author	Objective	Patients	Interventions	Results	Validation
van Schayck et al.(2009) Netherlands	To evaluate the efficacy of bupropion and nortriptyline compared with placebo in smokers with COPD risk	255 COPD risk	IG 1: Bupropion-12 weeks IG 2: nortriptyline -12 weeks CG: Placebo 12 weeks	Prolonged Abstinence: IG1:20.9%, IG2: 20%, G.C:13.5% Significant differences between bupropion and placebo [RR=1.6, 95% IC=0.8-3.0]	Cotinine in urine Self-reports
Tashkin et al. (2011)	To evaluate the efficacy of varenicline in patients with COPD	504 patients with mild and moderate COPD	IG: Varenicline + educational booklet on smoking cessation information and brief sessions (10 minutes) telephone counseling CG: placebo + educational booklet on smoking cessation information and brief sessions (10 minutes) telephone counseling	Continuous abstinence IG:42.3% CG:8.8% p<.0001	Self-reports Carbon monoxide in expired air
INTERVENTIONS FOR SMOKING CESSATION IN PATIENTS HOSPITALIZED FOR COPD					
Author	**Objective**	**Patients**	**Interventions**	**Results**	**Validation**
Sundblad, Larsson y Nathell (2008)	To evaluate a smoking cessation program	478 COPD patients	IG: hospitalization for 11 days were used to develop the motivation to quit smoking through information, exercise the option to take a nicotine replacement therapy, learning coping strategies and given personal support CG: usual care	Abstinence rates at 12 months IG: 52% vs. CG: 7% Abstinence rates at 3 years IG: 38% vs. CG: 10%	Self-reports Carbon monoxide in expired air
Borglykke, Pisinger, Jørgensen & Ibsen (2008)	To evaluate the effect of a smoking cessation group in hospitalized patients with COPD	223 hospitalized patients with COPD	IG: Participants attended group intervention sessions (two hours weekly for five weeks) NRT was used when necessary CG: usual care	Abstinence rates at 12 months IG:30% CG:13%	Self-reports Carbon monoxide in expired air

IG: Intervention Group; CG: Control Group; NRT: Nicotine Replace Therapy

Table 1. Interventions for smoking cessation in patients with chronic obstructive pulmonary disease (COPD).

Also, Borglykke, Pisinger, Jorgensen and Ibsen [40] evaluated the effect of a smoking cessation group in hospitalized patients with COPD. Patients were assigned to a control group (n = 102) or an intervention group (n = 121). In the first two sessions of the intervention, the group received information on smoking cessation and had to set a date to start the withdrawal that was supported NRT when necessary. At 1 year follow-up 36 (30%) patients in the intervention group remained abstinent compared with 13 (13%) patients in the control group [odds ratio (95% confidence interval): 2.83 (1.40 -5.74). A significant difference was observed between the intervention group and control group with respect to the self reporting of the phlegm production however no significant improvement was observed in terms of survival benefit at 3 years follow up period (intervention group 86% vs. control group 85%).Therefore, the authors conclude that this study showed that a group intervention for chronic patients made it possible to get high withdrawal rates. Furthermore, this intervention showed positive impact in hospitalization in survival and reducing phlegm.

9. Training of professionals who carry out interventions for smoking cessation

Ballbé et al. [41] assessed if the lack of promotion on the cessation of smoking in hospitals is due to deficits in professional training. In this study, knowledge, attitudes and action regarding the smoking behavior of 66 health professionals before and after training on brief intervention was evaluated. The performance of these professionals with 170 patients was compared before and another 170 training (patient's report). It was found was that the intervention training for smoking cessation increases knowledge of psychological skills by 23.3% and 27.1% of pharmacological resources. However no changes were observed with respect to the question of whether to smoke (30.8% before vs. 38.2% after training), to records the smoking status of patient medical history (73.4% vs. 65.9%), whether the patient want to quit (25% vs. 12.5%) or with respect to anti-smoking advice (21.9 % vs. 20.8%). This study shows that health care activity in hospitals tends to focus on treating specific diseases for which patients attend, and leave behind preventive interventions, even when the professionals have the training.

In a same line, Efraimsson, Fossum, Ehrenberg, Larson and Klang [42] tried to assess whether with a four-day training in motivational interviewing, a group of nurses will assume the communication style of motivational interventions (MI) for smoking cessation in primary care conducted with smokers with COPD. The nurses in their practice did not take the contents of the training they have received, which indicates that a course in motivational interviewing a few days was insufficient. It is concluded that training in communication methods should be integrated into the nursing curriculum, since the management of MI is a complex skill that requires a great workout.

In addition, sometimes personnel not sufficiently trained carry out the interventions. For example, Wilson et al. [27] obtained no differences between the interventions applied. The authors attribute the lack of success to patients and we must not forget that nurses who had received only 6 hours of training applied such interventions. It would be interesting to evaluate the results when intervention is performed by a psychologists with sufficient training in smoking cessation.

10. Discussion

The aim of this study was to conduct a review of the effectiveness of the treatments to quit smoking in patients with COPD, identifying the main difficulties to maintain abstinence and to propose strategies to eliminate such obstacles. As a result of the revision, we can say that although it is known how smoking affects COPD, the research attempting to demonstrate the benefits of quitting smoking on health in smokers diagnosed with COPD is insufficient. In addition, smoking history and the advice or counsel is not always a priority in hospitals. A large percentage of health professionals do not ask to patients if they smoke, therefore do not advise to quit, even though many of them have received formal training [41, 43-44]. Moreover, according to a survey, the majorities of patients are not offered help to quit smoking or are advised to make a follow-up with the physician or contact with a trained professional [43].

In addition, in the available reports, the interventions are very diverse both in relation to their content and in relation to their intensity. There are also differences in the professionals that conduct the interventions: physicians, nurses, psychologists, counselors or any other health personnel; this makes very difficult to compare results of different interventions. An important aspect to consider when analyzing the data obtained in present review is the difference in health staff that carried out the smoking cessation interventions, since their level of training was not considered; therefore, this could influence the results and the effectiveness of interventions. In some studies, nurses with little training to perform this task carried out the interventions [27]. It would be interesting to compare the results obtained in intervention carried by different professionals with no specialized training with those obtained by professionals who specializes in treating addictive behaviors.

In the studies reviewed, depending on the research involved, in some cases to calculate rates of abstinence only self-reports were used [e.g. 25], while in others to corroborate self-reported abstinence different biochemical test were used. This is another important aspect to consider when analyze and interpreting present findings.

Another problem that limits replication is that many studies do not describe the procedure followed in the psychological interventions, which could be central in the analysis of the results. That is, in most reports only the use of behavioral cognitive interventions is reported, but the techniques are not explained; therefore it is indispensable to specify and describe all the techniques used for patients who want to quit smoking and COPD.

A different area identified is the lack of assessment of psychological factors associated with relapse in the evaluation of different treatments, only side effects are evaluated with respect to the use of drug treatments and only evaluates both the level of depression with the "Beck Depression Inventory" and the level of motivation. Some reports suggest that depression and anxiety are present in patients with COPD, but do not mention if it is consequence of the disease or for quitting. It is known that lack of social support, depression, anxiety, anxiety sensitivity, negative affect, and deficiency of coping skills are factors associated with the ineffectiveness of interventions in smokers without the diagnosis of a disease, but little is known about the factors associated with relapse in the context of smoking cessation interventions in patients with COPD.

On the other hand, in terms of difficulties for smoking cessation in patients with COPD the review allowed to identify some factors:

- Many patients with COPD continue to smoke after diagnosis and those who manage to quit smoking have a high rate of relapse, for that reason many patients do not try quit again because their expectative is low.

- In general, smokers with COPD have characteristics that make difficult to quit, for example the level of dependency is severe, the number of cigarettes is high [45]; they are older and therefore have smoked for many years resulting in high dependency [46-47].
- A main barrier to quit smoking is the motivation. For example, in a study it was shown that patients with COPD stop smoking according the motivational state (precontemplation, contemplation, preparation, action), smokers in precontemplation associated significantly fewer advantages to quit smoking compared with smokers in contemplation or preparation stages. Smokers in preparation had significantly higher self-efficacy expectations about quitting than other smokers. Patients in preparation for quitting complained more about the symptoms associated with COPD. Smokers in contemplation and preparation to quit developed more plans to try to switch to action to stop smoking [48]. At this point, it is proposed to design an intervention for smokers with COPD motivated to quit and other unmotivated.
- The comorbidity with anxiety and depression is very high, particularly in women [49-50]. This difficulties to achieve the abstinence and justifies the use of psychological treatments to improve outcomes of smoking cessation treatments.
- Another factor that makes difficult to stop smoking is weight gain, particularly in women [45]. When patients stop smoking and gain weight, symptoms related with COPD are exacerbated and causes relapses.
- Social support between the moments the patients are diagnosed COPD and when decide to quit, is other factor. Some authors suggest that social support should be from a family member or someone close to the patient, instead of for example, another patient with COPD [46,51].

11. Conclusions

From present review about the interventions for smoking cessation and the identification of barriers to achieve and maintain abstinence, we suggest the inclusion of different techniques to overcome these barriers, since providing information about harm caused by smoking is not enough. It is imperative that patients with COPD to realize how smoking is decreasing their quality of life and deteriorating their health.

The motivational interviewing techniques [52-53] could be an effective method to support smoke cessation [42], but require significant training [54]. It is suggested the inclusion of motivational interviewing in the treatment for smoking cessation in smokers with COPD and personalized feedback with the use of measures of spirometry, Fletcher curve and to exploit the adverse events related to COPD to promote the decision of quitting [48]. En el patient with COPD the motivation for quitting increases if patients perceive that the respiratory symptoms are due to use of tobacco [55].

Problem-Solving Therapy helps patients to effectively deal with diverse problems from different learning strategies [56]. The objective of this therapy is to clearly define the problem, propose alternatives to solve the problem make decisions and implement solutions to assess the effectiveness of the alternative. For patients with COPD the strategies can be applied not only to the problems associated with quitting smoking, but also to emerging situations by the presence of the disease, such as social, physical and economic problems.

Functional analysis of problem behavior consists in the identification of the context of occurrence of the inadequate behavior and the consequences that maintain it. In treatments for smoking cessation implies the clear identification of the situation that triggers the consumption of cigarettes, and the positive and negative consequences of consumption, in order to plan and apply strategies that lead to abstinence from cigarettes [57].

Self-monitoring is a technique in which the patient is asked to record the duration, frequency and severity of the problem behavior. In the context of smoking cessation treatment, particularly in patients with COPD, it may ask the patient to record each cigarette consumed, the place of consumption, how it feels when smoke each cigarette, and to register the presence and severity of respiratory symptoms.

The proposal of a individualized plan for quitting would consist of two phases, one evaluation phase and the intervention phase that will include the techniques mentioned. In the evaluation phase, the goal would be to get specific information of psychological factors related with the consumption of cigarettes by the patient with COPD, to consider the individualized treatment.

Initially, it would be necessary to identify the stage of readiness to change [26], the pattern of consumption of cigarettes (daily average consumption per day, monthly consumption), identified the factors causing the consumption (moods, places, people or their combination) and the level of anxiety, depression, negative affection, social support, the level of dependency and the coping strategies of the patient.

From the results of the evaluation would be conducted a personalized feedback and decisional balance would be applied using the techniques of motivational interviewing (empathy, reflective listening, cognitive dissonance, without confrontation).

Based on the decisional balance the person must choose one of two strategies for reaching abstinence: 1) gradual reduction of the nicotine and tar consisting in the decline of 30 % of the initial consumption pattern every week until it reaches 0 %, or 2) abstinence.

To initiate strategies to abstinence from cigarettes consumption, start a record of a functional analysis of the behavior of smoking. This analysis include the negative effects of abstinence (nervousness, irritability, anxiety, depression, hunger, trouble sleeping) and the positive effects of abstinence, i.e. the registration of the reduction of the problems of the COPD from the change in the pattern of consumption (phlegm, breathing problems, cough).

Also, teach patients coping strategies for anxiety, depression, negative affect, and problem solving strategies to apply during periods in which the patient is still in situations or in the presence of factors (moods or people) that cause the consumption of cigarettes.

To summarize, the revisions point out that in COPD the smoking cessation programs should be intense, sustained over time and adapted to each patient individually. It also emphasizes the need of combining pharmacological and psychological treatments, particularly behavioral focused to the relapse prevention and stress management [58,59]. What is clear is that smoking intervention should be considered as a substantial part of the treatment of COPD. The psychological techniques mentioned previously, could help to eliminate barriers and provide personalized feedback to increase abstinence rates in patients with COPD.

Author details

Jennifer Lira-Mandujano[1], M. Carmen Míguez-Varela[2] and Sara E. Cruz-Morales[3]

1 Facultad de Psicología, Universidad Michoacana de San Nicolás de Hidalgo, México

2 Facultad de Psicología, Universidad de Santiago de Compostela, Spain

3 Psicofarmacología, UNAM-FES-Iztacala, México

References

[1] Global Strategy for the Diagnosis, Management and Prevention of COPD (revised 2011). Global Initiative for Chronic Obstructive Lung Disease (GOLD). http://www.goldcopd.org (accessed 22 June 2012).

[2] Celli BR., Halbert RJ., Isonaka S., Schau B. (2003). Population impact of different definitions of airway obstruction. European Respiratory Journal 2003; 22: 268–273. DOI: 10.1183/09031936.03.00075102

[3] Hardie JA., Buist AS., Vollmer WM., Ellingsen I., Bakke PS., Mørkve O. Risk of over-diagnosis of COPD in asymptomatic elderly never smokers. European Respiratory Journal 2002; 20 (5) 1117-1122.

[4] Pellegrino R., Viegi G., Brusasco V., Crapo RO., Burgos F., Casaburi R., Coates A., van der Grinten CPM., Gustafsson P., Hankinson J., Jensen R., Johnson DC., MacIntyre M., McKay R., Miller MR., Navajas D., Pedersen OF., Wanger J. (2005) Interpretative strategies for lung function tests. European Respiratory Journal 2005; 26(5) 948-968. DOI: 10.1183/09031936.05.00035205

[5] Akinbami LJ, Liu X. Chronic obstructive pulmonary disease among adults aged 18 and over in the United States, 1998–2009. NCHS data brief, no 63.

[6] Programa Nacional de Salud 2007-2012. [National Health Program 2007-2012] Secretaría de Salud. México,D.F. ISBN 978-970-721-414-9.

[7] Franchi M, ed. EFA Book on Chronic Obstructive Pulmonary Disease in Europe: Sharing and Caring. Brussels, European Federation of Allergy and Airways Disease, 2009. Available from: www.efanet.org/ documents/EFACOPDBook.pdf

http://dx.doi.org/10.5772/53265

[8] Montes A., Pérez M., Gestal JJ. Impacto del tabaquismo sobre la mortalidad en España [Impact of smoking on mortality in Spain]. Adicciones 2004;16(2 Suppl) 75- 82.

[9] U.S.D.H.H.S., editor. The health consequences of smoking: A report of the surgeon general. National Center for Chronic Disease Prevention and Health Promotion, Office of Smoking and Health; 2004.

[10] Godtfredsen NS., Lam TH., Hansel TT., Leon ME., Gray N., Dresler C., Burns DM., Prescott E., Vestbo J. COPD-related morbidity and mortality after smoking cessation: status of the evidence. European Respiratory Journal 2008;32(4) 844-853.

[11] Fletcher C., Peto R. The natural history of chronic airflow obstruction. British Medical Journal 1977; 1(6077) 1645-1648.

[12] Wise RA. The value of forced expiratory volume in 1 second decline in the assessment of chronic obstructive pulmonary disease progression. The American Journal of Medicine 2006;119 (10 Suppl 1) 4-11. DOI: 10.1016/j.amjmed.2006.08.002

[13] Hersh CP., DeMeo DL., Al-Ansari E., Carey VJ., Reilly JJ., Ginns LC., Silverman EK. Predictors of survival in severe, early onset COPD. Chest 2004;126(5) 1443-1451.

[14] Rabe KF., Hurd S., Anzueto A., Barnes PJ., Buist SA., Calverley P., Fukuchi Y., Jenkins C., Rodriguez-Roisin R., van Weel C., Zielinski J. Global strategy for the diagnosis, management, and prevention of chronic obstructive pulmonary disease: GOLD executive summary. American Journal of Respiratory and Critical Care Medicine 2007; 176(6) 532-555.

[15] Kanner RE., Connett JE., Williams DE., Buist AS. Effects of randomized assignment to a smoking cessation intervention and changes in smoking habits on respiratory symptoms in smokers with early chronic obstructive pulmonary disease: the lung health study. The American Journal of Medicine 1999, 106, 410-416.

[16] Makris D., Scherpereel A., Copin MC., Colin G., Brun L., Lafitte JJ., Marquette CH. Fatal interstitial lung disease associated with oral erlotinib therapy for lung cancer. BMC Cancer 2007; 150(7) 1-4. doi:10.1186/1471-2407-7-150

[17] Scanlon PD., Connett JE., Waller LA., Altose MD., Bailey WC., Buist, AS. Smoking Cessation and Lung Function in Mild-to-Moderate Chronic obstructive Pulmonary Disease. The Lung Health Study. American Journal of Respiratory and Critical Care Medicine 2000; 161 (2) 381-390.

[18] Jiménez-Ruiz C., Ruiz JJ., Cicero A., Riesco JA., Astral J., Guirao A. Implementation of smoking cessation services in respiratory medicine. Journal of Smoking Cessation 2001;2(1) 1-4.

[19] Tashkin DP., Kanner R., Bailey W., Buist S., Anderson P., Nides M., Gonzales D., Dozier G., Patel MK., Jamerson B. Smoking cessation in patients with chronic obstructive pulmonary disease: a double-blind, placebo-controlled, randomised trial. Lancet 2001;357(9268) 1571-1575.

[20] Tonnensen P., Carrozzi L., Fagerström KO., Gratziou C., Jimenez-Ruiz C., Nardini S., Viegi G., Lazzaro C., Campell IA., Dagli E., West R. Smoking cessation in patients with respiratory disease: a high priority, integral component of therapy. European Respiratory Journal 2007;29(2) 390-417. DOI: 10.1183/09031936.00060806

[21] Coronini-Cronberg S., Heffernan C., Robinson M. Effective smoking cessation interventions for COPD patients a review of the evidence. Journal of the Royal Society of Medicine Short Reports 2011; 78 (2) 1-12. DOI 10.1258/shorts.2011.011089

[22] Strassmann R., Bausch B., Spaar A., Kleijnen J., Braendli O., Puhan MA. Smoking cessation interventions in COPD: a network meta-analysis of randomised trials. European Respiratory Journal 2009; 34(3) 634-640. DOI: 10.1183/09031936.00167708

[23] Lancaster T., Stead LF. (2011). Individual behavioural counselling for smoking cessation. Cochrane database of systematic reviews. In: The Cochrane Library, Issue 06,30.07.2011, Available from http://cochrane.bvsalud.org/cochrane/main.php?lib=COC&searchExp=smoking&lang=pt (accessed 22 March 2012).

[24] van der Meer RM., Wagena EJ., Ostelo RW., Jacobs JE., van Schayk CP. (2009). Smoking cessation for chronic obstructive pulmonary disease. Cochrane Review. In: The Cochrane Plus Library Issue 1. Oxford:Update Softwre Ltd. Available from http://www.update-software.com

[25] Hilberink SR., Jacobs JE., Bottema BJ., de Vires H., Grol RP. Smoking cessation in patients with COPD in daily general practice (SMOCC): six months' results. Preventive Medicine 2005;41(5-6) 822-827.

[26] Prochaska JO., DiClemente C. Stages and Processes of Self-Change of Smoking: Toward an Integrative Model of Change. Journal of Consulting and Clinical Psychology 1983; 51(3) 390-395.

[27] Wilson J., Fitzsimons D., Bradbury I., Stuart J. Does additional support by nurse enhance the effect of a brief smoking cessation intervention in people with moderate to severe chronic obstructive pulmonary disease? A randomised controlled trial. International Journal of Nursing Studies 2006;45(4) 508- 517.

[28] Lira-Mandujano J. Cruz-Morales SE. (2011). Motivational Intervention and Nicotine Replacement Therapies for Smokers: Results of a Randomized Clinical Trial, Mostafa Ghanei (Ed.). Respiratory Diseases, Croatia: InTech. ISBN: 978-953-307-964-6

[29] Stead LF., Perera R., Bullen C., Mant D., Lancaster T. (2011). Nicotine Replacement Therapy for Smoking cessation. Cochrane database of systematic reviews. In: The Cochrane Library, Issue 06, Available from http://cochrane.bvsalud.org/cochrane/main.php?lib=COC&searchExp=smoking&lang=pt (accessed 22 March 2012).

[30] Molyneux A., Lewis S., Leivers U., Andreton A., Antoniak M., Brackenridge A., Nilsson F., McNeil A., West R., Moxham J., Britton J. Clinical trial comparing nicotine replacement therapy (NRT) plus brief counselling, brief counselling alone and minimal intervention on smoking cessation in hospital inpatients. Thorax 2003;58(6) 484-488.

[31] Simon J., Carmody T., Hudes E., Snyder E., Murray J. Intensive smoking cessation counseling versus minimal counseling among hospitalized smokers treated with transdermal nicotine replacement: a randomized trial. American Journal of Medicine 2003;114(7) 555-562.

[32] Tonnesen P., Mikkelsen K., Bremann L. Nurse-conducted smoking cessation in patients with COPD using nicotine sublingual tablets and behavioral support. Chest 2006; 130; 334-342. DOI 10.1378/chest.130.2.334

[33] Christenhusz L., Pieterse M., Seydel E., van der Palen J. Prospective determinants of smoking cessation in COPD patients within a high intensity or brief counseling intervention. Patient Education and Counseling 2007. 66(2), 162-166. DOI: 10.106/j.pec. 2006.11.006

[34] Wagena EJ., Knipschild PG., Huibers MJH., Wouters EFM., van Schayck CP. Efficacy of bupropion and nortriptyline for smoking cessation among people at risk for or with chronic obstructive pulmonary disease. Archives of Internal Medicine 2005; 165(19) 2286-2292.

[35] van Schayck CP., Kaper J., Wagena EJ., Wouters FM., Severens JL. The cost-effectiveness of antidepressants for smoking cessation in chronic obstructive pulmonary disease (COPD) patients. Addiction, 2009; 104(12) 2110–2117, DOI:10.1111/j. 1360-0443.2009.02723.x

[36] Tashkin D., Rennard S., Hays T., Ma W., Lawrence D., Lee T. Effects of vareniclina on smoking cessation in patients with mild to moderate COPD: A randomised controlled trial. Chest 2011; 139(3), 591-599. DOI 10.1378/chest.10-0865.

[37] Rigotti NA., Clair C., Munafo MR., Stead LF. Interventions for smoking cessation in hospitalized pacients (Cochrane Review). The Cochrane Library 2012; 5. Chichester, RU: Wiley and Sons, Ltd. DOI: 10.1002/14651858.CD001837.

[38] Salas J., Huergo A., Malmierca E., Santianes J., Bustillo E. Anamnesis de tabaquismo y consejo antitabaco a pacientes ingresados en un servicio de neumología [Clinical history of smoking and anti-smoking advice to inpatients in a pneumology department]. Prevención del Tabaquismo 2005;7(1) 6-10.

[39] Sundblad, B. M., Larsson, K. & Nathell, L. High rates of smoking abstinence in COPD patients: smoking cessation by hospitalization. Nicotine and Tobacco Research.2008; 10 (5): 883–90. DOI: 10.1080/14622200802023890

[40] Borglykke A., Pisinger C., Jørgensen T., Ibsen H. The effectiveness of smoking cessation groups offered to hospitalised patients with symptoms of exacerbations of chronic obstructive pulmonary disease (COPD). The Clinical Respiratory Journal 2008; 2 (3) 158-165. DOI:10.1111/j.1752-699X.2008.00055.x

[41] Ballbé M., Mondon S., Nieva G., Walter M., Saltó E., Gual A. Evaluación de un programa de formación de profesionales sanitarios sobre abordaje del tabaquismo en pacientes hospitalizados [Evaluation of a training program for healthcare professionals

about smoking cessation interventions in hospitalizad patients]. Adicciones 2008;20(2) 125-130.

[42] Efraimsson EO., Fossum B., Ehrenberg A., Larson K., Klang B. Use of motivacional interviewing in smoking cessation at nurse-led chronic obstructive pulmonary disease clinics. Journal of Advanced Nursing 2011;68(4) 767-782.

[43] Nieva G., Gual A., Mondon S., Walter M., Saltó E. Evaluación de la intervención mínima en tabaquismo en el ámbito hospitalario [Evaluation of brief intervention for smoking cessation in hospital inpatients]. Medicina Clínica 2007;128(19) 730-732.

[44] Wagena EJ., Zeegers PA., van Schayck CP., Wouters FM. Benefits and Risks of Pharmacological Smoking Cessation Therapies in Chronic Obstructive Pulmonary Disease. Drug Safety 2003; 26 (6) 381-403.

[45] Jiménez-Ruiz C., Luhning S., Buljubasich D. Smoking Cessation Treatment for Chronic Obstructive Pulmonary Disease Smokers. European Respiratory Disease 2011; 7(2) 106-110

[46] Tashkin DP., Murray RP. Smoking cessation in chronic obstructive pulmonary disease. Respiratory Medicine 2009;103(7) 963-974.

[47] Wagena EJ., Van Der Meer RM., Ostelo RJ., Jabobs JE., Van Schayck CP. The efficacy of smoking cessation strategies in people with chronic obstructive pulmonary disease: results from a systematic review. Respiratory Medicine 2004;98(9) 805-815.

[48] Hilberink SR., Jacobs EJ., Schlösser M., Grol R, de Vries H. Characteristics of patients with COPD in three motivational stages related to smoking cessation. Patient Education and Counseling 2006; 61 (3), 449-457. DOI: 10.1016/j.pec.2005.05.012

[49] Maurer J., Rebbapragada V., Borson S., Goldstein R., Kunik ME., Yohanes AM., Hanania NA. Anxiety and depression in COPD: Current understanding, unanswered questions, and research needs. Chest 2008;134(4 Suppl) 43S-56S.

[50] Wagena JE., Ludovic MSC., van Amelsvoort GMP., Ijmert K., Wouters EFM. Chronic Bronchitis, Cigarette Smoking, and the Subsequent Onset of Depression and Anxiety: Results From a Prospective Population-Based Cohort Study. Psychosomatic Medicine 2005; 67(4) 656-660. DOI: 10.1097/01.psy.0000171197.29484.6b.

[51] Hill K., Geist R., Goldstein RS., Lacasse Y. Anxiety and depression in end-stage COPD. European Respiratory Journal 2008; 31(3) 667–677. DOI: 10.1183/09031936.00125707

[52] Miller W. Enhancing Motivation for Change in Substance Abuse Treatment. Rockville: U. S. Department of Health and Human Services; 1999.

[53] Miller RW., Rollnick S. Motivational Interviewing. New York: Guilford Press;1991.

[54] Becoña E., Míguez MC. Group behavior therapy for smoking cessation. Journal of Groups in Addiction and Recovery 2008; 3(1-2) 63-78.

[55] Walters N., Coleman T. Comparison of the smoking behaviour and attitudes of smokers who attribute respiratory symptoms to smoking with those who do not. British Journal General Practice 2002;52(475) 132-134.

[56] O'Donohue W., Fisher EJ., Hayes CS. Cognitive Behavior Therapy. Applying Empirically supported techniques in your practice. New Jersey: John Wiley &Sons, Inc; 2003.

[57] O'Donohue W., Fisher EJ. General principles and empirically supported techniques of cognitive behavior therapy. New Jersey: John Wiley & Sons, Inc. 2009.

[58] Granda Orive JI., Jareño Esteban J., Roig Vázquez F. Tratamiento del tabaquismo en el EPOC: Revisión actualizada [Treatment of smoking in COPD: updated review]. Prevención del Tabaquismo 2011;13(3) 117-121.

[59] Effing TW., Bourbeau J., Vercoulen J., Apter AJ., Coultas D., Meek P., van der Valk P., Partridge MR., van der Palen J. Self-management programmes for COPD: Moving forward. Chronic Respiratory Disease 2012;9(1) 27-35. DOI: 10.1177/1479972311433574